Emergencies in Clinical Medicine

EDITED BY

H.J. KENNEDY
BSc, MD, MRCP
Lecturer, Department of Medicine,
Royal Hallamshire Hospital,
Sheffield

BLACKWELL SCIENTIFIC PUBLICATIONS

OXFORD LONDON EDINBURGH

BOSTON PALO ALTO MELBOURNE

© 1985 by
Blackwell Scientific Publications
Editorial offices:
Osney Mead, Oxford, OX2 0EL
8 John Street, London, WC1N 2ES
23 Ainslie Place, Edinburgh, EH3 6AJ
52 Beacon Street, Boston
  Massachusetts 02108, USA
667 Lytton Avenue, Palo Alto
  California 94301, USA
107 Barry Street, Carlton
  Victoria 3053, Australia

First published 1985

Photoset by Enset (Photosetting)
Midsomer Norton, Bath, Avon
and printed and bound
in Great Britain by
Biddles Ltd,
Guildford and King's Lynn

DISTRIBUTORS

USA
  Blackwell Mosby Book Distributors
  11830 Westline Industrial Drive
  St Louis, Missouri 63141

Canada
  Blackwell Mosby Book Distributors
  120 Melford Drive, Scarborough
  Ontario M1B 2X4

Australia
  Blackwell Scientific Book Distributors
  31 Advantage Road, Highett
  Victoria 3190

British Library
Cataloguing in Publication Data

Emergencies in Clinical Medicine.
  1. Emergency medicine
  I. Kennedy, H.J.
  616'.025   RC86.7

  ISBN 0-632-01051-7

Contents

List of Contributors

A.G. ARNOLD MD, MB, ChB, MRCP, *Consultant Physician, Hull Royal Infirmary, Hull*

J.K. ARONSON MA, DPhil, MB, ChB, MRCP, *Clinical Reader, Department of Clinical Pharmacology, Radcliffe Infirmary, Oxford*

J. BELL MB, MRCP, *Research Fellow, Nuffield Dept of Clinical Medicine, John Radcliffe Hospital, Oxford*

M.K. BENSON MD, MB, BS, FRCP, *Consultant Physician, Chest Unit, Churchill Hospital, Oxford*

R. BLACKWOOD MA, BM, BCh, MRCP, *Consultant Physician, Wexham Park Hospital, Slough, and Honorary Consultant Physician at Hammersmith Hospital, London*

L. BLUMHARDT MRACP, BSc, MB, ChB, *Senior Lecturer, Unit of Neurological Sciences, Walton Hospital, Rice Lane, Liverpool*

N.A. BOON MA, MB, BChir, MRCP, *Lecturer, Department of Cardiology, John Radcliffe Hospital, Oxford*

C.W. BURKE FRCP, *Consultant Physician, Department of Endocrinology, Radcliffe Infirmary, Oxford*

R.W.G. CHAPMAN BSc, MD, MB, BS, MRCP, *Senior Registrar, Department of Gastroenterology, John Radcliffe Hospital, Oxford*

L. COTTER MB, ChB, MRCP, *Consultant Cardiologist, Manchester Royal Infirmary, Manchester*

T.W. EVANS BSc, MB, ChB, MRCP, PhD, *Research Fellow, Department of Medicine, Hallamshire Hospital, Sheffield*

A. FISHER MB, BCh, FFARCS, *Consultant Anaesthetist, Department of Anaesthetics, John Radcliffe Hospital, Oxford*

R.C.D. GREENHALL DM, FRCP, *Consultant Neurologist, Radcliffe Infirmary, Oxford*

B. GRIBBIN MD, MB, BCh, FRCP, *Consultant Physician, Department of Cardiology, John Radcliffe Hospital, Oxford*

J.V. JONES PhD, MB, BChir, MRCP, *Consultant Cardiologist, Royal Infirmary, Bristol*

H.J. KENNEDY BSc, MD, MB, BS, MRCP, *Lecturer, Department of Medicine, Hallamshire Hospital, Sheffield*

G. PASVOL DPhil, MB, ChB, MRCP, *Senior Lecturer, Nuffield Department of Clinical Medicine, John Radcliffe Hospital, Oxford*

PRIDA PHUAPRADIT MD, MRCP, *Assistant Professor of Medicine, Ramathibodi Hospital, Mahidol University, Bangkok, Thailand*

A.E.G. RAINE DPhil, BA, MB, ChB, BMedSc, MRCP, *Lecturer, Nuffield Department of Medicine, John Radcliffe Hospital, Oxford*

R.C. ROBERTS MA, DPhil, BM, BCh, MRCP, *Lecturer, The National Hospital, Queen Square, London*

D.J. SHALE MD, BSc, MB, BS, MRCP, *Senior Registrar, Chest Unit, Churchill Hospital, Oxford*

H.A. SHEPHERD MA, MB, BChir, MRCP, *Senior Registrar, General Medicine and Gastroenterology, Southampton General Hospital, Southampton*

E.B.O. SMITH MB, BS, FRCP, FRCPsych, *Consultant Psychiatrist, Barnes Unit, John Radcliffe Hospital, Oxford*

J.A.R. SMITH MB, FRCS, *Senior Lecturer, Department of Surgery, Hallamshire Hospital, Sheffield*

P.J. TEDDY MA, DPhil, BSc, BM, BCh, FRCS, *Consultant Neurosurgeon, Department of Neurosurgery, Radcliffe Infirmary, Oxford*

D.F. TREACHER BA, MB, BS, MRCP, *Senior Medical Registrar, Intensive Care Unit, St Thomas's Hospital, Lambeth Palace Road, London*

J.M. TROWELL MB, BS, MRCP, *Honorary Consultant Physician and Lecturer, John Radcliffe Hospital, Oxford*

R.C. TURNER MD, MB, BChir, FRCP, *Clinical Reader and Honorary Consultant Physician, Radcliffe Infirmary, Oxford*

C.P. WARLOW MD, BA, MB, BChir, FRCP, *Consultant Neurologist, Department of Neurology, Radcliffe Infirmary, Oxford*

J. WATKINS BSc, MB, BS, MRCP, *Consultant Physician, Department of Cardiology, St Mary's Hospital, Portsmouth*

D.J. WEATHERALL FRCP, FRCPath, FRS, *Professor of Medicine, Nuffield Department of Clinical Medicine, University of Oxford*

G.K. WILCOCK BSc, DM, FRCP, *Professor of Care of the Elderly, Bristol University and Frenchay Hospital, Bristol*

Acknowledgements

Many thanks are due to Mr M.J.E. Ely of Becton Dickinson UK Ltd for providing support for both the series of lectures from which the concept of this book arose and the secretarial expenses incurred in preparing the manuscript.

Grateful thanks are also due to my wife for documenting the data on medical emergencies from the casualty records of an entire year, and to everyone at Blackwell Scientific Publications who have been of invaluable assistance.

H.J.K.

1 · Introduction and Survey of Emergency Admissions

H. J. KENNEDY

Introduction

The idea for this book arose from a series of lunch time lectures concerning the management of medical emergencies given to the junior medical staff at the John Radcliffe Hospital in Oxford. The aim of the lectures and subsequently of this book, is to consider the practical management of the acutely ill patients that are admitted and treated by physicians in a general hospital. The authors of the chapters have endeavoured not only to give a practical guide to the management of the emergencies but also to consider the current limitations in our knowledge and discuss the controversies in the management of these patients. Finally, they have also given the reasons for following their particular approach to the management. Therefore, the book is not primarily supposed to be a pocket guide but more to be an aid to physicians who already have a knowledge of the practical management of medical emergencies. Nevertheless, it is hoped that the book will also be useful to house officers, anaesthetists, general practitioners, medical students and other doctors involved in the care of patients with acute medical problems.

It has not been possible to consider the management of all medical emergencies but, as will be seen from the survey contained in this chapter, all the common problems are considered in detail. In addition, less frequent emergencies, such as some of the infectious and imported diseases are included, because they are becoming more frequent in the United Kingdom with the greater ease of travel. Moreover, it is important that they are recognized and treated promptly.

Survey of emergency admissions

A survey has been undertaken of all the patients who were admitted with acute medical problems by physicians at the John Radcliffe Hospital during a recent one year period in order to establish the approximate frequency of these emergencies in a busy general hospital in the United Kingdom.

The John Radcliffe is the district general hospital for Oxford and the surrounding area. It serves a population of approximately 300,000 people. It is the only hospital in the district with an accident and emergency department. It is also a teaching hospital and regional centre for several medical services. However, some specialties are centred at other hospitals in Oxford, such as the infectious diseases unit, the chest clinic, the renal unit and neurology wards. Each of these units takes some emergency admissions without the patients going to the John Radcliffe Hospital. Therefore, the survey given below does not include all the emergencies seen in Oxford and is somewhat biased as the emergency admissions to the specialized units are not included. Nevertheless, the survey does give some idea of the frequency of the various problems arising in the Oxford district.

There was a total of 4,161 admissions during the year. Many other patients were seen in the emergency area but they were allowed to go home. Therefore, they are not included. The frequency of admission was greater in the winter months and least during the summer. They ranged from 446 in January to 272 in June. The mean age of the patients, which includes the majority of emergency admissions of elderly people within the district, was 60.4 years (ranging from 14 to 99). Paediatric admissions were not included in this survey. The mean age would be significantly greater if the large number of patients who had taken an overdose were excluded; as they form a considerably younger population. The relative frequency of the various emergency admissions is given in Table 1.1. These data were obtained from the details recorded in the accident and emergency department record book.

Table 1.1. Frequency of the more common emergencies admitted by physicians to the John Radcliffe Hospital in one year

Emergency	Number of admissions in one year	Percentage of total admissions
Overdose	491	11.8
Myocardial infarction	482	11.6
Cerebrovascular accident	429	10.3
Chest pain	325	7.8
Heart failure	223	5.4
Collapse	212	5.1
Upper gastro-intestinal haemorrhage	202	4.9
Deep venous thrombosis	187	4.5
Pneumonia	146	3.5
Diabetic emergencies	137	3.3
Chronic airways obstruction and chest infection	135	3.2
Cardiac arrhythmias	127	3.1
Epilepsy	92	2.2
Haematological problems	79	1.9
Severe hypertension	27	0.6
Miscellaneous	867	20.8

Therefore, they do not represent the definitive diagnosis when the patients had been fully investigated. Moreover, the figures do not indicate the total number of any particular emergency occurring within the hospital. For example, cardiac arrest does not occur often in the emergency department but it does occur frequently within the hospital.

Several interesting points arise from the figures given in Table 1.1. First, patients who had taken an overdose of drugs were the most numerous of all the emergencies. This is a sad reflection on our society. Nevertheless, it demonstrates that it is a substantial problem for both the medical, psychiatric and social services. Obviously, it is vital that, not only should the immediate medical resuscitation be efficient but also that the underlying psychological and social problems of each individual should be investigated and as much help as possible given.

A second interesting point arising from the data in Table 1.1 is the high frequency of degenerative cardio-vascular disease. If 'chest pain', which is largely composed of suspected cardiovascular abnormality, is included then forty per cent of all the emergencies are caused by acute cardiovascular problems. It is ironical to think that as with the overdoses, a substantial proportion of these problems are likely to be related to social factors such as smoking and diet.

Nevertheless, patients with emergency medical problems continue to be seen in our hospitals in large numbers. They must be managed with skill and efficiency. Hopefully, this book may play a small part in furthering this objective.

2 · Common Clinical Presentations of Medical Emergencies

H. J. KENNEDY

The common clinical presentations discussed in this chapter are as follows:
- Coma (including a section on brain death)
- Breathlessness
- Chest pain
- Abdominal pain
- Severe headache

Transient loss of consciousness and funny turns are considered in detail in Chapter 17.

The approach to patients presenting with these problems will be discussed with particular reference to the clinical features, differential diagnosis and initial management. Guidelines are given in each section as to how to determine the most likely underlying diagnosis. The reader is referred to the other chapters of the book for considerations of the definitive diagnoses.

Coma

Normal alertness depends on a close interaction between the cerebral cortex and the reticular formation in the mid-brain and brain stem. Relatively minor abnormalities of the reticular formation may lead to unconsciousness as it is particularly sensitive to small areas of local damage and to drugs and metabolic disorders. More extensive diffuse abnormalities or large lesions raising intracranial pressure are required for coma to result from cortical damage.

The management of an unconscious patient and the diagnosis of the underlying abnormality may not be straightforward and requires an orderly approach. The main causes of coma are given in Table 2.1.

Immediate management

The first priority is to preserve vital functions. The airway must be maintained and adequate ventilation ensured. The mouth and pharynx are cleared of any debris or secretions. Intubation, mechanical ventilation and added oxygen may have to be instituted when they are indicated. The patient should be placed in the semi-prone position with the head lowered. If there is any possibility of a head injury, the patient must be handled with great care in case a spinal injury has been sustained. An intravenous infusion should be started. Convulsions are controlled and cerebral perfusion must

Table 2.1. Causes of coma

Supratentorial mass lesions	
Cerebral infarct, haemorrhage or embolism	
Cerebral tumour	
Cerebral abscess	
Extradural haematoma	
Subdural haematoma	
Subtentorial lesions	
Brain stem infarct, haemorrhage or embolism	
Cerebellar infarct, haemorrhage or embolism	
Tumour	
Diffuse disorders	
Hypoxia or Ischaemia	Reduced PaO$_2$ due to: respiratory failure, anaemia, poisoning etc.
	Reduced perfusion due to: cardiac arrhythmia, syncope, shock, pulmonary embolus, severe hypertension, disseminated intravascular coagulation, vasculitis etc.
Epilepsy and post–ictal states	
Drugs and toxins	e.g. alcohol, barbiturates, glutethemide, benzodiazepines, opiates, other analgesics and sedatives
Trauma	Concussion, contusion and laceration
Infection	Meningitis, encephalitis, cerebral malaria, typhoid, typhus and yellow fever
Subarachnoid haemorrhage	
Hypothermia and hyperpyrexia	
Metabolic disorders	
Hypoglycaemia and diabetic ketoacidosis	
Hepatic coma	
Uraemia	
Thyroid, pituitary and adrenal disease	
Fluid and electrolyte or acid:base disturbance	
Porphyria	
Thiamin and B12 deficiency	
Toxaemia of pregnancy	
Psychiatric disorders	
Malingering	
Hysteria	
Catatonia	

be maintained by establishing an adequate blood pressure. The plasma level of glucose may be estimated using a stick test, although blood must always be taken for accurate glucose measurement. Subsequently, 25 gm of 50% glucose should be given intravenously if there is any suspicion of hypoglycaemia.

Clinical assessment

History

After the initial supportive measures have been instituted, as detailed a history as possible should be obtained and a careful examination undertaken. Information may be gleaned from relatives, friends, passers-by, the patient's general practitioner (GP), the police and ambulance crew. Observers should be questioned about the mode of onset of the coma (e.g. fits, headache, chest pain or assault). Details of ingestion of drugs or alcohol should be obtained. The family or referring doctor should be asked to search for drugs in the patient's home. The previous medical history should be obtained from the family, GP and previous hospital records. In particular, a history of epilepsy, unconscious episodes, drug abuse and therapy, alcohol abuse, cardiovascular disease and diabetes should be sought.

Examination

A rapid but skilful general physical examination is required. First, the clothes and belongings of the patient need to be searched for any evidence of a previous medical history, such as warning cards for patients taking steroids or anticoagulants, and insulin in diabetics. Secondly, every patient should be examined for evidence of trauma, infection, drug administration (tablets in the mouth or injection sites), recent operations, swollen calves suggesting deep venous thrombosis, and so on. The cardiovascular, respiratory, gastrointestinal (including the liver), endocrine and urogenital systems must be examined carefully. The core temperature should be recorded with a low reading rectal thermometer.

Neurological examination in the comatose patient is quite different from a normal neurological assessment. The main points in the examination of the unconscious patient are: establishing the level of consciousness, examination of the pupils, eye movements, corneal responses, fundi, respiration and remaining motor functions. Neck stiffness and Kernig's sign are sought. We use the following assessment for grading conscious level:
0   Fully conscious.
1   Responds to questioning.
2   Responds to commands.
3   Responds only to painful stimuli.
4   No response to any stimulus.

Pressure on the nail bed and pinching the Achilles' tendon are good ways of exerting a painful stimulus. The value of examining the respiration, pupil reflexes, oculocephalic and oculovestibular reflexes and motor functions are summarized in Table 2.2.

Table 2.2. Neurological signs in coma

Neurology	Pupils	Oculocephalic and oculovestibular reflexes	Motor	Respiration
Unilateral supratentorial mass lesions	Ipsilateral 3rd nerve palsy develops with coning	Present. Become depressed if coning occurs	Hemiparesis	Periodic: Cheyne Stokes
Subtentorial	Asymmetrical initially	May be present initially but lost early	Asymmetric initially but progresses to symmetry	Irregularly irregular
Diffuse, metabolic and drugs	Well preserved but note specific drug effects: Opiates—constriction Atropine—dilates Barbiturates—fixed. **NB** When abnormal permanent damage is not indicated	Variable. Even when absent function may return	Symmetric abnormalities. Look for flapping tremor, convulsions common	Hyper- or hypo-ventilation

The size, symmetry and response to light of the pupils should be recorded. A unilateral large fixed pupil indicates a third nerve palsy on the same side as the lesion. Both pupils tend to be fixed in the mid-position when the mid-brain is damaged. When both pupils become fixed and dilated, extensive damage to the brain stem is likely. Bilateral small pupils usually result from a pontine lesion or from opiate administration. The other drugs that effect pupillary reflexes are atropine-like substances and barbiturates. Abnormal pupil reactions are common in metabolic and drug induced coma and it is important to realize that even fixed dilated pupils are reversible in these circumstances.

Doll's eye movements are not present in a conscious individual. They appear when diffuse cortical damage has occurred but when the brain stem is intact. Brain stem lesions result in the total or partial loss of the doll's eye movements. A further test of brain stem function is the caloric test. The tympanic membranes must be inspected before undertaking this test. Forty

ml of ice-cold water is instilled over 30 seconds; there is normally a con-
jugated deviation of the eyes towards the stimulated side. When the pons
and medulla have been destroyed there is no response in the eye movements
to either doll's eye or caloric stimulation.

The respiratory pattern is another useful marker for the level of remaining nervous function. Cheyne-Stokes respirations appear when there is
bilateral hemisphere disturbance. Hyperventilation may occur with mid-
brain dysfunction. Where the brain stem is damaged breathing becomes
irregularly irregular. Drug related or metabolic causes of coma may induce
either hyper- or hypo-ventilation.

Motor system functions have to be tested differently from those in a
conscious individual. Usually, spontaneous movements or movements in
response to painful stimuli may be observed. Motor responses to painful
stimuli are hemiplegic with hemispheric lesions. Decerebrate rigidity with
clenched jaw and extended neck, back and limbs occurs when the mid-brain
is damaged. The limbs are flaccid with brain stem dysfunction. Symmetrical
motor abnormalities are usually found with drug induced or metabolic
coma. Look for characteristic features such as asterixis (flapping tremor).

Investigations

There are some investigations which should be undertaken in every
comatose patient. Blood should be taken for measurement of blood glucose,
electrolytes, urea and creatinine, liver biochemical tests and full blood
count, platelets and prothrombin time. A sample should also be sent to the
laboratory to screen for drugs. Part of this sample should be stored for
further detailed analysis, should this become necessary. Similarly, specimens of any vomit or gastric lavage should also be saved. An arterial blood
sample should be taken for the measurement of pH, pO_2 and pCo_2. A chest
X-ray and electrocardiogram (ECG) are always required as is a specimen of
urine for sugar, ketone bodies, microscopy, culture and analysis for drugs.

Skull X-rays are sometimes required as are computerized tomographic
(CT) scans. Provided that there is no evidence of raised intracranial pressure
a lumbar puncture must be carried out if the patient is pyrexial, even if there
is little or no neck stiffness, as meningitis and encephalitis may present in this
manner.

Management

Immediate urgent measures were considered at the beginning of this
chapter. Usually, the diagnosis has become established when a full history
and examination have been undertaken and the results of the investigations

are available. When this is the case, the appropriate treatment should be instituted without delay; such as operation for subdural or extradural haemorrhage and fluid and electrolyte replacement with controlled insulin therapy in diabetic coma. When there are no localizing signs, no evidence of metabolic derangement and no signs of infection, an immediate diagnosis is not always possible. Drug overdose is the most common cause of coma in this situation. In any case, all unconscious patients must be nursed and supported with great care. The points of importance are given in Table 2.3.

Table 2.3 Management of the unconscious patient

1 Ventilation	Clear oropharynx, nurse in semi-prone position. If inadequate ventilation, intubate and ventilate.
2 Perfusion	Establish intravenous line. Treat any cause of shock, e.g. anaphylaxis, sepsis or hypovolaemia.
3 Blood sugar	Measure regularly and treat appropriately.
4 Clinical features	Obtain as detailed a history as possible. Examine and investigate as described in this chapter. Re-examine often to detect changing signs.
5 Establish diagnosis	Treat underlying condition.
6 Cough and gag reflexes	When no cough reflex is present, no food or fluid can be given orally. Consider intubation to protect airway. Keep oropharynx clear by regular suction. If cough reflex present but gag is absent, consider a fine bore naso-gastric tube for feeding.
7 Check corneal reflex	If absent place paraffin gauze over closed lids.
8 Two hourly turns	Turn to prevent pressure sores. Change bedding promptly if bedclothes become soiled. Consider Paul's tubing in men. May have to catheterize.
9 Monitoring	Regularly monitor: conscious level, temperature, pulse, blood pressure, respiration, blood sugar, fluid balance and weight if possible.
10 Physiotherapy	Start early physiotherapy to chest and limbs.
11 Drugs	**Do not give** steroids or antibiotics unless they are specifically indicated.

Brain death

Establishing the diagnosis of brain death has become very important with the development of artificial ventilation and other intensive care technology. It has also become important due to the advent of organ transplantation. The criteria for the diagnosis of brain death in the United Kingdom and United States have been considered in detail elsewhere (Pallis 1983; Black 1978).

A summary of the criteria is given in this section:

1   *Exclusion of reversible causes* of brain damage, such as hypothermia, drug overdose and severe metabolic disorder. The activity of muscle relaxants must be reversed.

2   Identification of the *definite cause* of brain death.

3   *No spontaneous respiration* even when stimulated by 5% carbon dioxide (Pa CO_2 must reach at least 6.65 kPa). Previous chronic obstructive airways disease, muscle relaxants, respiratory depressants and hyperventilation must be considered.

4   *No cerebral response* to any form of stimulation and *brain stem reflexes* must be *absent*. These include pupillary, oculocephalic, corneal, gag and vestibulo-ocular reflexes. Metabolic disorders, vestibular damage and drugs must be excluded. Testing of the oculovestibular reflex is discussed earlier in this chapter.

An electro-encephalogram (EEG) is neither reliable nor essential for the diagnosis of brain death, but it may be helpful in some difficult cases. Studies of cerebral blood flow using either isotope methods or carotid angiography may occasionally be helpful.

Breathlessness

Breathlessness is a frequent and distressing presenting symptom. The main causes are given in Table 2.4.

Clinical assessment

History

It is important to determine the duration of the breathlessness and whether it began in relation to any factor such as fumes, exertion, lying down (orthopnoea) or to a recent upper respiratory tract infection. Knowledge of whether the breathlessness began abruptly and if it is associated with other symptoms such as cough, chest pain, palpitations, syncope or paraesthesiae is also helpful. A past history of respiratory, cardiovascular, metabolic, neuromuscular or psychiatric disorder should be sought. The occupation and current drug therapy of the patient must be ascertained. Help with this information and with the history in general may often be obtained from relatives, friends, the patient's general practitioner and from previous hospital records.

Table 2.4 Causes of breathlessness

Cardiovascular
Myocardial infarction
Arrhythmias
Hypertension
Ischaemic heart disease
Mitral and aortic valve disease
Cardiomyopathy
Left ventricular aneurysm
Dissecting aneurysm
Cardiac tamponade
Congenital heart disease
Left atrial myxoma
Hyper- and hypothyroidism

Respiratory
Acute exacerbation of chronic airways
obstruction
Asthma
Pneumonia
Pneumothorax
Pulmonary collapse
Pleural effusion
Adult respiratory distress syndrome
Occupational pulmonary disease
Fibrosing alveolitis
Inhalation pneumonitis, e.g.
aspiration of stomach content, fumes etc
Allergic pneumonitis
Carcinoma of bronchus
Obstruction of upper airways
Acute laryngotracheo-
bronchitis in children
Acute epiglottitis

Embolic
Pulmonary embolism
Fat embolism
Amniotic fluid embolism

Miscellaneous
Metabolic eg. diabetic ketoacidosis,
uraemia
Shock
Neuromuscular diseases
Acute cerebrovascular disease
Psychological

Examination

General

The character of the dyspnoea should be observed. It may exhibit stridor in large airways obstruction, wheezing in asthma and be bubbly with pulmonary oedema or exudation. Patients with severe breathlessness usually sit upright with their hands holding the arms of the chair and their arms straight. This position allows the maximum use of the accessory respiratory muscles to aid respiration. When conditions such as massive pulmonary embolism, shock or severe left ventricular failure lead to hypotension then the patient has to lie down to maintain cerebral perfusion. This usually exacerbates the respiratory failure.

All breathless patients should be examined for central cyanosis and clubbing. Central cyanosis is only observed when five or more grams of haemoglobin are deoxygenated. Therefore, when anaemia is present central cyanosis may never appear despite a very low arterial oxygen tension. The presence or absence of a cough and sputum production may help in the diagnosis of dyspnoeic patients. Any available sputum should be examined. The mouth and pharynx should be carefully inspected for evidence of a foreign body.

Pulse, blood pressure and venous pressure

The pulse should be palpated to search for arrhythmias and abnormal pulse forms such as pulsus paradoxus or alternans. However, measurement of the blood pressure is the best way of determining the presence of these abnormal pulse forms. Pulsus paradoxus is said to exist when there is a fall in arterial blood pressure of 10 mm Hg or more. It is most commonly found in severe asthma or in cardiac tamponade. Examination of the neck veins is often difficult in dyspnoeic patients but can be very important. A raised venous pressure may help to distinguish between a massive pulmonary embolism and acute left ventricular failure. However, the pressure may be raised in acute left ventricular failure as well as after a massive pulmonary embolism. When a paradoxical blood pressure is present the jugular venous pressure falls on inspiration in asthma whereas it rises on inspiration in patients with cardiac tamponade (Kussmaul's sign).

The chest

This should be examined for abnormal movements, deviation of the trachea and displacement and abnormal character of the apex beat. This will help to elicit mediastinal shift and cardiac abnormalities. A double apex beat or an unusually diffuse apex beat may be detected when a left ventricular aneurysm is present.

On auscultation of the heart a mitral incompetent murmur may be heard after rupture of the chordae tendineae or be due to papillary muscular dysfunction. However, breathlessness in the presence of mitral incompetence is more commonly due to left ventricular failure in the presence of previous valve damage. The possibility of subacute bacterial endocarditis should always be considered. When a myocardial infarction is complicated by a rupture of the ventricular septum, a thrill and harsh pansystolic murmur are found. Other murmurs to keep in mind are the aortic regurgitation murmurs that may occur with aortic dissection or severe hypertension and the variable systolic and/or diastolic murmurs that may be found with an atrial myxoma. The chest should be examined for the classical signs of diminished breath sounds over fluid, bronchial breathing over consolidated lung, and so on. The chest must be examined carefully for signs of a pneumothorax, especially in patients with previous pulmonary disease, as even a small pneumothorax may cause respiratory difficulty in these patients.

There are several other points to remember. First, the breath sounds may be virtually absent with no rhonchi in severe asthma due to the very poor airflow. Secondly, widespread rhonchi may be produced in left ventricular failure and after a pulmonary embolus; this may cause diagnostic confusion if other signs are not carefully elicited. Thirdly, crepitations are produced by oedema in the alveolar walls. Therefore, crepitations are not only found with acute left ventricular failure but also in bronchopneumonia, allergic and fibrosing alveolitis and chemical pneumonitis. Finally, the possibility of breathlessness being due to metabolic, neuromuscular and psychiatric causes should not be forgotten.

Investigations

A good quality chest X-ray is the most important investigation in patients presenting with breathlessness. Inspiratory and expiratory films are necessary when a pneumothorax is suspected and a lateral film is required in most other patients. However, it must be stressed that an X-ray is not a substitute for a thorough physical examination. The classical appearances of the X-ray in pulmonary oedema, pneumothorax, pleural effusion and fibrosed, consolidated and collapsed lung are well known. The chest X-ray may also be helpful in making a diagnosis of pericardial effusion where the cardiac shadow is enlarged, pear-shaped and the left heart border is straight; as the normal appearance of the left atrial appendage and pulmonary artery are obscured. In addition, an unusually large or double aortic shadow may be seen in the presence of a dissecting aneurysm. The chest X-ray is usually normal immediately after both small and large pulmonary emboli. If a patient has had previous chest X-rays these may be very helpful in making a diagnosis.

An electrocardiogram should be carried out in all acutely breathless patients. This will help with the diagnosis of many causes of breathlessness such as cardiac arrhythmia, pulmonary embolism, left ventricular aneurysm and so on. Previous ECGs may be very useful for comparison. Similarly, arterial blood gas analysis should be undertaken in most patients. The changes found in the electrocardiogram and blood gas analysis in the different conditions are given in the relevant chapters of this book.

The other investigations which may be of value in acutely breathless patients are: a full blood count, biochemical profile, microbiological examination of the sputum, respiratory function tests, echocardiography and isotope ventilation and perfusion scans. Pulmonary, aortic and left ventricular angiography are of value in particular situations. For example, an arch aortogram may be required to confirm the diagnosis of a dissecting aneurysm.

Management

The emergency management of acutely breathless patients depends on a rapid and accurate diagnosis. This should be achieved by following the guidelines that have been outlined in this chapter. The patient should be allowed to maintain the posture which he finds to be most comfortable. An arterial blood sample for blood gas analysis should always be taken before beginning oxygen therapy. If oxygen has been given already, for example by the ambulance crew, the blood gases should still be determined urgently. This is vitally important in patients with any possibility of having airways obstruction and carbon dioxide retention. In such patients, 24 per cent inspired oxygen should be administered once the arterial blood gas sample has been taken. Serial blood gases should be undertaken in these patients; if the PaO_2 remains very low (<8.0 kPa) and there is no rise in the $PaCO_2$ then the inspired oxygen may be raised to 28 per cent. Continued careful monitoring of the PaO_2 and $PaCO_2$ must be maintained as carbon dioxide may be retained gradually. The management of respiratory failure is fully discussed in chapter 11. The management of other common causes of acute breathlessness, such as acute heart failure, asthma, pulmonary embolism and others given in Table 2.4 are considered in detail in the relevant chapters.

The management of three causes of breathlessness not considered elsewhere in this book are briefly discussed.

Acute upper airways obstruction

This is not common in adults but requires prompt action when it occurs. Debris and foreign bodies should be removed from the mouth and pharynx. Similarly, foreign material can be removed from the larynx by laryngoscopy. Humidification of inspired air may be helpful when there is inflammation of the larynx. Treatment for anaphylaxis (see anaphylactic shock, chapter 14) may help when angioneurotic oedema has occurred. An emergency tracheostomy may have to be undertaken in some patients with acute upper airways obstruction. When the situation is desperate, an intravenous cannula or needle may be inserted into the trachea in the midline immediately below the thyroid cartilage.

Cardiac tamponade

When a pericardial effusion is causing cardiac embarrassment, e.g. marked paradox or arterial hypotension, the fluid may have to be aspirated. Whenever possible, this should be undertaken by a cardiologist as it is not without risk. If feasible, the patient is seated so that the fluid accumulates in the lower pericardium. Either the epigastric or apical route may be used; the former tends to be safer. For this approach, the local anaesthetic needle is inserted below and to the left of the xiphisternum and advanced upwards and a little to the left at an angle of 30–40° to the abdominal wall. There is often a little give as the needle passes through the pericardium and straw coloured or blood stained fluid may then be obtained. When it is blood stained it may look like blood but it is dark due to oxygen desaturation, it does not clot as it is defibrinated and it has a low haematocrit. When undertaking pericardial aspiration it is helpful to connect the limb leads of an ECG in the usual way and to attach the chest lead to the aspiration needle. The ECG is set to record impulses from the chest lead as the needle is inserted; raised ST segments appear on the tracing if the needle touches the epicardium.

Massive pleural effusion

Large pleural effusions can cause unpleasant breathlessness. One litre of pleural fluid may be removed in the first instance; any more can lead to the development of pulmonary oedema in the expanding lung. The seventh or eighth intercostal space posteriorly is usually the best site for aspiration. An Abrams needle should be used when a pleural biopsy is required. The needle should be inserted just above the rib below as the neurovascular bundle runs along the lower rib margins. The fluid obtained should be sent for bacteriological, biochemical and cytological examination.

Chest pain

Chest pain is a common presenting symptom. Most patients are concerned that their pain is due to severe heart disease. The more common causes are given in Table 2.5.

Table 2.5. Causes of chest pain

Cardiac
Obstructive coronary artery disease
   Atherosclerosis: Angina pectoris
                Myocardial infarction
                Unstable angina
   Poliarteritis
   Syphilic aortitis
   Coronary embolism
Increased myocardial oxygen demand
   Aortic valve disease
   Hypertension
   Right ventricular hypertrophy
   Hypertrophic obstructive
   Cardiomyopathy
   Thyrotoxicosis
Mitral valve leaflet prolapse

Pericardial
Pericarditis
   Viral, bacterial, tuberculosis
   Myocardial infarction
   Post infarction syndrome
   Trauma, uraemia, connective tissue disease
   Neoplasm

Aortic
Dissecting aneurysm

Other intrathoracic causes
Pulmonary embolism
Tracheobronchitis
Pleurisy
Subphrenic abscess
Pneumothorax
Pneumomediastinum
Neoplasia

Gastro-intestinal
Oesophagus
   Reflux
   Abnormal motility
   Mallory Weiss Tear
   Tumour
Peptic ulceration
Pancreatitis
Cholecystitis
Biliary colic
Irritable bowel syndrome

Musculoskeletal
Muscle strain
Rib fracture
Arthritis
Tietze's syndrome
Barnholm's disease
Neoplasia

Neurological
Herpetic neuralgia
Root pain
Vertebral disease
Pancoasts tumour

Miscellaneous
Anaemia

Functional
Effort syndrome and neurosis

Clinical features

Severe central chest pain

Patients with severe persistent central crushing chest pain are often seen in hospital with a suspected diagnosis of myocardial infarction. Unstable angina, acute pericarditis, dissection of the thoracic aorta, pulmonary embolism, oesophageal spasm, an acute abdomen, such as acute pancreatitis and biliary colic, Tietze's syndrome, spinal pain and functional chest pain are the main differential diagnoses. A careful history from the patient or witnesses and a rapid but searching physical examination are essential. The main distinguishing clinical features are given below and in the appropriate chapters.

Angina pectoris

Patients presenting with retrosternal pain must be questioned closely concerning their symptoms because a diagnosis of angina pectoris must not be undertaken lightly. Conversely, it is equally important not to miss the diagnosis. Angina presenting in relation to exertion is usually easy to recognize but remember angina in relation to other situations such as cold, emotion or after a heavy meal. Relief by glyceryl trinitrate may aid the diagnosis.

Diabetes mellitus, hypothyroidism and hyperlipidaemias should be excluded in all cases of angina. The coronary arteries may be obstructed not only by atheroma but also by inflammation as in arteritis or the other diseases shown in Table 2.5. Other conditions causing increased oxygen consumption by the myocardium may also result in angina symptoms.

Mitral valve prolapse

This may lead to anginal type pain or atypical chest pain. It occurs particularly in young women but is found in patients of any age and either sex. Diagnosis is suspected by the presence of a systolic click or late systolic murmur. These may only appear on exercise and may vary with posture.

Functional chest pains

Most patients with functional chest pains consider that they have a cardiac disorder. The pain that these patients present with is often atypical and they frequently have symptoms of anxiety such as palpitations, dizziness and syncope. Nevertheless, it can be very difficult to distinguish between these patients and those with true myocardial infarction or angina. Particular care has to be taken in the investigation and management of such patients as they can easily become cardiac invalids.

Dissecting aneurysm (see chapter 10)

Pericarditis

Pain arising from the pericardium is usually located in the precordium and is burning in nature. There may be referred pain via C_3, C_4 and C_5 to the left shoulder. Upper abdominal and back pain may also occur which may mimic intra–abdominal problems, such as acute cholecystitis and pancreatitis. Typically, the pain is worse on lying in the left lateral position and may be exacerbated by respiration. It may be relieved by sitting forward. The presence of a pericardial rub is a helpful sign. However, the absence of a rub does not exclude pericarditis.

Chest pain from other intrathoracic causes

Massive pulmonary embolism may cause a crushing central chest pain that resembles myocardial infarction. Smaller emboli can result in peripheral pulmonary infarction leading to pleural inflammation causing pleuritic pain. Pulmonary embolism is discussed in chapter 8. Pleuritic pain is usually characteristic. However, it may cause inflammation of the diaphragmatic pleura which frequently leads to pain in the shoulders. Signs of the under-lying cause of inflammation, such as breathlessness and haemoptysis may facilitate in making the diagnosis. Finally, a brief sharp stabbing pain associated with breathlessness may occur with a spontaneous pneumothorax (chapter 15).

Chest pain of gastro-intestinal origin

Pain arising from the oesophagus is typically a retrosternal chest or neck pain, burning in nature, which comes on while lying down or bending over and is relieved by antacids. It may mimic angina pectoris or myocardial infarction making diagnosis difficult, especially as pain from oesophageal spasm may be relieved by glyceryl trinitrate in some patients. Oesophageal pain should be excluded in all cases of angina type pain when the diagnosis is in doubt. Pain arising from the oesophagus commonly results from inflam-mation due to reflux, abnormal oesophageal motility and spasm or some-times tumour. Several other gastro-intestinal problems may cause chest pain (Table 2.6). These may also cause diagnostic confusion and should not be forgotten when the differential diagnosis is considered.

Chest pain of musculoskeletal or neuromuscular origin

Pain arising from musculoskeletal and neurological sources may also cause diagnostic difficulty. In particular, Bornholm's disease, Tietze's syndrome and degenerative disease of the cervical and thoracic spine can mimic ischaemic cardiac pain.

Investigations

An ECG is the most useful investigation in patients presenting with 'angina type' pain. However, it may be normal in patients with angina and even initially in patients who have had a myocardial infarction. When angina is suspected an exercise ECG will show clear evidence of ischaemia in about 75 per cent of patients who are finally diagnosed as having angina pectoris. In patients with pericarditis the ECG characteristically shows widespread ST segment elevations that are concave upwards (in distinction from the convex ST segments found with myocardial injury). However, the absence of these abnormal ST segments does not exclude pericarditis. The ECG may also show characteristic patterns in patients who have suffered a pulmonary embolism (see chapter 8).

A plain chest X-ray, possibly with lateral or inspiratory and expiratory films is also of value in patients with chest pain. A chest X-ray may help in the diagnosis of a left ventricular aneurysm, pericardial effusion, aortic dissection and in most cases of chest pain caused by pulmonary or pleural pathology.

Echocardiography is also very useful in the diagnosis of chest pain. In particular, the diagnosis of mitral valve leaflet prolapse, other valve lesions, ventricular aneurysm, aortic dissection and pericardial effusion are often established by the findings at echocardiography.

When considering oesophageal abnormalities as a cause of chest pain, helpful investigations include a barium swallow and meal, with subsequent head down tilt, to look for abnormal motility and reflux. An upper gastro-intestinal endoscopy should be done to look for abnormalities including oesophagitis and oesophageal mucosal tear. Finally, the acid perfusion or Bernstein test may be useful, as can an acid reflux test.

Management

All patients suspected of having a myocardial infarction should be admitted to hospital, preferably to a coronary care unit, even if the ECG does not show definite signs of a myocardial infarction. It is wise to admit patients with suspected pericarditis for further investigation of the underlying causes (Table 2.5). The detailed management of the other main causes of chest pain

Table 2.6. Causes of abdominal pain

Abdominal	
Wall	Trauma, haematoma
Peritoneal inflammation	Pancreatitis, cholecystitis, appendicitis, Meckel's diverticulum, diverticulitis, ulcerative colitis, Crohn's disease, ischaemic colitis, pseudomembranous colitis, lymphadenitis, pyelonephritis, abscesses, endometriosis, salpingitis
Perforated viscus	Oesophagus, stomach, duodenum—ulcers, carcinoma and trauma
	Small intestine—trauma, diverticulum, typhoid Appendix, gallbladder
	Colon—diverticulum, carcinoma, toxic megacolon, trauma
	Uterus and fallopian tubes
Rupture of solid organ	Liver—trauma, hepatoma, hydatid cyst
	Spleen—trauma, splenomegaly, malaria, Kula Azar Ovarian cyst
Torsion of an organ	Stomach, gallbladder, bowel, ovarian cyst, fibroid, testicle
Obstruction	Stomach and intestine—paralytic, mechanical, strangulated
	Biliary tree, urinary tract
Motility disorder	Irritable bowel, constipation, uterine contraction
Vascular	Dissection of aorta, renal, hepatic and splenic infarction
	Vasculitis of bowel, polyarteritis, Buergers disease, collagen disease
	Hereditary angioneurotic oedema
	Henoch-Schoenlein purpura, haematoma, ischaemic colitis, migraine
	Hepatic congestion, mesenteric ischaemia, embolus and infarction
Miscellaneous	Gastro-enteritis, peptic ulceration, retroperitoneal tumours
Thoracic	
Pulmonary and pleural	Pleurisy, pneumonia, pneumothorax
Cardiac and vascular	Myocardial infarction
Oesophageal	Oesophagitis spasm and carcinoma
Neurological	Herpes Zoster, tabes dorsalis, abdominal epilepsy, radiculitis, nerve root compression
Metabolic	Uraemia, diabetes, porphyria, familial hyperlipidaemia, familial Mediterranean fever, hypercalcaemia, haemolytic crisis, adrenal insufficiency, venom, lead poisoning
Psychiatric	Munchausen's syndrome

are given in the relevant chapters of this book; myocardial infarction and unstable angina, chapter 4; pulmonary embolism, chapter 8; dissecting aneurysm, chapter 10; pneumothorax, chapter 15.

Abdominal pain

Abdominal pain is frequently thought of as a surgical problem. However, this is often incorrect and physicians must be skilled in assessing an acute abdomen. The causes of abdominal pain are given in Table 2.6.

Clinical features

A detailed history and skilled examination are essential in the management of acute abdominal pain. In many cases, the need for surgical intervention has to be judged largely on the clinical features as little further information is obtained by the investigations. The pain may be of either visceral type carried in the sympathetic fibres to the spinal cord segments from T_5-L_2, or parietal type when the peritoneum is irritated or inflamed. Pain from the peritoneum is carried in the somatic sensory fibres that innervate the abdominal wall.

History

The character, location, timing, radiation and aggravating and relieving factors of the pain are all helpful. Where was the patient and what was he doing when the pain began?. Symptoms of vomiting, bowel disturbance, food intolerance, urinary and gynaecological disorders should be sought. The patient should be questioned about his occupation, smoking, alcohol consumption, drug therapy and travel abroad.

Examination

A general inspection of the patient must be undertaken before approaching the abdomen. Otherwise extra-abdominal signs of both extra- and intra-abdominal pathology may be missed; for example, fever, anaemia, jaundice or an enlarged left supraclavicular lymph node associated with carcinoma of the stomach or a foetor associated with uraemia, diabetic keto-acidosis or chronic liver failure. The abdomen should be inspected carefully for any abnormality such as asymmetry, scars and abnormal movement with respiration. Palpation should be undertaken with skill so as to cause the minimum discomfort possible. However, areas of tenderness, rebound tenderness, rigidity and masses must be examined carefully. Examination of the hernial orifices and a rectal examination is carried out in all patients. The scrotum and testes must be examined. Vaginal examination is indicated in female patients when a gynaecological cause is suspected or there is the slightest doubt as to the diagnosis. Palpation and percussion of the intra-abdominal organs is essential and auscultation for bowel sounds and bruits is important. When assessing elderly patients it should be remembered that they may have few symptoms or signs when a serious event, such as perforation of a viscus has occurred.

Investigations

When the clinical features have been elicited carefully, often only simple investigations are required. Determination of the haemoglobin and white blood cell count are frequently useful. However, the haemoglobin concentration may be misleading in patients who are bleeding (chapter 23). The plasma electrolytes, creatinine, urea and sugar may be important in patients with a metabolic disturbance. Plasma and urinary amylase levels may be useful in the diagnosis of acute pancreatitis but they can be high in other causes of an acute abdomen, such as perforated peptic ulcer, cholecystitis and strangulated bowel. Moreover, the amylase levels are not always raised in patients with acute pancreatitis (chapter 26).

A chest X-ray and erect and supine abdominal films are often of value. Other radiological investigations, such as small bowel studies in mechanical obstruction of the small intestine or arteriography when vascular lesions are suspected, may be helpful. The advent of ultrasonography and flexible endoscopy has also enhanced the doctor's ability to make the correct diagnosis.

The use of computers to aid in the diagnosis of the acute abdomen has been advocated in recent years. When used correctly the computer appears to substantially enhance the diagnostic accuracy of the doctor.

Management

All patients admitted with acute abdominal pain are kept in bed and should not eat or drink until the diagnosis becomes established. An intravenous infusion is commenced in the presence of vomiting or dehydration. The pulse rate, blood pressure, temperature and fluid balance must be recorded. When vomiting persists, a nasogastric tube is inserted. When surgery is thought to be necessary it should not be delayed once the patient is in a stable condition. Nevertheless, it is important not to resort to surgery where the diagnosis and the need for operation is uncertain. It is preferable in these circumstances to monitor and support the patient for a few hours to observe their progress when the diagnosis will become apparent. Where infection is suspected, appropriate samples should be taken for culture and, usually, prophylactic antibiotics are given to cover the operation. These antibiotics should not be continued postoperatively unless there is a specific indication.

Severe headache

Headache is a common presenting symptom to general practitioners. It is relatively uncommon in emergency medical practice. However, when a patient is admitted with a severe headache it may indicate serious underlying pathology. The causes of headache are given in Table 2.7.

Table 2.7 Causes of headache

Intracranial	
Raised intracranial pressure	Cerebral tumour, primary or secondary
	Brain abscess
	Subdural haematoma
Meningeal irritation	Meningitis—Acute bacterial
	Viral
	Tuberculosis
	Syphilis cryptococcus
	Subarachnoid haemorrhage
Other intracranial	Encephalitis
Vascular disorders	Migraine
	Severe hypertension
	Cluster headaches
	Giant cell arteritis
Cranium and scalp	Pagets disease
	Herpes Zoster
	Secondary tumours
Extracranial	
Lesions of the eye	Iritis, glaucoma
Lesions of the ear	Otitis media and mastoiditis
Others	Nasal sinuses–infection, tumour
	Oral cavity and teeth
	Cervical spine and temporomandibular joints
Others	Toxic states, alcohol, general infections, uraemia, lead poisoning, carbon monoxide poisoning, post traumatic, trigeminal neuralgia
Psychogenic	Muscle tension
	Hysteria

Clinical features

History

The onset, character, location, timing and radiation of the pain and the presence of any associated symptoms are important. When a headache is of sudden onset, severe and associated with neurological signs then a serious underlying pathology is likely. The patient should be questioned about his age and previous history of headaches and other disease. In addition, details of alcohol consumption, drug ingestion, smoking habits and social situation are also required. These features are all likely to help in the diagnosis as most headaches have specific features, such as temporal arteritis which is found in more elderly patients with tenderness in the temporal region or the aura which often precedes the onset of migraine.

Examination

A thorough physical examination is essential. General inspection and examination is required first to exclude systemic, metabolic or cardiovascular disease. The head should be examined for local tenderness and swellings, the cranial arteries should be palpated and auscultation of the arteries, scalp and eyes should be undertaken. A detailed neurological examination and testing for neck stiffness and cervical spine mobility should also be carried out. Local disease of the eyes, ears, nose and mouth should not be forgotten.

Investigations

The investigations indicated depend on the suspected diagnosis. Many patients will require a skull X-ray and simple haematological and biochemical tests to help exclude metabolic disease. A lumbar puncture should not be undertaken when there is evidence of raised intracranial pressure, but sampling of the cerebrospinal fluid (CSF) is essential when meningitis is suspected (chapter 20). The value of a lumbar puncture in the diagnosis of subarachnoid haemorrhage is discussed in chapter 19. The use of computerized axial tomographic (CAT) scanners in many countries has aided the diagnosis of intracranial lesions considerably. However, on a world wide basis their availability is limited.

Management

In general, patients with a severe headache prefer to lie quietly in a darkened room. This desire should be respected providing that they can be properly observed and monitored. The temperature, pulse, blood pressure and conscious level should be recorded in all patients. Steroid therapy (40–60 mg of prednisolone daily) should be started immediately in patients with cranial arteritis and should not be delayed until a temporal artery biopsy has been undertaken. The abnormal histology of the artery is present for several days after steroid therapy is commenced. Any delay in treatment may lead to blindness. The management of the other conditions that cause patients to present as emergencies with severe headache are considered in the relevant chapters of this book; severe hypertension, chapter 7; stroke, chapter 16; subarachnoid haemorrhage, chapter 19; meningitis and encephalitis, chapter 20; subdural haematoma, chapter 33.

Further reading

Coma
Cartlidge N. (1983) Diagnosis and management of coma. *Medicine International* **1**, 1428–1431.

Brain death
Harrison M. (1983) Diagnosis of brain death. *Medicine International* **1**, 1432–1434.
Pallis C. (1983) *ABC of brain stem death*. British Medical Association, London.
Black P. McL (1978) Brain death. *New England Journal of Medicine.* **299** Part 1. 338–344, Part 2. 293–401.

Breathlessness
Ogilvie C. (1983) Dyspnoea. *British Medical Journal* **287**, 160–161.
Pearson S.B., Pearson E.M. and Mitchell J.R.B. (1981) The diagnosis and management of patients admitted to hospital with acute breathlessness. *Postgraduate Medical Journal* **57**, 419–424.

Chest pain
Schneider R.R. and Seckler S.G. (1981) Evaluation of acute chest pain. *Medical Clinics of North America* **65**, 53–66.

Abdominal pain
Saegesser F. (1981) The acute abdomen—differential diagnosis. *Clinics in Gastroenterology* **10**, 123–144.

Headache
Greenhall R.C.D. (1983) Headache and facial pain. *Medicine International* **1**, 1389–1393.

3 · Cardiac Arrest

JOHN WATKINS

When cardiac output abruptly ceases, 'cardiac arrest' is said to have occurred, whether or not it results primarily from a change in heart rhythm. Unless an effective cardiac output can be restored within 4–5 minutes, irreversible brain damage or death are almost inevitable. Since half of all the deaths from coronary heart disease occur within two hours of the onset of symptoms, it is incumbent upon *all* clinicians to be skilled in the management of cardiac arrest. Trained personnel can expect to successfully resuscitate 20–40 per cent of all victims of cardiac arrest (Scott 1981), with a 60 per cent five-year survival in those who leave hospital (Peatfield *et al* 1977). However, there is little room for complacency. A recent survey in a university hospital showed that the majority of junior doctors were incapable of initiating effective cardiopulmonary resuscitation (Lowenstein *et al.* 1981).

Causes of cardiac arrest

Arrhythmias associated with myocardial ischaemia or infarction account for most cases of cardiac arrest. However, it must be remembered that occasional potentially fatal arrhythmias result from other causes as indicated in Table 3.1.

Table 3.1. Causes of potentially fatal arrhythmias.

---

1. Myocardial ischaemia/infarction (coronary artery disease, aortic stenosis etc)
2. Electrolyte imbalance—hyper and hypokalaemia (eg diuretics)
          —hypocalcaemia (eg repeated blood transfusion)
          —hypomagnesaemia (eg chronic diuretic therapy)
3. Idiosyncratic or toxic drug reactions
          —digoxin, quinidine and any intravenously administered antiarrhythmic agent
          —general anaesthesia
4. Hypothermia
5. Cardiac trauma
6. Electrocution
7. Respiratory arrest leading to myocardial hypoxia and acidosis (raised intracranial pressure, stroke, drugs, tracheal foreign body etc.)
8. Congenital prolongation of the QT interval ($QT_c > 0.42$ s)

The other principle mode of cardiac arrest is electromechanical dissociation. That is the absence of cardiac output resulting from sudden pump failure or circulatory obstruction with no primary change in heart rhythm. This may arise as a result of myocardial rupture (usually the left ventricular free wall or the belly of a papillary muscle), pericardial tamponade, herniation of the heart (usually through a congenital pericardial defect), or massive pulmonary embolism. It occasionally follows the use of cardioplegic drugs and is not an uncommon terminal event in patients with global myocardial dysfunction from any cause.

Recognition of cardiac arrest

Sudden collapse in any individual must be considered a cardiac arrest until proved otherwise. Confirmation of the absence of an effective cardiac output is obtained by failure to feel a carotid or femoral pulse. Breathing may or may not have ceased, but the patient is usually apnoeic and universally cyanosed within a minute of a cardiac arrest. Likewise, the victim will rapidly become flaccid and unresponsive although, in the first few seconds, loss of consciousness may not be complete. Generalized convulsions and incontinence are common.

It is important to consider upper airways obstruction (for example, by the aspiration of food or dentures) as the cause of a cardiorespiratory arrest, especially if the victim was eating at the time. Initial management of such patients is obviously rather different, being directed towards relief of the respiratory obstruction.

Initial management

The key aspects of cardiopulmonary resuscitation are embraced in the mnemonic ABC:
Airway,
Breathing,
Circulation.

Except where upper airways obstruction is suspected as the cause of the cardiac arrest, initial attention should be directed towards the *circulation*. Once it is established that there is no effective cardiac output:

1. Strike the mid-sternum forcibly with the clenched fist

If the patient is asystolic or in complete heart block, this may initiate an idioventricular rhythm (Don Michael and Stanford 1963; Semple *et al.* 1968). Rarely, even ventricular tachycardia and ventricular fibrillation are terminated by this manoeuvre (Bornemann and Scherf 1969; Barrett 1971).

If this is not successful:

2. Defibrillate the unmonitored patient with a 400 Joule direct current shock

Do not wait for an electrocardiographic (ECG) diagnosis. Any delay will reduce the chances of successful cardioversion of ventricular tachycardia or fibrillation. A single shock will not be harmful if the patient is asystolic or suffering from electromechanical dissociation. Likewise, defibrillate the monitored patient who is in ventricular tachycardia or ventricular fibrillation. Do not use low energy shocks for ventricular fibrillation, since its abolition depends upon simultaneous depolarization of the entire myocardium. If this does not produce a palpable pulse:

3. Institute external cardiac massage

This should precede step two if the defibrillator is not immediately to hand. If the patient is not on a cardiac bed, insert fracture boards under his chest or place him on the floor. Start cardiac massage at a rate of sixty compressions per minute. The heel of one hand should be placed over the lower half of the patient's sternum with the other hand on top and at 90° to the first. With straight arms, depress the sternum by about two inches (for a more detailed description see 'Standards and guidelines for CPR . . . '1980).

A new form of cardiopulmonary resuscitation has been described in which simultaneous cardiac massage and lung inflations are performed forty times per minute (Chandra et al. 1980). This appears to have certain theoretical advantages over the conventional technique but its utility and safety in clinical practice have yet to be established.

Effective cardiac massage should produce a pulse that is easily palpable (systolic pressure > 60 mm Hg). This should give adequate cerebral perfusion and may even restore consciousness if initiated immediately. The inability to produce a good pulse with proper external cardiac massage usually means that there has been a cardiac catastrophe such as ventricular rupture. If this is unlikely in the clinical context, it may occasionally be justified to perform open chest cardiac massage through a left thoracotomy.

4. Check airway and start artificial respiration

If more than one person is present at the cardiac arrest, this should be started immediately. This should also precede step two if a defibrillator is not immediately available. Remove dentures and any other foreign bodies from the patient's mouth and pharynx. If vomiting has occurred, clear the pharynx with a sucker. Put the patient on his back and expose the chest and neck. Extend the head backwards by putting one hand behind the patient's neck and lifting, while pressing on the forehead with the other hand. If the airway is still apparently obstructed, place two fingers behind the angle of the jaw on each side and pull the mandible forward, holding the mouth open with the thumbs.

If spontaneous breathing does not resume, start mouth-to-mouth artificial respiration by inflating the chest with four deep breaths in rapid succession. Thereafter, inflate the chest twelve times per minute, that is once for every five sternal depressions. Pinch the nose shut and be sure that an airtight seal is formed over the patient's mouth by your own. (For a more detailed description, see 'Standards and guidelines...' 1980). Very occasionally, laryngeal or tracheal obstruction will render mouth-to-mouth artificial respiration impossible. If an endotracheal tube is not available or cannot be passed, an emergency tracheostomy will then be necessary.

5. Establish an intravenous line

Ideally, this should be in the subclavian or jugular veins or in a large peripheral vein. It is rarely necessary to cut down on the saphenous vein and, in practice, this is a poor access site to the circulation. If more than one minute has elapsed since the cardiac arrest, approximately one meq/kg of 8.4 per cent sodium bicarbonate should be infused and half of this dose should be repeated every fifteen minutes while resuscitation efforts continue.

Further management

Certain administrative points must be considered once the resuscitation attempt is under way. If possible, establish:
(a) the time of the arrest;
(b) the circumstances surrounding the arrest;
(c) that all necessary personnel have been summoned;
(d) that all necessary equipment has been sent for;
(e) that the patient has not been designated 'not for resuscitation' because of his clinical condition prior to the cardiac arrest. If there is any doubt about this point, continue the resuscitation attempt and send for one of the patient's own medical attendants.

1. Establish optimal ventilation

As soon as possible, a cuffed endotracheal tube should be passed (size eight or nine for an average sized adult). This will guard the patient's airway during the continuing resuscitation attempt and will enable 100 per cent oxygen rather than expired air to be used for inflating the lungs. If an endotracheal tube is not available or cannot be passed, 100 per cent oxygen can sometimes be delivered by using a bag-valve-mask system held over the mouth with an oropharyngeal airway in place. However, in practice it is often hard to fully inflate the lungs by this technique, in which case mouth-to-mouth resuscitation should be restarted.

2. Establish cardiac rhythm

Connect the patient to a monitor or an ECG machine. Alternatively, it is possible on some defibrillators to display the ECG by using the paddles held against the chest wall as electrodes. However, it must be remembered that any movement may result in an electrocardiographic artefact that simulates ventricular fibrillation.

3. Treat arrhythmias

(a) Ventricular fibrillation

Give a 400 joule direct current (DC) shock. Place one paddle at the base of the heart and the other at the apex. Ideally, use gel defibrillator pads to ensure good skin contact and to minimize skin burns. If electrode jelly is used, ensure none gets on the skin between the paddles. It is your responsibility to ensure that no-one but the patient receives the 400 joules!

If ventricular fibrillation persists after two shocks, or if it recurs within a few minutes, give lignocaine 100 mg as an intravenous bolus before giving further shocks. This procedure may be repeated as necessary.

If there is *fine* ventricular fibrillation (amplitude of fibrillatory waves < 5 mm), or if DC shock precipitates asystole or an agonal rhythm of slow, broad ventricular complexes, give one ml of a 1:1,000 adrenaline solution *via a central venous line or by direct intracardiac injection* and repeat defibrillation. Repeat adrenaline as necessary after five minutes.

If still unresponsive, ventricular fibrillation may sometimes be abolished by varying the position of the defibrillator paddles. Particularly in obese patients, more of the delivered energy will reach the heart if the 'fore and aft position' is adopted (anterior paddle to left of mid-sternum, posterior paddle below left scapula).

If all the above fail, try an intravenous bolus of bretylium tosylate (5 mg/kg), as this is the only drug which has been shown to terminate ventricular fibrillation in man (Sanna and Arcidiacono 1973).

Finally, consider a specific remediable cause such as continuing acidosis, hypokalaemia or hypothermia. If and when an effective rhythm is restored, an intravenous lignocaine infusion (2 mg/minute) should be maintained for the next twenty-four hours if it can be tolerated.

(b) Ventricular tachycardia

If the patient is pulseless the treatment is as for ventricular fibrillation, except that a 200 joule shock will usually suffice. If there is a weak pulse and the patient has not completely lost consciousness, a brief trial of intravenous lignocaine is sometimes justified (100 mg initially followed by a further 50–100 mg bolus after fifteen minutes).

(c) Asystole

Asystole is sometimes due to profound vagotonia as in acutely raised intracranial pressure or inferior myocardial infarction. Under these circumstances, 1.2 mg of intravenous atropine sulphate may induce sinus or junctional rhythm. However, more commonly, asystole is the result of a more generalized severe cardiac insult and is unresponsive to atropine. The aim of drug therapy in this situation is to induce an idioventricular rhythm or ventricular fibrillation which might then be amenable to DC cardioversion.

Give either one ml of 1:1000 adrenaline or 5–15 μg of isoprenaline via a central line or directly into the heart and repeat as necessary after five minutes. Try 10 ml of 10 per cent calcium gluconate if there is no response to the catecholamines. Remember, none of these drugs should be given into the sodium bicarbonate infusion. Finally, if all these manoeuvres are ineffective, consider a trial of transvenous or transoesophageal pacing as is discussed in the next section. It is far more likely to be effective if the asystole has been transient rather than persistent. Pacing will merely produce electromechanical dissociation if the asystolic episode is a reflection of massive myocardial damage.

(d) Other bradyarrhythmias

Sinus or nodal bradycardia, complete heart block or idioventricular rhythm may all lead to a 'cardiac arrest' if the ventricular rate is sufficiently slow. Temporary pacing is then indicated. Pacing is most rapidly achieved with a transoesophageal electrode if screening facilities are not available. Some 20–30 volts are usually required to depolarize the left ventricle. This is a temporary measure and transvenous pacing should be substituted as soon as possible if the bradycardia persists.

An alternative approach is the use of a balloon tipped, flow guided, transvenous pacing electrode, which is advanced blindly into the right heart until ventricular pacing is established.

(e) Other tachyarrhythmias

Supraventricular arrhythmias with ventricular rates in excess of 180 beats per minute may sometimes lead to a clinical state indistinguishable from 'cardiac arrest'. This is particularly true where there is ventricular pre-excitation. As a general rule, any tachyarrhythmia that causes impaired consciousness should be immediately terminated by DC shock.

Check metabolic state

At the first opportunity, take an arterial blood sample for the determination of pH, PO_2 and PCO_2 as they are important measures of the effectiveness of the resuscitation technique. If resuscitation was started immediately and 100 per cent oxygen given, the PO_2 and pH should be normal or only slightly reduced. Gross hypoxia or acidosis suggest that ventilation may be inadequate for some reason such as a pneumothorax, aspiration, or if the endotracheal tube is in the oesophagus. Ideally, the haemoglobin and blood glucose should also be checked and corrected as appropriate.

Indications for terminating a resuscitation attempt

This should be a unanimous decision and should ideally be taken in consultation with the patient's own physician. The implication is that no reasonable hope for recovery remains. The following factors should be considered before terminating a resuscitation attempt.

1. What is the likely underlying cause?

Clearly, if the circumstances suggest cardiac rupture, resuscitation attempts might reasonably be discontinued sooner than they would be in a patient whose cardiac arrest was thought to be due to digoxin toxicity.

2. Has the attempt continued long enough?

While it is not possible to generalize about this, at least 30–45 minutes of cardiopulmonary resuscitation should be tried before considering terminating the attempt. Remember that victims of freshwater drowning, hypothermia and certain drugs may recover after many hours, so that prolonged resuscitation attempts are mandatory in such circumstances.

3. Have all therapeutic options been applied?

For example, has the cardiac massage resulted in a palpable pulse? If not, do the clinical circumstances warrant an attempt at open chest cardiac massage? Similarly, has the artificial respiration led to appropriate chest movement and regression of cyanosis? If not, is there a case for tracheostomy? Have all possible adverse metabolic factors been corrected and is there an adequate circulating blood volume?

4. Have all objective parameters of recovery been properly assessed?

The presence of fixed dilated pupils is clearly a grave prognostic sign but it may have been drug induced. Stop resuscitation briefly and watch carefully for spontaneous respiratory efforts. Listen to the heart as well as feeling both carotid and both femoral pulses. Finally, check that the straight line on the ECG monitor is not a lead displacement artefact!

Further reading

Barret J.S. (1971) Letter to the Editor. *New England Journal of Medicine* **284**, 393.

Bornemann C. and Scherf D. (1969) Paroxysmal ventricular tachycardia abolished by a blow on the precordium. *Diseases of the Chest* **56**, 83–84.

Chandra N., Rudikoff M.T. and Weisfeldt M.L. (1980) Simultaneous chest compression and ventilation at high airway pressure during cardiopulmonary resuscitation. *Lancet* **1**, 175–8.

Don Michael T.A. and Stanford R.L. (1963) Precordial percussion in cardiac asystole. *Lancet* **1**, 699.

Lowenstein S.R., Libb S., Mountain R.D., Hansbrough J.F., Hill D.M. and Scoggin C.H. (1981) Cardiopulmonary resuscitation by medical and surgical house officers. *Lancet* **11**, 679–81.

Peatfield W.C., Sillett R.W., Taylor D. and McNicol M.W. (1977) Survival after cardiac arrest in hospital. *Lancet* **1**, 1223–5.

Sanna G. and Arcidiacono R. (1973) Chemical ventricular defibrillation of the human heart with bretylium tosylate. *American Journal of Cardiology* **32**, 982–7.

Scott R.P. (1981) Cardiopulmonary resuscitation in a teaching hospital. A survey of cardiac arrests occurring outside intensive care units and emergency rooms. *Anaesthesia* **36**, 526–30.

Semple T., Al Badran R.H. and Boyes B.E. (1968) Physical stimulation of the heart. *British Medical Journal* **1**, 224.

Standards and guidelines for cardiopulmonary resuscitation (CPR) and emergency cardiac care (ECC) (1980) *Journal of the American Medical Association* **244**, 453–509 (Supp).

4 · Myocardial Infarction and Unstable Angina

R.A. BLACKWOOD

Changes in the care of patients with a myocardial infarction have been considerable in the last ten years. The length of hospital stay has decreased, early ambulation is much more common and patients are informed more about their condition. Routine anticoagulant therapy has declined while the use of prophylactic anti-arrhythmic drugs has increased (Wenger *et al.* 1982). The idea that jeopardized myocardium might be salvageable has led to endless trials of beta-blockers, nitrates, etc. Post infarction exercise testing is almost commonplace now and although there is a clearer picture of the evolution of a myocardial infarction, numerous controversies still exist.

Although this chapter deals with hospital management, care of the patient begins at home and hospital doctors must be aware of the controversies which exist in the pre-hospital phase.

The pre-hospital phase

Forty per cent of all deaths from acute myocardial infarction occur within the first hour. Therefore, speedy medical assistance is very important and has led to coronary care ambulances as well as teaching of the public in cardio-pulmonary resuscitation. The doctor at the bedside of the patient at home must give an analgesic, possibly an anti-arrhythmic agent, and summon an ambulance, if appropriate, as soon as possible. He should stay with the patient until he is satisfied no danger exists.

The pre-hospital phase—controversies

1. *Which analgesic should be used?*

Morphine given intravenously, or one of its analogues, is the drug of choice. It lowers peripheral resistance, reduces left atrial filling pressure and also reduces left ventricular end diastolic pressure. Although this is beneficial, the cardiac output may fall a little and the patient should be kept supine. Pentazocine should not be used as it raises peripheral resistance and increases the load on the heart. Morphine also has the advantage of euphoria and sedation.

2. *Are prophylactic anti-arryhthmic drugs of value?*

There is some evidence that intramuscular or intravenous anti-arrhythmic drugs given prophylactically at home may affect mortality (Wyman *et al.* 1974; Lie *et al.* 1974). More recently Lignocaine has not been shown to be of significant benefit but this may be because adequate blood levels were not achieved. Up to 300 mg of Lignocaine may be needed in some patients (Lie *et al.* 1978). Mexilitene is currently on trial but no results are yet available. Atropine may be very useful if the patient appears to be vasovagal.

3. *Home care or hospitalization?*

Three trials conducted in Newcastle, Nottingham and Bristol showed no difference in mortality between home and hospital (roughly 12 per cent in each group) (Mather *et al.* 1976; Hill *et al.* 1978; Dollipriana *et al.* 1977; respectively). However, there are serious problems with these trials. The Newcastle trial was retrospective, the others were prospective and random. There were large numbers of patients who dropped out of the trials for various reasons. In addition, the number of patients included in the trials was a tiny percentage of the total number of patients suffering from a myocardial infarction in each district. In the Nottingham trial a team went to the house and only randomized the patient if he was not in need of urgent treatment after one hour. It is this time which is most critical. These trials cannot be taken as a true indication of whether home or hospitalization treatment is appropriate. A patient who presents forty-eight hours after his pain will receive little benefit from a Coronary Care Unit and patients over sixty-five will probably do just as well at home.

4. *Do coronary care ambulances reduce mortality?*

The high mortality of myocardial infarction in the first few hours prompted the setting up of Coronary Care Ambulances. Ambulancemen trained in recognition of arrhythmias and resuscitation respond to calls as rapidly as possible and effectively take coronary care to the home. Results are encouraging and suggest that this practice should be more widespread. (McIntosh *et al.* 1978; Luxton *et al.* 1975). Up to five per cent of the patients in these trials have ventricular fibrillation in the ambulance from which they recover.

Hospital phase

Attention for the patient should be available as soon as he arrives at hospital. In some hospitals admission may be direct to the Coronary Unit, but in most the patient with chest pain arrives in Casualty. It is most important that the patient should be in a place where he can be monitored and if necessary resuscitated if he has a suspected myocardial infarction. Ideally, this will be a Coronary Care Unit. The patient should remain in Casualty for only 15–30 minutes. A brief history and examination followed by an electrocardiogram (ECG) is sufficient in Casualty. Full history taking can wait until later. An intravenous route should be established immediately (i.v. drip or Venflon) and Morphine or an analogue given if the patient has not received analgesia. The patients should be attached to an ECG monitor and should remain so during transfer. It is very difficult to achieve such care for the coronary patient but it is undoubtedly of benefit.

ECG monitoring, measurements of blood pressure and vital signs are the routine management of the Coronary Care Unit. ECGs and enzyme estimations are performed daily on patients for the first three days in order to confirm the diagnosis. The majority of patients will leave the Unit without any serious complications but 70 per cent will have had some sort of arrhythmia. The usual length of stay in a Coronary Care Unit is forty-eight hours, i.e. until the risk of arrhythmias is minimal but this depends on the individual patient.

Only about 60 per cent of all patients admitted to a C.C.U. will have had a true myocardial infarction. Some of the others will have had angina and others will never be diagnosed. A few patients will have gall bladder or gastro-intestinal diseases and oesophageal spasm is popular but almost impossible to prove. Musculoskeletal pains will account for others and only rarely do pleuritic pains filter into a C.C.U. The diagnoses which mimic cardiac pain more accurately are massive pulmonary embolism (often giving an inferior infarct pattern) or pericarditis. The latter should be obvious by a friction rub and its relation to posture. Pericardial pain is normally better sitting up and worse lying down. A massive pulmonary embolism should be more apparent by shock, cyanosis and dyspnoea in the absence of left ventricular failure.

There are two major complications of a myocardial infarction: arrhythmias and myocardial failure. The former has received enormous attention in recent years with numerous anti-arrhythmic agents available. The latter continues to be a bad prognostic sign with attempts at prophylaxis being one of the advances of the last few years. The other complications are: rupture of the ventricle, septum or mitral valve, systemic and pulmonary emboli, pericarditis, the post myocardial infarction syndrome and the development of a left ventricular aneurysm. Prompt treatment of these complications at the earliest possible stage is highly desirable and this is, of course, the function of the Coronary Care Unit.

Hospital phase—problems

1. *Arrhythmias*

The treatment of arrhythmias is given in detail in chapter 5. An outline is given below.

	Arrhythmia	*Management*
Ectopics	Atrial } Junctional	No treatment
	Ventricular	Lignocaine (Mexilitene, Disopyramide, Procainamide, Phenytoin and a beta-blocker can be used if Lignocaine fails in this order)
Tachycardias	Atrial } Junctional	Digoxin, Disopyramide, Amiodorone, Verapramil, Beta-blockers
	Ventricular	Cardioversion/Lignocaine (and anti-arrhythmics as for ventricular ectopics)
	Ventricular fibrillation	Direct current shock
Bradycardia	Sinus bradycardia	Atropine
	Sinus arrest	Atropine, then pacemaker if necessary
	Second and third degree heart block	Pacemaker
	First degree heart block and Wenckebach	Wait
	Right bundle branch block and left anterior hemiblock	Pacemaker
	Right bundle branch block and left posterior hemiblock	Pacemaker

Any of the tachyarrhythmias may need cardioversion if the arrhythmia is dangerous or the patient is developing left ventricular failure. The order in which anti-arrhythmics are used for treating ventricular arryhthmias is a personal one, but few patient need more than a bolus and infusion of Lignocaine. Pacemaker insertion for bifasicular block is only necessary if it develops after the initial infarction. Pre-existing bifasicular block is not necessarily paced.

Certain arrhythmias can be described as premonitory. Bundle branch block may predispose to asystole, complete heart block to ventricular fibrillation, ventricular ectopics to ventricular tachycardia and atrial ectopics to atrial tachyarrhythmias.

2. Myocardial failure

(i)   Mild. A diuretic is usually sufficient.
(ii) Moderate. A diuretic and digoxin may be necessary.
(iii) Severe (cardiogenic shock).
Approximately 12% of patients with acute myocardial infarction develop cardiogenic shock and the mortality is over 80% per cent. The definition of cardiogenic shock is usually a systolic blood pressure of 85 mm Hg or less, oliguria, confusion and cold clammy skin. The treatment shown in Fig. 4.1 is only possible if pressure monitoring is available in the Coronary Care Unit.

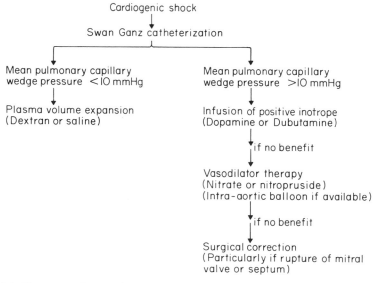

Fig. 4.1. Treatment for cardiogenic shock

3. Other complications

(i)   Systemic emboli: removal of embolus if possible and full anti-coagulation.
(ii) Pulmonary emboli: full anticoagulation.
(iii) Rupture of ventricle: little can be done in this situation; if the ventricle is leaking slowly, echocardiography will reveal an effusion and this can be tapped, followed as appropriate by surgical repair.

(iv)   Rupture of mitral valve cusp: this may be mild but if severe and the patient survives the initial disaster, surgical repair should take place about six weeks post infarction. Mortality is very high (about 80 per cent at six weeks). Some degree of mitral insufficiency will occur in 10–20 per cent of patients.

(v)   Rupture of septum: repair at six weeks post infarction is necessary if the patient can be kept alive (mortality about 80 per cent at six weeks).

(vi)   Pericarditis: symptomatic treatment alone is necessary. It may occur in 20–30 per cent of transmural infarctions.

(vii)   Post myocardial infarction syndrome: symptomatic treatment is necessary and only rarely are steroids needed.

(viii) Left ventricular aneurysm: it is not usually necessary to excise a left ventricular aneurysm and then only for symptoms, i.e. chest pain, left ventricular failure and arrhythmias.

Hospital phase—controversies

1. *How long should the patient stay in the Coronary Care Unit?*

The risk of arrhythmias falls rapidly and should be minimal by forty-eight hours. Factors which are associated with a poor short term prognosis are age and extensive infarction. The latter may be indicated by large enzyme levels, left ventricular failure or cardiogenic shock, recurrent arrhythmias, continued pain and hypertension. These patients may need to stay longer (Thompson *et al.* 1979).

2. *Is oxygen routinely indicated?*

In patients where pulmonary oedema has developed or is developing it is necessary to give oxygen. In uncomplicated myocardial infarction its value would be to limit infarct size. Oxygen delivered to the myocardium certainly increases but added oxygen may cause arterial vasoconstriction which can cause a fall in cardiac output and a rise in arterial pressure. This latter effect would increase myocardial oxygen consumption. Infarct size with and without oxygen inhalation has been compared in both dogs and man. Results have so far been conflicting (Maroko *et al.* 1975; Madias *et al.* 1976; Rawles and Kenmore 1976). It does not yet appear that routine treatment of myocardial infarction with oxygen is justified particularly because it is very irritating to the patient.

3. *Is Digoxin dangerous in the early stages of myocardial infarction?*

Digoxin increases myocardial oxygen consumption but this has not been found to alter infarct size (Morrison *et al.* 1980). Digoxin may also increase the risk of ventricular arrhythmias. However, the risk is small and in the failing heart it is safe to give.

4. *Is routine low dose anticoagulation necessary?*

This is justified in all patients with a myocardial infarction as long as they are on bed rest and is particularly important if cardiac failure is present (Thompson and Robinson 1978). Heparin 5,000 units b.d. or t.d.s. should be used.

5. *Which enzyme should be measured?*

Figure 4.2 shows the release of the different cardiac enzymes after a myocardial infarction. Misinterpretation of enzyme results can occur. A single intramuscular injection may increase creatine phosphokinase (CPK) by tenfold although the myocardial isoenzyme of CPK (MB CPK) is not affected (Kuster 1972). Alcohol ingestion causes a rise in aspartate trans-aminase (AST) from the liver and CPK from muscle and as many as 10 per cent of patients who are admitted to a Coronary Care Unit will have been drinking alcohol (Lafair and Myoson 1968). CPK, lactate dehydrogenase (LDH) and AST rise after exercise. However, the MB CPK remains normal

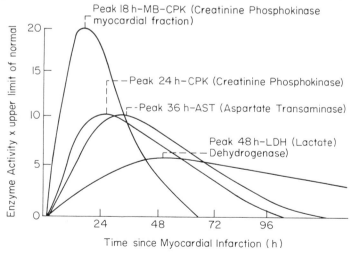

Fig. 4.2. Enzyme changes after a myocardial infarction.

unless the exercise is very severe. Thirty minutes of exercise is enough to raise the CPK activity. Because MB CPK is largely unaffected by other conditions and because it rises rapidly after an infarction, it is currently the most useful enzyme to measure.

6. *What conditions, other than myocardial infarction, cause a rise in enzymes?*

Myocarditis and a dissecting aneurysm cause significant rises in all cardiac enzymes (Choresis and Leonidus 1962). A persistent tachycardia lasting several hours may result in a small rise in enzymes and the LDH rises in 50–80 per cent of patients with a pulmonary embolus. A single DC shock can cause a twofold rise in CPK and multiple shocks a higher rise. Closed chest cardiac resuscitation will increase the CPK activity.

7. *Should an arrhythmia be treated before it appears?*

All patients could receive a prophylactic anti-arrhythmic when they arrive in the Coronary Care Unit. Lignocaine given within four hours of the onset of a myocardial infarction appears to decrease the risk of ventricular fibrillation (Lie *et al.* 1974). However, only a small proportion of patients arrive in a Coronary Care Unit within this time. Since there is no way of predicting those who are going to develop ventricular fibrillation (VF) it would be reasonable to give all patients a bolus of Lignocaine followed by an infusion. There are no recent reports on this procedure and some centres hardly use Lignocaine at all. Therefore, this question is still open and is a decision for the unit concerned.

8. *Should ventricular ectopics be treated?*

The frequency and shape of ventricular ectopics is not helpful in predicting those who will develop ventricular fibrillation. The rationale is that ventricular ectopics represent ventricular irritability and this may lead to ventricular fibrillation. Since some of these patients do develop ventricular fibrillation it is reasonable to treat ventricular ectopics under certain circumstances:
(i) If heart rate < 50 beats/min. Ventricular ectopics may occur here as escape beats. Treatment with Atropine is thought appropriate and may abolish the ectopics.
(ii) If heart rate > 50 beats/min. Treat with Lignocaine if frequency > 10/min., or multifocal, or R wave near to previous T wave, or more than two in a row.

9. *How long are anti-arrhythmics necessary?*

Only if arrythmias are severe or continued need appropriate therapy be continued out either on discharge from the Coronary Care Unit or the hospital. If Lignocaine is used to suppress ventricular ectopics in the first few hours of an infarction it is not necessary to follow this up with oral anti-arrhythmics. A patient who has suffered ventricular fibrillation may need long term anti-arrhythmic therapy particularly if there are signs of cardiac failure.

10. *Is it possible to limit infarct size?*

A myocardial infarction evolves over about twenty-four hours (Yusef *et al.* 1978). In its initial phase, there is a zone of necrosis surrounded by a zone of potentially salvageable ischaemic tissue. If this tissue can be preserved until collateral flow develops the infarct will be kept to a minimum size. It is very difficult to measure infarct size because enzyme estimations and ECG changes do not always correspond to the area of necrosis. Trials to assess if infarct size is limited are of mainly academic value because it is long term mortality which is more important.

(a) Beta-blockers. These drugs reduce myocardial oxygen demand by negative inotropism and chronotropism, reduce catecholamine induced lipolysis and therefore oxygen consumption and ventricular arrythmias. In addition, they may block potassium efflux from myocardial cells during ischaemia thus reducing the risk of ventricular fibrillation. Propranolol (Norris *et al.* 1978) and Atenolol (Yusef *et al.* 1980) have both been shown to reduce infarct size in man.

(b) Vasodilators. Vasodilators may diminish either afterload or preload or both and thus reduce left ventricular oxygen consumption. Nitroglycerin has been shown to reduce myocardial ischaemia in patients with left ventricular failure and in others (Borer *et al.* 1975; Chattarjee *et al.* 1973). Other vasodilators, notably nitroprusside have been used but have not yet been found to be of value (Brown *et al.* 1976). The major problem with vasodilators is the drop in systemic pressure which may be detrimental to the myocardium. Therefore, careful haemodynamic monitoring is essential.

(c) Intra-aortic balloon counter pulsation (IABC). IABC lowers systolic arterial pressure thus reducing afterload and the left ventricular wall tension. It also increases diastolic pressure and hence myocardial oxygen supply. Although results suggest a benefit whilst pulsation is present ischaemia appears to return afterwards and the benefit may be lost (Gold *et al.* 1976). The particular value of IABC is maintaining a patient in a suitable condition until surgery is possible, e.g. repair of ruptured interventricular septum.

(d) Hyaluronidase. Hyaluronidase maintains collateral flow to ischaemic tissue, presumably by increasing passive diffusion. Trials in dogs, rats and man suggest it may be helpful but further trials, currently underway, are necessary (Maroko *et al.* 1972; Maroko and Braunswald 1973).

(e) Others. Heparin (Saliba *et al.* 1976), glucose-insulin-potassium (Stanley and Prather 1978), corticosteroids (Morrison *et al.* 1976), Mannitol (Powell *et al.* 1976), anti-inflammatory agents (McLean *et al.* 1978), and oxygen may all limit infarct size. However, none of the data is yet convincing enough for any of these agents to be used routinely. In practice, steroids may 'mummify' cells and lead to a tendency to ventricular aneurysm (Kloner *et al.* 1978).

In summary, both beta-blockers and vasodilators appear very promising in limiting infarct size, but whether this will influence long term mortality or morbidity remains to be seen.

11. *Is coronary artery bypass grafting to be considered after an acute myocardial infarction?*

Urgent revascularization within 6–8 hours of an acute myocardial infarction may be of benefit (Berg *et al.* 1975), However, a controlled trial has not been performed and patients who can stand an operation may well survive anyway. In cardiogenic shock, surgery after IABC may be of value (Mundth 1976). Revascularization such as this is dependent on urgent angiography and surgery which is rarely available to Coronary Care Units.

The post coronary care unit phase

After forty-eight hours in the Coronary Care Unit most patients move to a hospital ward. They may sit out on the third day and go to the bathroom on the fourth or fifth day. Discharge home is usually from the seventh to tenth day. No particular monitoring is necessary and at this stage the patient should have a clear understanding of what he must do when he goes home. Any complications which develop, e.g. left ventricular failure or chest pain must be carefully treated and usually keep the patient in hospital a little longer.

The post coronary unit phase—controversies

1. *Is ECG monitoring in the ward of value?*

The majority of patients who die in the week following their discharge from the Coronary Care Unit do so from myocardial failure even though this may be associated with arrhythmias. Therefore, ECG monitoring is of little value (Reynell 1975). Certain patients, e.g. those with pacemakers *in situ* may need to be closely monitored, but the cessation of monitoring is usually a psychological boost for the patient.

2. *How quickly should a patient be mobilized?*

In the 1950s many patients with myocardial infarction lay on their backs for six weeks. Emboli were common. Patients have been mobilized more and more quickly and the worry that they would develop left ventricular aneurysms has not been confirmed. Rapid mobilization is excellent psychologically, but just how quickly is not yet determined.

The post hospital phase

The uncomplicated myocardial infarction patient should gradually increase his mobilization until six weeks after the initial event. A decision should be made about his immediate return to work even if part-time. An outline programme is shown below but it is very variable according to the individual patient.

Week 1   In house only.
         Downstairs in the morning, upstairs to bed in evening only.
         Baths not too hot.
Week 2   House and garden only.
Week 3   House, garden and up and down road outside house about 200
         yards.
Week 4   Walking up to ½–1 mile per day.
         Can drive—check with general practitioner first.
Week 6   Return to out-patients. Full check-up.
         Return to work if fit.
         Should be walking 1–2 miles/day.

Intercourse may restart at 2–3 weeks with patient's regular partner!

When the patient visits the out-patients department at six weeks post infarction, secondary prevention is the important factor. There are three aspects of this:

1. Symptoms: angina (chest pain), left ventricular failure (dyspnoea etc.) and recurrent arrhythmias (palpitations etc.) are bad prognostic signs and must be dealt with vigorously.

2. Risk factors: The patient must be advised carefully regarding smoking, obesity and exercise. If hypertension, hyperlipidaemia or diabetes are found, they must be treated accordingly.

3. Drugs: There are three groups of drugs to consider. Firstly, the patient may need an appropriate anti-arrhythmic for recurrent arrhythmias. Secondly, recent evidence suggests that beta-blockers may improve prognosis and should be considered. Thirdly, 'antiplatelet' drugs of various kinds have also undergone trials for secondary prevention and these too must be considered.

After the initial follow up in the out-patients six weeks post-infarction, the uncomplicated patient need not be followed further if the general practitioner is happy to continue care. There is a growing tendency to subject all patients to an exercise treadmill test about six weeks to three months post-infarction. This may isolate those at greater risk and perhaps those who need surgery.

The post hospital phase—controversies

1. *Is psychotherapy useful to the post-infarction patient?*

One study suggests that psychotherapy helps patients to re-establish their self image, but there is no evidence that this improves mortality (Mayou 1979). Since relatives are often over protective counselling them may be of benefit.

2. *Is routine anti-arrhythmic therapy helpful?*

Phenytoin and procainamide have been used in trials as long term pro-phylaxis against lethal arrythmias (Peter *et al.* 1978; Kowsowsky *et al.* 1973). Neither drug has been shown to be significantly helpful.

Endless beta-blocker trials have been instituted and recently have sug-gested decreased mortality in those taking the drug. Whether this is due to suppressing arrhythmias or another factor is not clear and the recent Timolol study (Norwegian Multicentre Study Group 1981) suggests arrhythmias were just as common. Therefore, there is no evidence that long term anti-arrhythmic therapy is of value. The incidence of side effects may be very high, e.g. with Procainamide it was 60 per cent.

3. *Should all patients be given a beta-blocker?*

This question has received enormous attention and more than thirty trials have now taken place. No trial has suggested that beta-blockers are detri-mental and the number of patients developing severe side effects are small. Practolol (no longer available), Alprenolol (not available in this country), Timolol, Metoprolol and possibly Propranolol have all shown an improve-ment in mortality at one year of between 20–40 per cent. Rigorous cross examination of these trials has not changed these figures (Mitchell 1981) and although more trials are expected, many physicians are evolving towards their routine use.

4. *Are 'antiplatelet' drugs useful post-infarction?*

The action of these drugs is based on the assumption that sudden death and re-infarction depend on the coagulation of platelets and the spasm of the arteries. This may not be true. Prostaglandin synthesis may result in the formation of prostacyclin (PGI_2) which inhibits platelet coagulation and vasospasm or Thromboxane (TX) which encourages platelet coagulation and vasospasm.

Aspirin, Dipyridamole and Sulphinpyrazone affect the production of prostaglandin (PGI_2) and it is not certain whether this lowers the effective balance of thromboxane and prostacyclin. Results to date are somewhat conflicting and there is certainly no clear indication for their use (Anturan Research Group 1978; Elwood et al. 1974).

5. Is routine exercise testing post-infarction essential?

Some centres perform limited exercise testing on the day before the patient is discharged as a prognostic indicator (Theroux et al. 1979). Those who perform badly will be treated differently from the uncomplicated patient and this is of benefit because the risk of re-infarction is greatest within the first three months of the initial event. This is rarely practical in many centres. A modified exercise test later may also be of similar value particularly if they are strongly positive. These patients must be considered for early surgery.

Unstable angina

The various names given to this condition indicate its imprecise definition. Unstable angina exists somewhere between stable angina and myocardial infarction. It includes rapidly increasing angina, angina developing at rest, prolonged chest pain similar to a myocardial infarction or any similar combination. However, there are no enzymatic or ECG changes of myocardial necrosis. The term pre-infarction angina was used for this condition but in practice less than 10 per cent actually go on to develop an infarction during the acute phase (Conti and Curry 1979).

Management of this condition is initially medical, based on the evidence of the relatively low early rate of infarction and death and the lack of their alteration by emergency bypass grafting (Unstable Angina Study Group 1978). In addition, results suggest that surgery is optimally performed after clinical stabilization has been achieved (Weintrant et al. 1979).

Medical management is therefore:

(a) Bed rest, oxygen, analgesia, sedation.
(b) Coronary care unit monitoring.
(c) Drugs to reduce risk of infarction:
 (i) Vasodilators—sublingual, oral or i.v. nitrates.
 (ii) Beta–blockers.
 (iii) Calcium antagonists.

These drugs seem to be very helpful in reducing the risk of infarction (Fish et al. 1973; Hill et al. 1981) and the calcium antagonists may reduce coronary vasospasm (Hugenholz et al. 1981). Heparin may also be useful in reducing the size of infarction. My own practice is to put the patient on a beta-blocker, calcium antagonist and a nitrate.

If medical therapy fails (i.e. pain continues) for more than 24–48 hours, surgical intervention must be considered. The patient must be able and appropriate to undergo emergency cardiac catheterization and then coronary artery bypass grafting.

Other methods of treating unstable angina include intra-aortic balloon pumping (Amsterdam *et al.* 1981) and percutaneous transluminal coronary angioplasty (Williams *et al.* 1981).

Further reading

Amsterdam E.A., Awan N.A., Lee G., Low R., Joye J.A., Forester J., Randig S., Mason D.T. (1981). Intra-aortic balloon counterpulsation. Rationale, application and results in Rackley, C.E., Editor. *Critical Care Cardiology.* F.A. Davis Co. Philadelphia p. 79.

Anturan Reinfarction Trial Research Group (1978) Sulphinpyrazone in the prevention of cardiac death after myocardial infarction. *New England Journal of Medicine* **298**, 289–295.

Berg R., Kendall R.W., Duvoisin C.E., Ganji J.H., Rudy L.W., Everhart F.J. (1975) Acute myocardial infarction a surgical emergency. *Journal of Thoracic and Cardiovascular Surgery* **70**, 432–439.

Borer J.R., Redwood D.R., Levitt B., Cagin N., Bianchi C., Vallin H., Epstein S.E. (1975) Reduction in myocardial ischaemia in nitroglycerin or nitroglycerin plus phenyleptrine administered during acute myocardial infarction in man. *New England Journal of Medicine* **293**, 1008–1012.

Brown T.M., Matthews O.P., Walter P.F. (1976) Assessment of affect of vasodilator therapy upon haemodynamics and ischaemic injury of acute myocardial infarction. *American Journal of Cardiology* **37**, 123.

Chattarjee K., Parmley W.W., Ganz W., Forrester J., Walisky P., Croyellus C., Swan H.T.C. (1973) Haemodynamic and metabolic responses to vasodilator therapy in acute myocardial infarction. *Circulation* **48**, 1183–1193.

Choresis C., Leonidas J. (1962) Serum transaminases in diphtheric myocarditis. Their relation to electrocardiographic findings. *Acta Paediatrica* **81**, 293.

Conti C.R., Curry R.C. Jr. (1979) Therapy of unstable angina pectoris. Coh P.F., Editor. *Diagnosis and therapy of coronary artery disease.* Little, Brown and Co. Boston, (p. 333).

Dollipriana A.W., Coling W.A., Donaldson R.J., McCormack P. (1977) Teeside Coronary Survey. Fatality and comparative severity of patients treated at home, in hospital ward and in the coronary care unit after myocardial infarction. *British Heart Journal* **39**, 1172–1178.

Elwood P.C., Cochrane A.L., Burr M.L., Sweetnam P.M., Williams G., Welshy E., Hughes S.J., Renton R. (1974) A randomized control trial of acetylsalicylic acid in the secondary prevention of mortality from myocardial infarction. *British Medical Journal* **1**, 436–440.

Fish I.S., Gorlin R., Herman M.V. (1973) The intermediate coronary syndrome: Clinical, angiographic and therapeutic aspects. *New England Journal of Medicine* **288,** 1193.

Gold H.K., Leinbach R.C., Brickley M.J., Mundth E.D., Daggeh W.M., Austen W.G. (1976) Refractory angina pectoris. Follow up after intra-aortic balloon pumping and surgery. *Circulation,* **54,** (Suppl. III) 41–46.

Hill J.D., Hampton J.R., Mitchell J.R.A. (1978) A randomized trial of home versus hospital management for patients with suspected myocardial infarction. *Lancet* **1,** 837–841.

Hill N.S., Antaman E.M., Green L.H., Alpart J.S. (1981) Intravenous nitroglycerin. A review of pharmacology, indications, therapeutic effects and complications. *Chest* **79,** 69.

Hugenholz P.G., Michels H.R., Serruys P.W., Brower R.W. (1981) Nifedipine in the treatment of unstable angina, coronary spasm and myocardial ischaemia. *American Journal of Cardiology* **47,** 163.

Kloner R.A., Fishbein M.C., Braunwald E., Maroko P.R., Lew M. (1978) Mummification of the infected myocardium by high dose corticosteroids. *Circulation* **57,** 56–63.

Kowsowsky H.D., Taylor J., Lown B., Ritchie R.F. (1973) Long term use of procainamide following acute myocardial infarction. *Circulation* **47,** 1201–1204.

Kustar K. (1972) Increased creatinine kinase concentration after intramuscular injection of 'Diazepam'. *General Medicine* **2,** 154.

Lafair J.S., Myoson R. (1968) Alcoholic myopathy with special reference to creatinine phosphokinase. *Archives of Internal Medicine* **122,** 417.

Lie K.I., Wollens H.J., Van Capelle F.J., Durrer D. (1974) Lidocaine in the primary prevention of ventricular fibrillation. *New England Journal of Medicine* **291,** 1324–1326.

Lie K.I., Liem K.L., Louridtz W.L.J., Janse M.T., Willebrands A.F., Durrer D. (1978) Efficacy of Lidocaine in preventing primary ventricular fibrillation within one hour after a 300 mg. intramuscular injection. *American Journal of Cardiology* **42,** 486–488.

Luxton M., Peter T., Harper R., Hunt D., Sloman G. (1975) Establishment of the Melbourne mobile intensive care service. *Medical Journal of Australia* **1,** 612–615.

Madias J.E., Madian N.E., Hood W.B. (1976) Praecordial segment mapping II. Effect of oxygen inhalation on ischaemic injury in patients with acute myocardial infarction. *Circulation* **53,** 411–417.

Maroko P.R., Libby P., Blear C.M., Sobol B.E., Braunwald E. (1972) Reduction by hyalurinidase of myocardial necrosis following coronary artery occlusion. *Circulation* **46,** 430–437.

Maroko P.R. and Braunwald E. (1973) Modification of myocardial infarction size after coronary occlusion. *Annals of Internal Medicine* **79,** 720–733.

Maroko P.R., Radrancy P., Braunwald E., Hale S.L. (1975) Reduction of infarct size by oxygen inhalation following acute coronary occlusion. *Circulation* **45,** 1160–1175.

Mather M.G., Morgan D.C., Pearson N.G., Read K.L.Q., Shaw D.B., Steed C.R., Thorne M.G., Lawrence C.J., Riley I.S. (1976) Myocardial infarction: A comparison between home and hospital care for patients. *British Medical Journal* **1,** 925–929.

Mayou R. (1979) Psychological reactions to myocardial infarction. *Journal of the Royal College of Physicians of London* 13, 103–105.

McIntosh A.F., Crabbe M.E., Grainger R., Williams J.H., Chamberlain D.A. (1978) The Brighton resuscitation ambulances, a review of 40 consecutive survivors of out of hospital cardiac arrest. *British Medical Journal* 1, 1115–1118.

McLean D., Fishbein M.C., Braunwald E., Maroko P.R. (1978) Long term preservation of ischaemic myocardium after experimental coronary artery occlusion. *Journal of Clinical Investigation* 61, 541–581.

Mitchell J.R.A. (1981) Timolol after myocardial infarction: an answer or a new sort of questions? *British Medical Journal* 282, 1565–1570.

Morrison J., Reduto L., Pizzarollo R., Geller K., Malery T., Galotta S. (1976) Modification of myocardial injury in man by cortico steroid administration. *Circulation* 53, (Suppl. 1) 200–203.

Morrison J., Coronilas J., Robbins M., Onj L., Eisenberg S., Reiser P., Scherr L. (1980) Digitalis and myocardial infarction in man. *Circulation* 62, 8–16.

Mundth E.D. (1976) Mechanical and surgical interventions for the reduction of myocardial ischaemia. *Circulation* 53, (Suppl. 1) 176–183.

Norris R.M., Samuel N.L., Clarke E.D., Smith W.M., Williams B. (1978) Protective effect of Propranolol in threatened myocardial infarction. *Lancet* 2, 907–909.

Norwegian Multicentre Study Group (1981) Timolol induced reduction of mortality and reinfarction in patients surviving acute myocardial infarction. *New England Journal of Medicine* 304, 801–807.

Peter T., Ross D., Duffield A., Luxton M., Harper R., Hurst D., Sloman G. (1978) Effect on survival after myocardial infarction of long term treatment with phenytoin. *British Heart Journal* 40, 1356–1360.

Powell W.T., Dibona D.R., Flores T., Leaf A. (1976) The protective effect of hyperosmotic mannitol in myocardial ischaemia and necrosis. *Circulation* 54, 603–615.

Rawles J.M., Kenmore A.C.F. (1976) Controlled trial of oxygen in uncomplicated myocardial infarction. *British Medical Journal* 1, 1121–1123.

Reynell P.C. (1975) Intermediate coronary care—A controlled trial. *British Heart Journal* 37, 166–168.

Saliba M.T., Kuzman W.T., Mash D.T., Lazry J.E. (1976) Effect of Heparin in anticoagulant doses on the electrocardiogram and enzymes in patients with acute myocardial infarction. A cervical pilot study. *American Journal of Cardiology* 57/58, (suppl. II) 61.

Stanley A.W., Prather J.W. (1978) Glucose–insulin–potassium patient mortality and acute myocardial injury in man by cortico steroid administration. *Circulation* 53, (Suppl. 1) 200–203.

Theroux P., Ross J., Franklin D., Kemper W.S., Sasayana S. (1979) Prognostic value of exercise testing soon after myocardial infarction. *New England Journal of Medicine* 301, 341–345.

Thompson P.L., Fletcher E.E., Katarahis V. (1979) Enzymatic indices of myocardial necrosis. Influence on short and long-term prognosis after myocardial infarction. *Circulation* 59, 113–119.

Thompson P.L., Robinson J.S. (1978) Stroke after acute myocardial infarction. *British Medical Journal* 2, 457–459.

Unstable Angina Pectoris Study Group: Unstable angina pectoris. National Co-operative Study Group to compare medical and surgical therapy. Parts I & II *American Journal of Cardiology* **37**, 896 (1976) & **42**, 839 (1978).

Weintrant R., Aroesty J.M., Pailin S., Levine F.H., Makis J.E., La Raia P.J., Cohen S.I., Kuland G.F. (1979) Medically refractory angina pectoris: Long-term follow up of patients undergoing intra-aortic balloon counterpulsation and operation. *American Journal of Cardiology* **43**, 877.

Wenger N.K., Hellerstarin H.K., Blackburn H., Castranova S.J. (1982) Physician practice in the management of patients with uncomplicated myocardial infarction: Changes in the past decade. *Circulation* **65**, 421–427.

Williams D.O., Riley R.S., Singh A.K., Gerlinitz H., Most A.S. (1981) Evaluation of the role of coronary angioplasty in patients with unstable angina pectoris. *America Heart Journal* **182**, 1.

Wyman M.H., Hammersmith L. (1974) Comprehensive treatment plan for the prevention of primary ventricular fibrillation in acute myocardial infarction. *American Journal of Cardiology* **33**, 661–667.

Yusef S., Lopoz R., Maddison A., Sleight P. (1978) Electrocardiographic and enzyme evolution of infarct size in man. *Circulation* **57**, **58** (Suppl. II) 172.

Yusef S., Ramsdale D., Peto R., Furse L., Bennett D., Bray C., Sleight P. (1980) Early intravenous Atenolol treatment in suspected acute myocardial infarction. *Lancet* **ii**, 273–277.

5 · Cardiac Arrhythmias

BRIAN GRIBBIN

Cardiac performance is governed in part by the rate of the heart and the synchrony of atrial and ventricular contraction. Individuals with normal cardiac function can tolerate wide fluctuations in heart rate and even rhythm changes without the significant haemodynamic impairment which is implicit in the term 'emergency'. Therefore, when faced with an emergency, one has to consider those arrhythmias which by themselves can cause a severe fall in cardiac output and vital organ perfusion. Extreme bradycardia or periods of cardiac standstill consequent upon sino-atrial disease or atrio-ventricular nodal disease are examples, as are ventricular fibrillation and fast ventricular tachycardia. In addition, the Wolff–Parkinson–White syndrome may allow fast supra-ventricular rhythms, such as atrial flutter and atrial fibrillation, to be conducted one to one to the ventricles.

Arrhythmias are more common in patients with underlying heart disease. The more severe the heart disease, the more likely that considerable clinical deterioration will follow the onset of an abnormal heart rhythm. For example, it is well recognized that pulmonary oedema and loss of consciousness may occur in patients with mitral stenosis when atrial fibrillation intervenes. It is less well known that suppression of frequent single ventricular ectopic beats can lead to improved cardiac output in patients with severe left ventricular disease. The last example emphasizes the point that arrhythmias may produce their effects not only by altering heart rate but also by nullifying the benefits of atrial contraction and synchronized ventricular depolarization.

If faced with an emergency due to an arrhythmia, appropriate therapeutic action may have to be taken immediately. However, a careful history plus physical examination and standard twelve lead electrocardiogram (ECG), often offer a clue to the likely diagnosis. Exercise testing or ambulatory twenty-four hour ECG monitoring may provide evidence regarding the nature of the arrhythmia. In addition, a member of the family may be asked to record the patient's pulse during an attack. This may, at least, provide a diagnosis of cardiac standstill. Every attempt should be made to procure an ECG diagnosis of the arrhythmia and if necessary, provocation during intra-cardiac electrophysiological studies should be attempted.

Modes of treatment available

There are certain well recognized arrhythmogenic influences which must be considered in any patient presenting with symptomatic arrhythmias. Hypokalaemia, acidaemia, thyroid overactivity and drug toxicity should be considered and, if confirmed, appropriate management should be instituted. However, in general there are four main approaches to arrhythmia control. These are drug treatment, cardioversion by direct current (DC) shock, pacing and ablative techniques including cardiac surgery.

Drug treatment

The large number of anti-arrhythmic drugs available underlines the difficulty in predicting their effectiveness in any one situation. Nevertheless, a pattern of usage has been built up based on knowledge of the electrophysiological properties of the drugs and clinical experience. When this information is added to an understanding of the mechanism of the arrhythmia, effective control is more likely. The possible mechanisms are illustrated in Fig. 5.1. For example, a supraventricular tachycardia incorporating an A-V nodal re-entry pathway is likely to respond to a drug

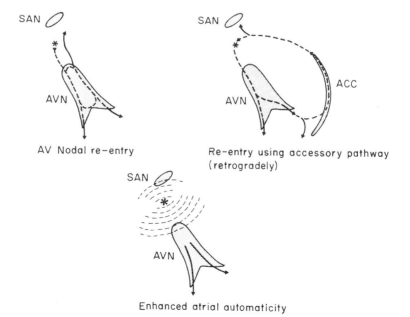

Fig. 5.1. Different mechanisms of supraventricular tachycardia. The asterisk represents the ectopic focus which initiates the tachycardia. SAN = sino-atrial node, AVN = atrioventricular node, ACC = accessory pathway.

such as Verapamil which alters conduction through the node. However, this drug is unlikely to terminate paroxysmal atrial tachycardia due to enhanced automaticity in atrial muscle, although it can still be used to slow the ventricular response. Despite these considerations uncertainty may still exist. In the presence of a recurrent and potentially dangerous arrhythmia the effectiveness of various drugs can be tested by attempting serial provocation of the arrhythmia during intra-cardiac studies. Under these circumstances, once a drug, given intravenously, has been shown to prevent a tachyarrhythmia it is important to ensure that oral treatment results in similar therapeutic blood levels.

DC cardioversion

This form of treatment has a major role to play in the termination of serious tachyarrhythmias. It has the advantage of rapid action with few side effects when used correctly. The mode of action is the instantaneous depolarization of all myocardial cells with concomitant interruption of re-entry pathways. Hopefully, the sino-atrial node recovers first and takes over the rhythm of the heart. Whenever possible the current should be synchronized with the R wave of the ECG so that random application of electrical energy does not fall during the vulnerable period of the cardiac cycle around the apex of the T wave. At this time the myocardial cells are in varying degrees of refractoriness and ventricular fibrillation can be induced.

Cardioversion is the treatment of choice for patients who are in a state of circulatory collapse as a result of a tachyarrhythmia. The energy required in an adult varies, being of the order of 25 joules for atrial flutter and 200 joules for ventricular fibrillation. When dealing with emergencies it is usually best to cardiovert as soon as possible. However, thought should always be given to the acid:base state, the presence of electrolyte abnormalities, the provision of adequate oxygenation and the possibility of drug toxicity or underlying sino-atrial disease. For example, digitalis toxicity increases the risk of cardioversion because of the danger of inducing ventricular fibrillation. Nevertheless, if the clinical circumstances dictate, cardioversion at low energy levels should be tried together with the use of an anti-arrhythmic agent, such as Lignocaine, which is given in an attempt to reduce the risk of ventricular fibrillation. Patients taking digitalis without evidence of toxicity can have standard cardioversion procedures. More recently internal cardioversion, using low energy discharges via an electrode catheter has been used to terminate sustained ventricular tachycardia and supraventricular tachycardias in patients refractory to drug treatment. At present, this form of treatment is in the experimental stage as is the automatic implantable defibrillator which is designed to detect and terminate ventricular tachycardia and ventricular fibrillation.

Pacing

Pacemakers have a logical and well tried place in the management of patients with symptomatic bradyarrhythmias. Right ventricular pacing is usually sufficient to prevent severe symptoms in patients with intermittent or sustained bradycardia. However, there are patients whose overall cardiac performance can be considerably worse at a pacing rate of seventy beats per minute than during a sinus bradycardia of fifty beats per minute. These patients include those with marked left ventricular hypertrophy, left ventricular outflow obstruction or poor left ventricular function who require atrial contraction to fill a non compliant left ventricle. When atrial contraction is required an attempt should be made to institute either atrial pacing (if A-V nodal conduction is normal) or a form of atrio-ventricular (A-V) sequential pacing. When the latter is compared to ventricular pacing in patients with AV block, it has been shown to improve cardiac output at rest and especially during exercise (Kruse, 1982). Emergency physiological pacing is also available with the recent development of an A–V sequential temporary electrode. The heart can also be paced from an electrode passed down the oesophagus. This technique offers more reliable atrial than ventricular pacing, and in the past rather large voltages have been required causing discomfort to the patient. However, Gallagher *et al.* (1982) have provided evidence that by widening the duration of the pacing stimulus the applied current can be reduced. This allows effective atrial pacing without significant side effects. If this is confirmed, this mode of pacing may have a wider application as a form of emergency treatment.

Pacing techniques are also of considerable use in the emergency treatment of tachyarrhythmias. A re-entry pathway can be interrupted and the arrhythmia terminated if a well placed pacing stimulus can gain entry to the re-entry pathway and render refractory the tissues ahead of the advancing wave front. The chance of success is greater, especially with the fast tachycardias if the pacing electrode is placed close to the re-entry circuit and a train of impulses rather than a single stimulus is given. As a temporary measure pacing is most often used to terminate atrial flutter and ventricular tachycardia. A number of techniques have been used; underdrive pacing consists of asynchronous (fixed rate) pacing at about eighty to ninety beats per minute. It can be applied either to the atrium in an attempt to abort atrial or ventricular tachycardia, or to the right ventricle in an attempt to abort the latter. By chance, one or more of the pacing stimuli may produce a conduction block in the re-entry circuit. Pacing faster than the rate of the tachycardia is termed overdrive pacing. Applied to the right atrium it can be particularly effective in the management of recurrent atrial flutter with the atrial pacing rate gradually being reduced until sinus rhythm takes over. Obviously, detrimental haemodynamic consequences may result from ventricular overpacing and so a modification is used. In this, a burst of four to fifteen impulses stimulate the right ventricle at a rate faster than the tachycardia. It should be remembered that in cases of ventricular tachycardia, if overpacing is unsuccessful, an increase in the unpaced tachycardia rate can result. In these circumstances it may be necessary to carry out DC cardioversion.

More experience is being gained in the use of permanent pacemakers to terminate tachyarrhythmias and in particular supraventricular tachycardias. A demand ventricular pacemaker can be switched to the asynchronous mode by application of a magnet, thus allowing activation of underpacing by the patient. Other units revert automatically to the asynchronous mode if a tachycardia is sensed. Others can be programmed to produce burst pacing or to 'hunt' for the coupling interval which allows a stimulus to interrupt the re-entry mechanism (Spurrell et al. 1982). However, it has to be emphasized that the decision to use permanent pacing systems to control tachycardias must follow intracardiac electrophysiological studies so that the mechanism of the arrhythmia is not in doubt.

It is recognized that tachyarrhythmias are more likely to occur if there is an underlying sinus bradycardia. In these circumstances, temporary or permanent pacing can be an effective way of preventing the single ectopic which may lead to a re-entry tachycardia. An example is sino-atrial disease with alternating periods of marked bradycardia and supraventricular tachycardia. Lastly, mention should also be made of the value of temporary pacemakers in improving the haemodynamic status of patients despite failing to terminate or prevent the arrhythmia. One example is the use of overdrive atrial pacing in supraventricular tachycardia. The faster atrial rate, by increasing A-V block, results in a fall in ventricular rate. However, this technique carries a risk of inducing atrial fibrillation. Therefore, it must be certain that the patient does not have an accessory A-V pathway with a short refractory period (Wolff-Parkinson-White syndrome) because in this situation atrial fibrillation could be conducted one to one to the ventricles.

Ablation of conducting pathways and surgery

Surgical treatment of tachyarrhythmias is seldom required and is best carried out in those few centres experienced in the necessary investigative and surgical techniques. Its use may be considered in patients who have recurrent disabling or life threatening arrhythmias despite adequate medical therapy. Occasionally, surgical treatment may be advised in a young symptomatic person with the Wolff–Parkinson–White syndrome who is reluctant to consider long term drug therapy. It is in this latter condition that most surgical success has been achieved. Preliminary and intra-operative electrophysiological studies are necessary to map the spread of activity and to identify the exact position of the accessory pathway. If practicable, surgical transection or cryoblation of the myocardium through which the tract passes offers a good chance of preventing further re-entry supra-ventricular rhythms. Surgical isolation of the atrial focus producing par-oxysmal atrial tachycardia has also been carried out (Anderson *et al.* 1982), although atrial tachycardias, due to enhanced automaticity or a re-entry A–V node mechanism are not usually suitable for direct surgical attack. Nevertheless, relief from refractory tachycardias of this kind can follow ablation of the A-V node and the implantation of a permanent pacemaker. Different ablative techniques have been used. The least damaging and most effective of the surgical methods is cryoablation which allows the operator to confirm interruption of the conducting pathway before proceeding to irreversible damage by a more prolonged application of the cryoprobe (Camm *et al.* 1980). Intracardiac ablation has also been carried out as a closed chest procedure in patients with refractory supraventricular tachy-cardias by passing high energy DC shocks through an electrode positioned adjacent to the bundle of His or close to an accessible bypass tract (Gallagher *et al.* 1982). Lastly, we have to consider the difficult problem of recurrent ventricular tachycardia, usually in patients with ischaemic heart disease and often in those with severe ventricular damage or a ventricular aneurysm. The mechanism is probably micro re-entry within the border zone of endocardial injury and the pervenous catheter technique has been used to ablate the focal origin of a ventricular tachycardia (Hartzler 1983). However, because the potential exists for multiple re-entry pathways, localized ablation is unlikely to be effective in the majority of patients. There have been two main surgical approaches to this problem. First, an indirect one in which the source of the arrthymia is considered to be a ventricular aneurysm or infarcted area which is then resected without pre- or intra-operative mapping. Coronary artery revascularization also may be used with or without resection of damaged myocardium. Secondly, a more direct approach in which mapping of the tachycardia wave front, as it passes through the myocardium, is used as a way of identifying its source. Surgical removal of the source has had rather unpredictable results. For that reason, recent surgical procedures have attempted either to isolate the whole border zone capable of sustaining tachycardia as in the operation of encircling endocardial ventriculotomy (Guiraudon *et al.* 1978) or, to remove it by a more localized endocardial resection procedure (Josephson *et al.* 1979). The former operation involves making an incision through most of the wall thickness along a boundary between fibrotic and normal myocardium and as a consequence may result in deterioration of overall left ventricular function with the risk of postoperative cardiogenic shock. Endocardial resection surgery appears to be safer. In general, the direct approaches based on mapping techniques are more effective in preventing ventricular tachy-cardia.

Recognition and management of individual arrhythmias

Atrial tachyarrhythmia is a generic term used to describe a number of tachycardias which originate above the bundle branches and hence typically have a narrow QRS complex on the ECG. They include atrial fibrillation, atrial flutter, A-V nodal re-entry tachycardia, atrio-ventricular re-entry tachycardia associated with an accessory bypass tract and enhanced automaticity or micro re-entry causing atrial or junctional tachycardias.

Atrial fibrillation

This is a common arrhythmia rarely causing severe symptoms unless associated with underlying heart disease. Characteristically, the ECG shows an irregularly irregular ventricular rate with fibrillatory waves of atrial activity visible, although with fast heart rates they may not be obvious (Fig. 5.2). Ventricular rates are often at their highest, up to 280 beats per minute, at the onset perhaps due to associated sympathetic nervous activity. Faster ventricular rates can occur in patients with pre-excitation. In this situation, ventricular fibrillation is a real risk and Digitalis should not be given because of the possibility that it might shorten the refractory period of the bypass tract resulting in a faster ventricular response.

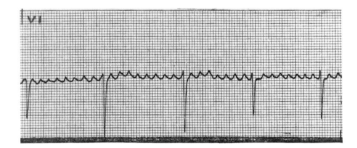

Fig. 5.2. Atrial fibrillation with slow ventricular response.

In an emergency situation synchronized DC cardioversion should be carried out without delay using 100 joules. Intravenous Verapamil 5 mg over one minute or 10 mg over five minutes can be relied upon to slow the ventricular response. It can be repeated at intervals until Digoxin, given intravenously initially and then orally, controls the ventricular rate. Recurrent atrial fibrillation may be prevented by a beta blocking drug or intravenous Amiodarone or Disopyramide with subsequent oral administration. Care should be taken to avoid giving a combination of Verapamil and a beta-blocker or Disopyramide because of the serious fall in cardiac contractility which may result.

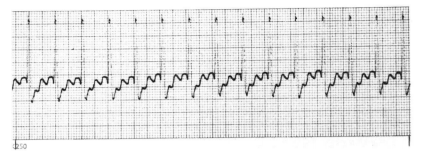

Fig. 5.3. Atrial flutter with 2 :1 A–V block.

Atrial flutter

This arrhythmia is diagnosed by the ECG features of rapid and regular atrial activity at 250 to 350 beats per minute shown as 'saw tooth' flutter waves particularly in leads II, III and AVF. Usually, the atrial rate is close to 300 beats per minute with 2:1 A-V block giving a ventricular rate of 150 beats per minute, which is well tolerated unless the cardiac reserve is low (Fig. 5.3). Flutter is unusual in patients without obvious heart disease and can be treated with Digoxin with a good chance of reverting to sinus rhythm or to atrial fibrillation. Care must be taken when using drugs such as Diso-pyramide, Procainamide and Quinidine which may alter a situation in which one has an atrial rate of 300 beats a minute with 2:1 A-V conduction to one in which the atrial rate is 200 beats per minute with 1:1 conduction. In these circumstances, Digoxin or a beta-blocker should be added to slow A-V conduction. Emergency treatment consists of low energy synchronized DC cardioversion (25–50 joules) or Verapamil given to increase A-V block and slow the ventricular rate. If there is a recurrence, then atrial overpacing, as outlined above, may be effective. The right atrium can be paced at rates of about 130 per cent of the atrial tachycardia rate for twenty seconds or so with the rate and duration of pacing being increased, if necessary, until the

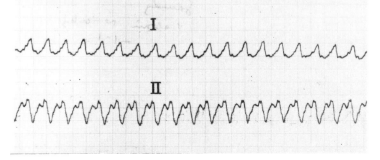

Fig. 5.4. Atrial flutter with 1:1 A–V conduction. Ventricular rate 250/minute.

arrhythmia is terminated. Atrial flutter with 1:1 A-V conduction raises the possibility of pre-excitation with anterograde conduction down the accessory pathway (Fig. 5.4). Circulatory collapse is then more likely requiring DC cardioversion. Digoxin should be avoided because of the risk of inducing atrial fibrillation with shortening of the refractory period of the bypass tract and acceleration of the ventricular rate. A useful drug under these circumstances is Amiodarone given intravenously and then orally. This slows conduction down the accessory pathway and may revert atrial flutter to sinus rhythm. Long-term treatment may be better judged following an electrophysiological study.

Atrial flutter with 1:1 A-V conduction down a bypass tract not responding satisfactorily to drug treatment and especially in the young is one condition in which ablation of the tract should be considered.

Atrio-ventricular nodal re-entry tachycardia

This is relatively common and often unassociated with heart disease and so rarely leads to an emergency situation. The mechanism is a re-entry circuit within the A-V node (Fig. 5.1) initiated by an ectopic beat and perhaps due to longitudinal functional dissociation within the node. Because retrograde activation of the atria often occurs at about the same time as anterograde ventricular depolarization the P waves are buried in the QRS complexes (Fig. 5.5). Less commonly, conduction through the retrograde V-A limb of the circuit is slow in which case the P waves occur after the QRS complexes with the RP interval greater than the PR. Electrophysiological work has shown that a proportion of patients with re-entry supra-ventricular tachycardias have a concealed accessory pathway; that is one which can only conduct retrogradely. In this the P wave also follows the QRS complex but the RP interval is usually less than the PR (Fig. 5.6). In either circumstance, the A-V node is part of the tachycardia circuit and vagal manoeuvres and drugs which alter conduction through the A-V node are likely to terminate the arrhythmia. Thus carotid sinus massage or a valsalva manoeuvre may be

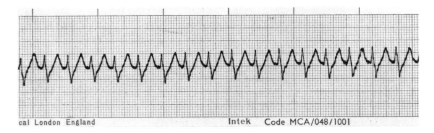

cal London England   Intek   Code MCA/048/1001

Fig. 5.5. A–V nodal re-entry tachycardia. The P wave is buried within the QRS.

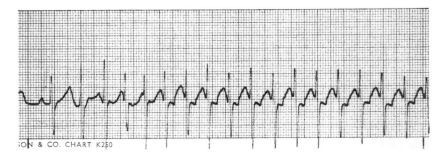

Fig. 5.6. A–V re-entry tachycardia. The first beat is sinus then an atrial ectopic starts a reciprocating tachycardia with negative P waves after each QRS.

effective. Verapamil, given intravenously, is the drug of choice. If it is found to be ineffective the diagnosis of A-V nodal tachycardia should be reconsidered. Digoxin or a beta-blocker is likely to be effective as a form of prophylactic treatment.

Pre-excitation syndromes

The requirement for these conditions is one or more extra connections of specialized heart muscle cells lying between the atria and ventricles. The properties and anatomical relationship of these tracts to the A-V node vary but they provide the setting for re-entry tachyarrhythmias and for rapid atrio-ventricular conduction. The ECG may show a short PR interval representing anterograde conduction down an accessory pathway and slurred R waves, as occurs in Wolff–Parkinson–White syndrome. A short PR interval and a normal QRS complex is seen in the Lown–Ganong–Levine syndrome with enhanced A–V nodal conduction or an A–V extra-nodal bypass tract. The hazards of these conditions and their management have been considered already.

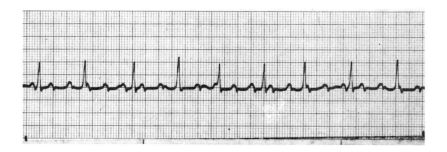

Fig. 5.7. Paroxysmal atrial tachycardia with variable A–V block.

Paroxysmal atrial and junctional tachycardias

These arrhythmias are often associated with heart disease or severe lung disease and particularly with Digitalis toxicity. Atrial tachycardia tends to be paroxysmal with a narrow QRS complex and an atrial rate of 150–250 beats per minute usually with a degree of A-V block (Fig. 5.7). Initially, the ventricular rate may accelerate and P waves may be clearly seen before the QRS complex. In junctional tachycardia, atrial activity may occur before, during or after ventricular activity. Occasionally, retrograde atrial spread from the junctional focus is blocked, in which case sinus rhythm or even atrial fibrillation may control the atria with an occasional fortuitous capture of the ventricles. However, the overall ventricular rhythm is governed by the junctional tachycardia at rates of about 130 beats per minute. Because of the relatively slow heart rate in junctional tachycardia (Fig. 5.8) emergency treatment is rarely required and it is enough to stop Digoxin and correct hypokalaemia and acid:base abnormalities. This approach is also indicated for atrial tachycardia but in this condition the ventricular rate may be fast and emergency treatment may be required. Because of the frequent association with digoxin toxicity cardioversion may not be the initial treatment of choice. However, if the patient is in a critical condition low energy synchronized DC shock (20 joules) can be used after Lignocaine is given intravenously. Phenytoin has also been used to control Digitalis induced fast tachyarrhythmias and Verapamil can be given to increase A-V block and slow the ventricular rate. Atrial overdrive pacing may be effective in terminating attacks. Even if it is unsuccessful, more rapid atrial pacing is likely to result in increasing atrio-ventricular block with a beneficial reduction of ventricular rate. In the absence of Digitalis toxicity, adequate Digoxin treatment is likely to be effective as is the use of Quinidine, Disopyramide or Amiodarone.

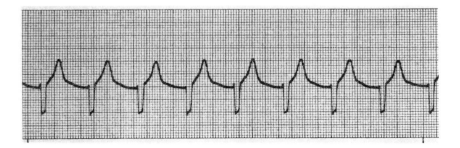

Fig. 5.8. Junctional rhythm. The retrograde P wave probably lies within the QRS.

Ventricular tachyarrhythmias

Emergency treatment is likely to be required for ventricular tachycardia and ventricular fibrillation. The latter is discussed in the chapter on cardiac arrest.

Ventricular tachycardia

This is defined as a run of three or more ventricular ectopic beats (Fig. 5.9). Its sinister reputation is based on the risk of it evolving into ventricular fibrillation and its association with severe heart disease such as acute myocardial infarction and left ventricular aneurysm. In addition, pronounced haemodynamic deterioration may occur as a consequence of the fast ventricular rate, loss of synchronized atrial contraction and the abnormal activation sequence of the ventricles. The ECG shows widened and abnormal complexes but other causes of broad QRS complex tachycardias must also be considered. Examples of these are supraventricular tachycardia with aberrant conduction, supraventricular tachycardia with prior left bundle branch block and when a supraventricular tachycardia is conducted anterogradely down an accessory pathway. Typically, ventricular tachycardia is characterized by a regular rhythm with capture beats, fusion beats and A-V dissociation. The latter may be detected clinically by observing intermittent cannon waves in the jugular venous pulse occurring when atrial and ventricular contraction coincide. However, when none of these helpful features is present some reliance may be placed on studies in which intracardiac electrophysiological data have allowed comparison of the 12-lead ECG characteristics of ventricular tachycardia and supraventricular tachycardia with aberrant conduction. For example, Wellens *et al.* (1982) showed that the QRS complex duration was usually greater than 0.14 seconds and left axis deviation was common in ventricular tachycardia. Nevertheless, these criteria could not differentiate ventricular tachycardia

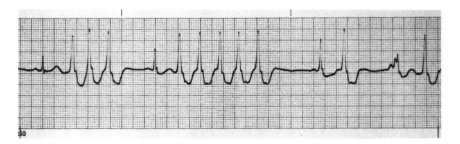

Fig. 5.9. Ventricular tachycardia. The first beat is sinus, the 5th, 11th and 13th are fusion beats.

from supraventricular tachycardia with prior left bundle branch block. For this reason it can be an advantage to have an ECG recorded during sinus rhythm or to record atrial activity using an oesophageal electrode and so confirm V–A dissociation in ventricular tachycardia.

Severely ill patients with sustained rapid ventricular tachycardia should be treated with DC cardioversion using 100 joules. If this is unsuccessful then 200 joules should be effective. Subsequently, the need for prophylactic treatment has to be considered. When ventricular tachycardia occurs early after acute myocardial infarction it is usual to give Lignocaine initially as an intravenous bolus followed by an infusion for twenty-four hours. Patients with ventricular tachycardia occurring some days after myocardial infarction often have severe myocardial damage and appropriate emergency treatment should be followed by oral maintenance therapy. The effectiveness of any one drug or combination of drugs cannot be guaranteed in the treatment of ventricular tachycardia. However, it is becoming apparent that the efficacy of long-term treatment can often be predicted by studying the effect of drugs, such as Flecainide, given acutely during intracardiac electrophysiological studies but this is not true of Amiodarone. Sotalol has been advocated because in addition to its beta-blocking activity it has a lengthening effect on the duration of the action potential. Adequate drug dosage should be confirmed by measuring plasma levels whenever difficulty is found in controlling bouts of ventricular tachycardia. Temporary overdrive pacing can be very useful, in these patients, as it allows time to find an effective drug regime. Eventually, if all else fails, the patient should be considered for cardiac surgery and referral made to a specialized centre.

Torsade de pointes

This is an unusual form of ventricular tachycardia diagnosed by the ECG appearances of a shifting QRS axis with a periodicity of five to twenty beats (Fig. 5.10). It can lead to ventricular fibrillation and may be associated with sinus bradycardia and prolongation of the QT interval. The latter implies an

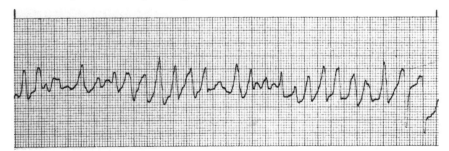

Fig. 5.10. Torsade de pointes.

inhomogeneity of ventricular repolarization and consequently a predisposition to re-entry tachycardia. It usually occurs in patients with ischaemic
heart disease. However, the possibility of electrolyte abnormalities, in
particular hypokalaemia and hypocalcaemia and drug toxicity with Quinidine, Disopyramide, tricyclic anti-depressants or phenothiazines should be
considered. Drugs which prolong the QT interval should not be given. DC
cardioversion can be used and overdrive pacing is usually the best way of
preventing a recurrence. Overdrive pacing should be continued until any
reversible abnormality has been corrected. Lignocaine may shorten the QT
interval in some patients and has been used to terminate an attack.

Congenital QT prolongation

Jervell and Lange–Neilsen (1957) described the condition of familial high
tone deafness, episodes of loss of consciousness and QT prolongation.
Although this condition is exceedingly rare, another inherited long QT
syndrome described by Romano (1965) and Ward (1964) must be taken into
consideration when faced with episodes of sudden loss of consciousness in
young people. Typically, the attacks occur at times of physical or emotional
stress. Enquiry into the family history may reveal first degree relatives with
syncopal attacks, perhaps treated inappropriately for years with anticonvulsant drugs. The resting ECG is normal apart from a long QT interval and
perhaps sinus bradycardia (Fig. 5.11). Physical examination is normal. The
mechanism is thought to be an imbalance in sympathetic drive to the heart
with dominance of the left sympathetic chain supply. This results in a
variable and fragmented pattern of myocardial repolarization and hence in
refractory period. It is assumed that a single ventricular ectopic beat initiates
a re-entry ventricular tachycardia which in turn progresses to ventricular
fibrillation. Certainly, ventricular tachycardia and fibrillation have been
documented during attacks. The prognosis in symptomatic individuals is not
good with a risk of sudden death and so life-long treatment is advised.

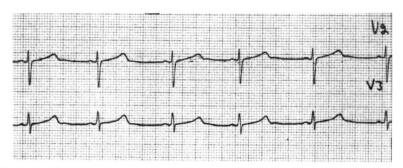

Fig. 5.11. From a patient with long QT syndrome.

Adequate beta-blockade and the use of Amiodarone appear to be effective in abolishing attacks. In addition to the beta-blockade those patients with co-existing sinus bradycardia may benefit from permanent pacemaker implantation. In the past and in cases of failed medical treatment left stellate sympathectomy has been recommended. Lastly, there are patients, usually children or young adults, who present with a typical history of the long QT syndrome but with normal ECGs. They appear to have catecholamine induced arrhythmias which may respond to therapy with beta-blocking agents.

Symptomatic bradyarrhythmias

Severe symptomatic bradyarrhythmias may arise as a result of disease of any part of the conducting system from the sino-atrial node, to the bundle branches. The fall in cardiac output and hence the severity of symptoms is governed by the rate of the bradycardia, the loss of atrial kick and the severity of underlying heart disease. The patient may be cold, clammy, confused and hypotensive but perhaps more common are recurrent episodes of loss of consciousness usually associated with periods of self-limiting cardiac standstill. The management of more sustained cardiac arrest is discussed in another chapter. Obviously, adequate cardiac output should be established as soon as possible and the means of effecting this will vary with the circumstances. For example, marked sinus bradycardia occurring early after acute myocardial infarction may improve with pain relief. However, it is unwise to accept a slow heart rate if accompanied by hypotension or symptoms. In this situation, Atropine can be given intravenously to increase the ventricular rate to sixty to seventy beats per minute. As the pulse rate increases, the blood pressure usually rises to an acceptable level. As a temporary expedient, atrial and sometimes ventricular pacing may be initiated by an electrode passed down the oesophagus. However, pervenous endocardial pacing is the treatment of choice and a skilled operator can insert a temporary pacing electrode quickly if adequate radiographic screening facilities are available.

Sino-atrial disease

This is a common disorder in which sinus bradycardia, sinus arrest and atrial tachyarrhythmias occur. Severe symptoms result from a delay in the onset of an escape rhythm after sinus arrest and this implies a coexistent conduction disorder in the A–V node or bundle of His. Atropine or Isoprenaline can be used intravenously. If a beta-blocking agent has been given then the Beta$_1$ agonist Prenalterol may lead to improvement in sinus rate. Symptomatic patients with sino-atrial disease should be treated with temporary pacing.

Permanent pacing is required if there is no evidence of an acute and possibly reversible cause. Anti-arrhythmic drug treatment may be given to suppress atrial tachyarrhythmias.

A–V block

Complete A–V block may be associated with intermittent cardiac standstill, marked bradycardia and related ventricular tachyarrythmia. Patients are often elderly and without other forms of serious heart disease. Atropine and Isoprenaline may be used initially but the risks of the latter causing ventricular tachyarrhythmia should be recognized. Temporary and then permanent pacing should be carried out.

Further reading

Anderson K.P., Stinson E.B. and Mason J.W. (1982) Surgical exclusion of focal paroxysmal atrial tachycardia. *The American Journal of Cardiology* **49**, 869–874.

Camm J., Ward D.E., Spurrell R.A.J. and Rees G.M. (1980) Cryothermal mapping and Cryoablation in the treatment of refractory cardiac arrhythmias. *Circulation* **62**, 67–74.

Gallagher J.J., Smith W.M., Kerr C.R., Kasell J., Cook L., Reiter M., Sterba R. and Harte M. (1982) Esophageal pacing: A diagnostic and therapeutic tool. *Circulation* **65**, 336–341.

Gallagher J.J., Svenson R.H., Rasell J.H., German L.D., Bardy G.H., Broughton A. and Critelli G. (1982) Catheter technique for closed chest ablation of the atrioventricular conduction system: a therapeutic alternative for the treatment of refractory supraventricular tachycardia. *New England Journal of Medicine* **306**, 194–200.

Guiraudon G., Fontaine G., Frank R., Escade G., Etievent P. and Cabrol C. (1978) Encircling endocardial ventriculotomy: a new surgical treatment for life-threatening ventricular tachycardia resistant to medical treatment following myocardial infarction. *The Annals of Thoracic Surgery* **26**, 438–444.

Hartzlet G.O. (1983) Electrode catheter ablation of refractory focal ventricular tachycardia. *Journal of the American College of Cardiology* **2**, 1107–1113.

Jervell A. and Lange-Nielsen F. (1957) Congenital deaf-mutism, functional heart disease with prolongation of the Q.T. interval and sudden death. *American Heart Journal* **54**, 59–68.

Josephson N.E., Harken A.H. and Harowitz L.N. (1979) Endocardial excision: a new surgical technique for the treatment of recurrent ventricular tachycardia. *Circulation* **60**, 1430–1439.

Kruse I., Arnman K., Conradson T.B. and Ryden L. (1982) A comparison of the acute and long-term haemodynamic effects of ventricular inhibited and atrial synchronous ventricular inhibited pacing. *Circulation* **65**, 846–855.

Romano C. (1965) Congenital cardiac arrhythmia. *Lancet* , 658–659. (letter).

Spurrell R.A.J., Nathan A.N., Bexton R.S., Hellenstrade K.J., Nappholz T. and Cramm A.J. (1982) Implantable automatic scanning pacemaker for termination of supraventricular tachycardia. *The American Journal of Cardiology* **49**, 753–760.

Ward O.C. (1964) A new familial cardiac syndrome in children. *Journal of the Irish Medical Association* **54**, 103–106.

Wellens H.J.J., Bar F.W.H.M., Vanagt E.J.D.M. and Brugada P. (1982) Medical treatment of ventricular tachycardia: Considerations in the selection of patients for surgical treatment. *The American Journal of Cardiology* **49**, 186–193.

6 · Acute Heart Failure

LAWRENCE COTTER

Acute heart failure is present whenever sudden severe malfunction of the heart occurs. Commonly this is manifest as cardiac arrest or cardiogenic shock. These subjects are discussed in the appropriate chapters, as is the only common form of acute right heart failure, namely that due to acute massive pulmonary embolism. Occasionally acute right heart failure occurs following myocardial infarction, usually accompanying acute left heart failure. When right heart failure occurs in isolation following myocardial infarction it is diagnosed by the presence of a markedly elevated jugular venous pressure in the presence of radiologically and clinically clear lung fields. The most important precept in its management is the avoidance of over-diuresis, causing low left sided filling pressures and a low output state. This may be very difficult and monitoring of right heart and pulmonary artery wedge pressures using a Swann–Ganz balloon tipped flotation catheter is often necessary. The mortality is high even when the condition is diagnosed accurately and managed optimally. Fortunately it is uncommon. By contrast, acute left heart failure manifest as cardiogenic pulmonary oedema, is one of the commonest of all medical emergencies.

Cardiogenic pulmonary oedema

Clinical features

Acute pulmonary oedema is a dramatic medical emergency which requires prompt and effective treatment. The patient is often unable to talk because of severe breathlessness. If he can talk, he may complain of the severe chest pain of an accompanying myocardial infarction. However, often little history is obtainable from the patient, although relatives may describe the sudden onset of severe dyspnoea, sometimes with the eventual production of pink frothy sputum—making the diagnosis obvious. There may or may not be a previous history of cardiac symptoms. On examination the patient is breathless, often desperately so, and using accessory muscles. There may be sweating and sometimes cyanosis. Initially the blood pressure is often elevated and the heart rate increased. Indeed, absence of tachycardia suggests a different diagnosis, unless the patient is beta-blocked. The jugular venous pressure is often elevated but not always so, and peripheral oedema is sometimes present due to more long standing fluid retention.

Clinically palpable pulsus alternans is uncommon. The heart sounds may be altered due to valvular heart disease and a gallop may be heard. Murmurs of underlying causative valvular heart disease may be present, but the most commonly heard murmur is that of 'functional' mitral regurgitation due to left ventricular and mitral ring dilatation. Bilateral and widespread crepitations are usually found on auscultation of the lung fields but occasionally severe bronchospasm alone is present with no crepitations.

The only investigations which are essential quickly are an electro-cardiogram and a chest X-ray. There are no electrocardiographic signs of pulmonary oedema but there may be signs of ventricular hypertrophy due to long standing hypertension or valvular heart disease, or evidence of myo-cardial ischaemia or infarction. The chest X-ray shows congested lung fields with hilar 'batswing' shadowing in classical severe cases, upper lobe blood diversion, sometimes 'Kerley B lines' and often an abnormal cardiac silhouette due to the underlying heart disease. Absence of cardiomegaly with pulmonary oedema is most commonly due to ischaemic heart disease, followed by mitral stenosis and tachyarrhythmias. Echocardiography is extremely helpful in diagnosing the cause of pulmonary oedema and may be indicated urgently especially if valvular regurgitation is possible. This is particularly true when a prosthetic valve is present, as severe paraprosthetic regurgitation may be present with no murmur. However, echocardiography is not necessary to diagnose the presence of pulmonary oedema and should not be performed until initial therapy has begun.

Differential diagnosis

The most common causes of acute severe breathlessness other than pulmonary oedema are bronchial asthma, pulmonary embolism and spontaneous pneumothorax (Ogilvie 1983).

Pulmonary embolism is not usually a likely differential diagnosis in the patient with pulmonary oedema, in particular the lung fields are usually clear and the chest X-ray shows either normal or underfilled lung fields. Spontaneous pneumothorax, sufficient to cause severe breathlessness, may show under expansion on the affected size with hyper-resonance, again without crepitations or wheeze. If a tension pneumothorax is present, mediastinal shift may be evident. The chest X-ray reveals the diagnosis.

'Cardiac asthma' due to pulmonary oedema may be extremely difficult to separate from bronchial asthma. The most useful clinical sign is the presence of a gallop rhythm in pulmonary oedema. However, right ventricular and left ventricular disease are also common in chronic obstructive lung disease. Furthermore, patients with chronic obstructive lung disease not infre-quently also have ischaemic heart disease with pulmonary oedema. The most useful arbiter in difficult cases is undoubtedly the chest X-ray.

Sometimes treatment is reasonably initiated with frusemide and amino-phylline before the X-ray is available (Pearson *et al.* 1981).

Finally, of course, cardiogenic pulmonary oedema has to be differen-tiated from other, much rarer causes of pulmonary oedema (Rubin, Cross and Zelis 1973) and shock lung (Chapter 14).

Management of cardiogenic pulmonary oedema

As soon as the diagnosis is reached, two questions need to be asked.

1. Are there precipitating causes of the pulmonary oedema and if so can they be reversed (Table 6.1)?

Table 6.1. Precipitating factors in cardiac pulmonary oedema

1 Infection
2 Arrhythmias
3 Endocarditis
4 Pulmonary embolism
5 Cessation of medical treatment, e.g. diuretics
6 Sodium load:
(a) increased intake orally or iv
(b) sodium retaining drug
7 Anaemia
8 Thyrotoxicosis

2. What is the aetiology of the heart disease, is there a surgically correctable condition present (Table 6.2)?

Table 6.2. Indications for cardiac surgery in pulmonary oedema

1 Acute severe aortic regurgitation
secondary to (a) infective endocarditis
(b) blunt chest trauma
(c) dissecting aneurysm of aorta
2 Critical aortic stenosis
3 Acute severe mitral regurgitation
secondary to (a) chordae tendinae rupture
(b) papillary muscle rupture or dysfunction
4 Severe mitral stenosis
— usually due to onset of atrial fibrillation
5 Ruptured interventricular septum
6 Left ventricular aneurysm
7 Prosthetic valve 'dysfunction'
due to (a) paravalvular leak
(b) prosthetic stenosis $2°$ to clot or vegetations
(c) prosthetic valve failure $2°$ to strut fracture
(d) biological valve degeneration etc.

As these question are being asked and answered, so specific therapy can be initiated (Table 6.3).

Table 6.3. Emergency treatment of cardiogenic pulmonary oedema

1 Sit patient up, administer oxygen.
2 Morphine iv.
3 Frusemide iv.
4 Consider: aminophylline
          digitalis
          vasodilators
5 Repeat morphine and frusemide.
6 Consider phlebotomy.
7 Consider ventilation.
8 IS THERE A ROLE FOR SURGERY?

Improvement in ventilation and oxygenation?

The patient with pulmonary oedema adopts a sitting position whenever possible and this should be facilitated. In the sitting position the venous return to the right atrium is diminished with reduction in pulmonary blood flow and congestion, the vital capacity is increased (Ramirez and Abelman 1974) and the work of breathing is reduced. These factors all help to diminish dyspnoea.

Tissue hypoxia is a fundamental result of, and correlates with, the degree of pulmonary oedema (Fillmore *et al.* 1970). It is substantially reduced by the administration of supplementary oxygen and its metabolic consequences and resultant downward spiral may be prevented. In addition, dyspnoea and the reduction in pulmonary capillary permeability due to hypoxia also may be improved with added oxygen.

Normal arterial oxygenation is not possible in the presence of pulmonary oedema due to impairment of diffusion across the alveolar-capillary membrane. This is exacerbated by the lower cardiac output which necessitates the peripheral tissues to extract more oxygen resulting in a lower oxygen content in the mixed venous blood. This abnormally deoxygenated blood passes through the intrapulmonary right to left shunts caused by ventilation perfusion mismatch and consequently exacerbates any arterial hypoxaemia (Kelman *et al.* 1967).

Oxygen should be administered in as high a concentration as possible. This usually means via a disposable face mask at a flow rate of 6–8 litres/ minute to deliver a concentration of 40–60 per cent oxygen. It is neither necessary nor desirable to limit the concentration of oxygen to 24 per cent unless the patient has a history suggesting respiratory failure with carbon dioxide retention. If a face mask proves unacceptable then nasal spectacles should be tried. Later, when the initial emergency is over, the concentration of oxygen should be reduced. Gas exchange may be considered to be satisfactory when the P_{CO_2} is normal at 4.6–5.3 kPa (35–40 mmHg) and the P_{O_2} is above 10.5 kPa (80 mm Hg) with a normal pH (Biddle and Yu 1980).

Morphine

Opiates, given intravenously, usually produce a rapid improvement in cardiac pulmonary oedema and are the most important and effective drug in its treatment. The benefits accrue in several ways. Which of these is most important remains controversial.

Morphine causes venodilation with reduction of the venous return and the pulmonary capillary hydrostatic pressure (Zellis *et al.* 1970). This reduces pulmonary blood pooling directly and also results in a decrease in myocardial oxygen consumption. Morphine diminishes the work of breathing by several other mechanisms. The responsiveness of the brain stem centres to increases in CO_2 retention is diminished and the pontine and medullary respiratory centres are also depressed. Apart from exerting this direct central effect, morphine is a powerful anxiolytic so that the hyperventilatory response to the discomfort itself is also diminished. Thus the work of breathing and its accompanying discomfort and distress are reduced. Furthermore, this decrease in stress results in a decrease in sympathtic outpouring and arteriolar tone so that peripheral resistance falls with accompanying beneficial results.

An average sized adult should be given 10 mg of morphine intravenously accompanied by an anti-emetic such as cylizine 50 mg or perchlorperazine (Stemetil) 12.5 mg. Further doses can be given when necessary. Whenever morphine is given, naloxone should be available in cases of profound respiratory depression.

Diamorphine, omnopon and cyclomorph are metabolized to morphine and are equally useful and favoured by some. Pentazocine should never be substituted for opiates in this circumstance.

Diuretics

Diuretics are used in pulmonary oedema to reduce the circulating plasma volume. This decreases the left atrial pressure, and although it is not likely that alveolar or interstitial fluid is mobilized quickly, any continued elevation of pulmonary capillary pressure is prevented.

The 'loop' diuretics frusemide, ethacrynic acid and bumetamide act by inhibiting chloride transport in the ascending limb of the loop of Henle along with sodium and thus water. In addition, more proximal sites may be involved and sodium re-absorption may also be inhibited in the distal tubule.

Urinary salt and water excretion increases within five minutes of intravenous frusemide, peaks within ten minutes and generally ceases within thirty minutes.

In pulmonary oedema, 40 to 80 mg of frusemide should be given intravenously. Almost immediate improvement sometimes occurs, well before any possible diminution in circulating blood volume is feasible via substantial increase in urine production. This is caused by the venodilator activity of these diuretics (Dikshit *et al.* 1973) and possibly some effect on after-load (Wilson *et al.* 1981). This also explains why hypotension may occasionally occur and how even anuric patients may derive some initial benefit from frusemide.

Bumetamide and ethacrynic acid have no advantages over frusemide in the acute situation.

If no improvement has occurred within thirty minutes, the diuretic should be repeated in an increased dosage with or without additional morphine. The diuretic action may be further enhanced by the addition of aminophylline if necessary and appropriate.

Aminophylline

The well known bronchodilating action of aminophylline via smooth muscle relaxation is particularly valuable in the treatment of pulmonary oedema when bronchospasm is present. The relaxation of vascular smooth muscle which may contribute in reducing left ventricular pre- and after-load is readily understood but other effects are more difficult to explain.

Aminophylline and other theophyllines have a positive inotropic effect, the mechanism of which is far from clear, but which is independent of its positive chronotropic effect (Marcus *et al.* 1972). This may be due to the reduction of the breakdown of cyclic AMP which aminophylline causes by inhibiting phosphodiesterase activity. This has the effect of potentiating the actions of catecholamines on the myocardium (Rall and West 1963). However, xanthines lengthen the duration of contraction while the direct action of catecholamines is to shorten the duration of contraction, so that a direct effect increasing myocardial cell calcium uptake may be the most likely explanation (Blinks *et al.* 1972).

The direct myocardial cellular action of aminophylline makes its effects independent of beta-adrenergic receptor activity and this may be useful when prior use of beta-blockers may be contributing to the myocardial problems. (When beta-blockers are definitely a major factor in the genesis of the pulmonary oedema, the powerful beta receptor agonist prenalterol may be particularly useful.)

Finally, aminophylline has a diuretic action. This is partly due to renal vasodilation, partly due to a direct inhibitory action on renal tubular reabsorption of sodium and, of course, partly due to its beneficial effects on cardiac output improving renal perfusion.

The heart rate is usually increased by aminophylline and not surprisingly arrhythmias may result. Therefore, it is sensible to avoid its use in acute myocardial infarction unless bronchospasm is severe and unresponsive to diuretics, morphine and oxygen. Nausea and hypotension are occasional side effects.

The dosage of aminophylline is 6 mg/kg body weight, given intravenously over 15–20 minutes. If more prolonged use is required (unusual in this context) 0.9 mg/kg/minute should be given in 5 per cent dextrose.

Digitalis

The use of digitalis glycoside in the treatment of pulmonary oedema is undisputed when atrial fibrillation with a rapid ventricular rate is present, particularly if there is mitral stenosis. However, its use in patients with sinus rhythm has remained a matter of controversy, despite 200 years of use since William Withering's treatise. Although the debate continues, recent controlled trials have currently swung the pendulum towards the use of digitalis as a positive inotrope (Smith 1982). The suggested beneficial haemodynamic effects of digitalis may be effected at a cellular level by inhibition of membrane sodium-potassium ATPase. This results in an increase in intracellular sodium, which itself increases intracellular calcium (and myocardial contractility) via a sodium-calcium exchange carrier mechanism. Other mechanisms are also active and indeed may even predominate (Noble 1980).

The use of digitalis has important negative features. Any positive inotrope must tend to increase myocardial oxygen consumption. Digitalis has a notoriously small therapeutic window between ineffectual homeopathy and dangerous toxicity, so that overdosage side effects are common. This is particularly true in acute myocardial infarction, where an increase in myocardial irritability may be disastrous. Furthermore, any increase in oxygen uptake is particularly unwelcome in acute infarction, as an increase in the size of the infarct may result. If the digitalis is given too rapidly these effects may be magnified with systemic and coronary vasoconstriction, and even ischaemic pain (Balcon, Hoy and Sowton 1968). When possible it is sensible to avoid the use of digitalis when pulmonary oedema is secondary to acute myocardial infarction with sinus rhythm.

Digitalis is most likely to be useful in sinus rhythm when cardiomegaly and gallop rhythm are present. Then the end diastolic volume may be reduced and thus systolic wall tension and myocardial oxygen consumption may also be reduced (Karliner and Braunwald 1972).

When improvement has not occurred following oxygen, morphine and diuretics then digoxin should be given intravenously in a dosage of 500 micrograms in 50 ml of 5 per cent dextrose over thirty minutes. This may be followed by 500 micrograms over one hour and if necessary a third dose may be given over two hours (assuming a normal sized adult with good renal function and no previous digitalis).

Vasodilators

Vasodilators should be used whenever possible in the treatment of heart failure (Massie and Chatterjee 1979). They are far more likely to produce marked improvement in acute pulmonary oedema than digitalis, although the latter is more frequently prescribed. When appropriately administered they lead to a marked improvement in the myocardial oxygen supply/ demand equation and also lead to improvement in symptoms.

A cardinal factor in the assessment of myocardial oxygen demand is the impedence to ejection from the left ventricle. This is reflected in the arterial blood pressure and can be reduced using arteriolar vasodilators—'after-load reduction'. Not only is the myocardial oxygen balance improved but the cardiac output increases with its consequent benefit, particularly on renal perfusion. Clearly it is not useful to reduce the blood pressure to the extent that the gradient across the coronary circulation is diminished, with reduction in coronary blood flow and exacerbation of any ischaemia.

Vasodilators acting on the venous system cause a 'pharmacological phlebotomy'. The venous pooling reduces the volume of blood returning to the heart—the 'pre-load', thus diminishing myocardial work and oxygen consumption. This reduction in the effective circulating blood volume causes a fall in left ventricular filling pressure and pulmonary capillary pressure, so that pulmonary congestion is also improved. However, if the filling pressure is reduced too much a degree of relative hypovolaemia results and the cardiac output may fall.

Numerous vasodilators have been used in patients with heart failure. These can be broadly classified as venodilators, arterial dilators and so called 'balanced' vasodilators with significant effects on both vascular beds.

Where the patients' problems are due to pulmonary congestion with manifest fluid overload indicated by elevation of the jugular venous pressure as well as lung crepitations, a venodilator is likely to be helpful. The most convenient and familiar are probably the nitrates. These are principally venodilators, although they also have some effect on the arteriolar side. Oral or cutaneously administered glyceryl trinitrate, isosorbide dinitrate or isosorbide mononitrate are effective but circumstances often require intravenous administration. Nitroglycerin may be started at 10 μg/minute, or isosorbide dinitrate at 5 mgm/h, and increased every twenty minutes or so.

Nitroprusside is a much more powerful arteriolar vasodilator than the nitrates and also has an important venodilating effect. It is the vasodilator which has been most extensively studied, particularly following myocardial infarction (Guiha *et al.* 1974; Massie and Chatterjee 1979). It is of most obvious benefit where an elevated systemic blood pressure is contributing to left ventricular problems with consequent pulmonary congestion. Nitro-prusside acting on the arterioles may increase cardiac output and reduce myocardial oxygen requirements even when systemic blood pressure is normal. It must be protected from light as it is unstable and becomes ineffective. It should only be administered to patients in an intensive care area, preferably with continuous monitoring of pulmonary artery wedge pressure and arterial pressure using intravascular lines. Initially 10 μg/minute is given, increasing by 5 μg/minute every five minutes until the pulmonary oedema is relieved or systemic pressure falls below about 100 mmHg (in a previously normotensive patient). The half life of nitroprusside is two minutes so that if hypotension is caused the infusion should be stopped and the bed tipped. The infusion can then be restarted at a lower dosage when the blood pressure returns to normal. Most patients require 50 to 150 μg/minute.

Determination of the optimum dose of vasodilators required in pulmon-ary oedema is greatly facilitated by the insertion of a flow-directed, balloon-tipped (Swan–Ganz) catheter into the pulmonary artery (PA) so that the pulmonary capillary wedge pressure, reflecting the left atrial pressure can be measured. A PA wedge pressure of around 18 mmHg is probably optimal. Measurement of the PA wedge pressure is invaluable in patients with resistant pulmonary oedema or pulmonary oedema associated with a low output state (Bayliss *et al.* 1983).

Venesection

Removal of 300–500 ml of venous blood is an extremely effective method of reducing the circulating blood volume and 'pre-load'. Furthermore, this reduction of pre-load may be accompanied by arteriolar vasodilation and an increase in cardiac output (Howarth, McMichael and Sharpey–Shafer 1946). Where conventional initial drug therapy has produced no improve-ment it can be life-saving. This is particularly true when renal impairment is present. Clearly it is likely to cause deterioration if the patient is hypo-volaemic. Venesection should only be performed when the central venous pressure is obviously elevated and the arterial blood pressure is adequate.

The technique of using rotating tourniquets to produce venous pooling in the limbs is not to be recommended (Editorial 1975). In acute on chronic heart failure a diminution in venous distensibility is present, so limiting the amount of venous pooling which is possible using this method. Habakuk *et al.* (1974) found it possible to produce a useful effect in only six of sixteen patients whom they studied, none of whom had previously been treated with opiates or diuretics. It is unlikely to be effective if other methods of treatment have failed in such patients and may deflect energy and thought away from more valuable therapeutic manoeuvres.

Assisted ventilation in pulmonary oedema

The alveolar-arterial oxygen difference in patients with acute myocardial infarction is usually abnormal and lung water has been shown to correlate well with the left atrial pressure (Yu 1971). In frank pulmonary oedema, hypoxaemia demonstrates that the disturbance in gas transfer across the alveolar capillary gap is extreme. This is not simply due to intra-alveolar fluid. Bronchospasm reflecting peribronchial oedema may occur with premature airway closure; this results in areas of atelectasis and veno-arterial shunting which contribute to the hypoxaemia. The hypoxaemia so produced in pulmonary oedema deleteriously affects left ventricular function so that a vicious circle results. This is compounded by the excessive work required to breathe with such stiff non-compliant lungs.

Intermittent positive pressure ventilation helps break the vicious pulmonary oedema—left ventricular dysfunction cycle by improving alveolar-capillary gas exchange. However, ventilating such patients is not without negative aspects, in particular cardiac output often falls. This is largely due to the increased resistance to venous return, an effect which may be exacerbated by the use of positive end expiratory pressure (PEEP). Hence PEEP should not be used unless clearly necessary. In addition of course, any patient who is intubated and ventilated is automatically exposed to all the inherent dangers of those procedures, notably pneumonia, atelectasis, pneumothorax, endotracheal trauma, as well as operator and machine dysfunction (Zwillich *et al.* 1974).

The decision regarding ventilation or not needs careful consideration. Half of the fifty patients studied by Aberman and Fulop (1972) were sufficiently hypoxaemic with P_{O_2} less than 6.6 kPa (50 mm Hg) to be in severe respiratory failure. Certainly such patients may well need ventilating, particularly if they have sustained a myocardial infarction. However, intubation should not be performed merely as a reflex action to unattractive blood gas tensions. Rather, intubation should be performed when the patient with severe pulmonary oedema fails to respond to, or deteriorates in spite of conventional therapy, particularly if the patient is becoming physically exhausted or mentally obtunded (Grossman and Aberman 1976).

Treatment of acidosis

The large proportion of patients with pulmonary oedema are acidotic despite hyperventilation. Some have carbon dioxide retention and an important number have lactic acidosis, due to hypoperfusion (Aberman and Fullop 1972). The general measures taken to improve the patient with pulmonary oedema will effect an improvement in the metabolic derangement. Indeed, persisting acidosis may be an indicator of inadequate general treatment. It is not necessary or advisable to try correcting the acidosis with intravenous bicarbonate.

Improvement of perfusion allows metabolism of the lactic acid and generation of endogenous bicarbonate within hours, while the usual hyperosmolar solutions of sodium bicarbonate may cause severe deterioration due to the expansion of circulating blood volume (Grossman and Aberman 1976).

Intra-aortic balloon counterpulsation

Most patients who have pulmonary oedema have left ventricular disease and may benefit greatly from vasodilator therapy. Patients with severe mitral or aortic regurgitation or acquired ventricular septal defects may also improve markedly if their arterial impedence is reduced. This occurs because added to the benefit of improved overall left ventricular performance, the proportion of blood flowing forward is increased compared to the abnormal flow through the mechanical defect.

Such patients with mechanical defects, particularly following myocardial infarction, are likely to benefit from intra-aortic balloon counterpulsation. This manoeuvre involves the placing of a balloon-tipped catheter into the descending aorta. The inflation of the balloon in early diastole helps augment flow down the ascending aorta into the coronary arteries. Its deflation immediately systole begins allows the left ventricle to eject blood into an aorta with a very low pressure.

Although the use of such a device may be useful in any patient with pump failure, its most important use is as a holding manoeuvre until corrective cardiac surgery can be performed on a remediable mechanical problem.

Surgery for pulmonary oedema

It is axiomatic that all patients with acute left heart failure should be considered candidates for corrective surgery. In fact, few patients with ischaemic heart disease have marked improvement in left ventricular performance following surgery. The important exceptions are those with mechanical defects, such as mitral regurgitation or ventricular septal rupture, and some patients with left ventricular aneurysms.

Any patient with acute valvular regurgitation, for example aortic regurgitation due to endocarditis or mitral regurgitation secondary to ruptured chordae or any other cause, must always be considered for acute valvular replacement.

Finally, the patient with a prosthetic heart valve who goes into pulmonary oedema should always be considered to have surgically correctable prosthetic valve dysfunction until proven otherwise as failure to recognize a surgically remediable cause for pulmonary oedema is always a tragedy (Table 6.2).

Conclusion

'Acute heart failure' is most commonly due to 'left heart failure' and this needs to be distinguished from noncardiogenic pulmonary oedema. Causes are many, but the essentials of acute management are largely similar involving the administration of oxygen, opiates and diuretics initially, together with vaso-dilators if possible, and other agents if necessary. With current pharmacological agents and life support systems no patient should die in the agony of pulmonary oedema. Finally, of vital importance is the underlying need to understand the cause of the problem in case early cardiac surgery is required.

Further reading

Aberman A. and Fulop M. (1972) The metabolic and respiratory acidosis of Acute Pulmonary Oedema. *Annals of Internal medicine* **76**, 173–184.

Balcon R., Hoy J. and Sowton E. (1968) Haemodynamic effects of rapid digitalisation following myocardial infarction. *British Heart Journal* **30**, 373–376.

Bayliss J., Norell M., Ryan A., Thurston M. and Sutton G.C. (1983) Bedside haemodynamic monitoring experience in a general hospital. *British Medical Journal* **287**, 187–190.

Biddle T.L. and Yu P. (1980) Acute Pulmonary Oedema in Chung E.K. (ed) *Cardiac Emergency Care* p. 8. Lea and Febiger, Philadelphia.

Blinks J.R., Olson C.B., Jewell B.R. and Braveny P. (1972) Influence of caffeine and other methyl xanthines on mechnical properties of isolated mammalian heart muscle: Evidence for a dual mechanism of action. *Circulation Research* **30**, 367–392.

Dikshit K., Vyden J.K., Forrester J.S., Chatterjee K., Prakush R. and Swan H.J.C. (1973) Renal and extrarenal haemodynamic effects of frusemide in congestive hert failure after acute myocardial infarction. *New England Journal of Medicine* **288**, 1087–1090.

Editorial (1975) Rotating Tourniquets for Left Ventricular Failure. *Lancet* **1**, 154.

Fillmore S.J., Shapiro M. and Killip T. (1970) Arterial oxygen tension in acute myocardial infarction. Serial analysis of clinical state and blood gas changes. *American Heart Journal* **79**, 620.

Grossman R.F. and Aberman A. (1976) Emergency Management of Acute Pulmonary Oedema. *Annals of Internal Medicine* **84**, 488.

Guiha N.H., Cohn J.N., Mikulic E., Franciosa J.A. and Limas C.J. (1974) Treatment of refractory heart failure with infusion of nitroprusside. *New England Journal of Medicine* 1, 587–592.

Habakuk P.A., Mark A.L., Kioschos J.M., McRaven D.R. and Abboud F.M. (1974) Effectiveness of congesting cuffs ('rotating tourniquets') in Patients with Left Heart Failure. *Circulation* **50**, 366–371.

Howarth S., McMichael J. and Sharpey–Shafer E.P. (1946) Effects of venesection in low output heart failure. *Clinical Science* **6**, 41–60.

Karliner J.S. and Braunwald E. (1972) Present status of digitalis treatment of acute myocardial infarction. *Circulation* **45**, 891–902.

Kelman G.F., Nunn J.F., Prys–Roberts C. and Greenbaum R. (1967) The influence of the cardiac output on arterial oxygenation: A theoretical study. *British Journal of Anaesthesia* **39**, 450–458.

Marcus M.L., Skelton C.L., Graner L.E., and Epstein S.E., (1972) Effects of theophylline on myocardial mechanics. *American Journal of Physiology* **222**, 1361–1365.

Massie B.M. and Chatterjee K. (1979) Vasodilator therapy of pump failure complicating acute myocardial infarction. *Medical Clinics of North America* **63**, 25–51.

Nixon P.C.F. (1968) Pulmonary Oedema with low left ventricular diastolic pressure in acute myocardial infarction. *Lancet* **2**, 146–147.

Noble D. (1980) Review: Mechanism of action of therapeutic levels of cardiac glycosides. *Cardiovascular Research* **14**, 495–514.

Ogilvie C. (1983) Dyspnoea. *British Medical Journal* **287**, 160–161.

Pearson S.B., Pearson E.M. and Mitchell J.R.B. (1981) The diagnosis and management of patients admitted to hospital with acute breathlessness. *Postgraduate Medical Journal* **57**, 419–424.

Rall T.W. and West T.C. (1963) The potentiation of cardiac inotropic responses to norepinephrine by theophylline. *Journal of Pharmacology and Experimental Therapeutics* **179**, 331–337.

Ramirez A. and Abelmann W.H. (1974) Cardiac decompensation. *New England Journal of medicine* **290**, 499–501.

Rubin E.D., Cross C.E. and Zellis R. (1973) Pulmonary Oedema. *New England Journal of Medicine* **288**, 292–304.

Smith T.W. (1982) Medical treatment of advanced congestive heart failure: digitalis and diuretics in Braunwald E., Mock M.B. and Watson J.T. (eds) *Congestive Heart Failure* p. 271 Grune and Stratton, New York.

Wilson J.R., Reichek N., Dunkman W.B. and Goldberg. S. (1981) Effect of diuresis on the performance of the failing left ventricle in man. *American Journal of Medicine* **70**, 234–239.

Yu P.N. (1971) Lung water in congestive cardiac failure. *Modern Concepts of Cardiovascular Disease* **50**, 27–35.

Zelis R.F., Mason D.T., Spann J.F. and Amsterdam E.A. (1970) The effects of morphine on the venous bed in man. Demonstration of a biphasic response. *American Journal of Cardiology* **25**, 136.

Zwillich C.W., Pierson D.J., Creagh C.E., Sutton F.D., Schatz E. and Petty T.L. (1974) Complication of assisted ventilation: A prospective study of 354 consecutive episodes. *American Journal of Medicine* **57**, 161–170.

7 · Malignant Hypertension

JOHN VANN JONES

Compared to some of the other medical emergencies described in this book malignant hypertension is uncommon. It occurs in about one per cent of known hypertensives and is the initial presentation of hypertension in an even smaller number of patients. The various forms of renal hypertension are more prone to develop the malignant phase. Renal damage is invariably present when the extreme elevation of pressure has developed even if the initiating cause has not involved the kidney.

Patients with malignant hypertension are usually symptomatic. They may have headaches, blurring of vision, be nauseated or even vomit. The level of consciousness may be altered from increased sleepiness to frank confusion and disorientation. If this is particularly marked and possibly associated with focal neurological defects or even loss of consciousness, then 'hypertensive encephalopathy' has developed.

Blood pressure is, of course, extremely high. The systolic pressure is usually above 200 mm Hg and the diastolic pressure is at least 130 mm Hg. Often both the systolic and diastolic pressures are much higher than these levels. Fibrinoid necrosis is present in the blood vessels and clinically this is seen to result in haemorrhages and exudates in the optic fundi. Papilloedema is also present. The damage to the blood vessels in the kidneys results in proteinuria and haematuria (Pickering 1968).

Very high blood pressures are often recorded as patients are brought into the Emergency Department. This is due to a defence or alerting reaction and is physiological rather than pathological (Folkow and Neil 1971). It is uncommon for any symptoms to be directly referable to such pressure elevation and it usually settles rapidly as the patient becomes used to his new environment. Similarly, some patients suffering from severe pain, such as that caused by a fractured bone or ruptured viscus, are found to have a high blood pressure. This high pressure settles with treatment of the primary condition and with analgesia.

Drug interactions may elevate the blood pressure, for example this occurs after the ingestion of cheese in patients taking monoamine oxidase inhibitors. Sudden withdrawal of clonidine therapy causes a rebound hypertension. Steroids, the contraceptive pill and carbenoxolone can all raise the blood pressure markedly although more usually their effect is slight. In addition, certain catecholamine containing cold cures can cause hypertension when used to excess or in overdosage.

Patients with an acute cerebrovascular accident may have very high initial blood pressures. Since high blood pressure predisposes to stroke, it can often be difficult to sort out the cause and effect. However, these patients should be monitored carefully for a few hours without being given any anti-hypertensive therapy as almost invariably the blood pressure settles spontaneously. Examination of the optic fundi and of the urine in such patients fails to show the usual changes found in malignant hypertension.

Raised intracranial pressure may elevate the blood pressure and also be associated with altered consciousness. Papilloedema may be present. In these circumstances, urinalysis is often normal and the eye changes are usually less florid than in the patient with malignant hypertension. Where there is still some doubt, the electrocardiogram often shows left ventricular hypertrophy or a strain pattern and the chest radiograph may show cardiomegaly in patients with established hypertension.

Therefore, in most situations it is possible to be fairly certain whether the patient is suffering from malignant hypertension or not. Occasionally, some people do present with high blood pressure that requires to be lowered more or less immediately. Patients with hypertensive encephalopathy, dissecting aortic aneurysm, eclampsia with fits and hypertensive left ventricular failure all come into this category (Bannan *et al.* 1980). It is seldom necessary to use parenteral therapy to lower blood pressure. In the past, intravenous boluses of 300 mg diazoxide have been used but this tended to cause precipitous falls in the blood pressure (Ledingham and Rajagopalan 1979). As a result, a few patients suffered neurological damage caused by hypotension and underperfusion of the cerebral circulation. Smaller boluses (50 mg) appear to be safer and more easily managed.

Diazoxide, nitroprusside, labetolol and phentolamine may all be given by continuous intravenous infusion. When used in this way, the dose of the drug should be titrated against a simultaneously measured arterial blood pressure. Therefore, both intravenous and intra-arterial lines have to be inserted and careful supervision of drug administration is required.

In practice, the time taken to make the necessary arrangements is considerable and close monitoring facilities may not be available. In my opinion it is better to start reducing the blood pressure immediately by giving 10 mg of hydrallazine either intramuscularly, intravenously or as a bolus. This causes a gentle reduction in blood pressure. Further 10 mg doses may then be administered hourly until the diastolic blood pressure is 100–110 mm Hg. At this stage, the parenteral therapy may be replaced by an oral beta-blocking agent and oral hydrallazine. In this way, the initial very high blood pressures are gradually reduced to reasonable levels. Later the pressure can be reduced further by changes in dose or the addition of another agent, such as a diuretic.

Oral atenolol has been advocated in the treatment of severe hyper-

tension and appears to work quite quickly (Bannan and Beevers 1981).
However, twenty to thirty per cent of people do not respond to beta-
blockers and valuable time would be lost. The use of calcium antagonists, for
example nifedipine and verapamil, has been advocated and they may be
useful as first line choices in the future. At present they are relatively
untried.

It may be important to be more aggressive in blood pressure control in
patients with a dissecting aneurysm. For several reasons such a patient who
also has malignant hypertension ought to be in an intensive therapy unit
where intra-arterial blood pressure can be monitored. When such a patient
is admitted to hospital the pressure reduction can be started with hydrallazine, as described above, together with a beta-blocking agent. With better
monitoring, parenteral labetolol could be titrated against the blood
pressure.

All patients with malignant hypertension should be on bed rest which
itself helps to quieten the patient and to lower the blood pressure. Some
analgesia or opiate may be required in patients with a dissecting aneurysm or
left ventricular failure. However, in patients with hypertensive encephalopathy, sedation is best avoided. Beta-blocking agents should not be used in
the initial treatment of hypertensive left ventricular failure. In general, in
malignant hypertension lowering the blood pressure is the fundamental step
that will save the patient and protect his circulation. However, it is important not to be too aggressive and in this way substitute one potential hazard
to the cerebral circulation (cerebral haemorrhage) with another (ischaemic
infarction). Strandgaard *et al.* (1973) clearly showed that hypertensive subjects do not tolerate blood pressure reductions to levels that would be quite
safe for previously normotensive individuals. In this situation, cerebral
perfusion deteriorates at higher blood pressure levels than normal, resulting
in cerebral ischaemia and even in brain damage. Similarly, with the kidneys,
too rapid a reduction of blood pressure can cause oliguria, anuria and acute
renal failure (Woods and Blythe 1967). The blood pressure should be
reduced but to some intermediate level between normal and high. Later,
further reduction is better tolerated and the treatment can be increased
accordingly.

Further reading

Bannan L.T., Beevers D.G. and Wright N. (1980) ABC of blood pressure reduction:
    Emergency reduction, hypertension in pregnancy and hypertension in the elderly.
    British Medical Journal **281**, 1120–1122.
Bannan L.T. and Beevers D.G. (1981) Emergency treatment of high blood pressure
    with oral atenolol. *British Medical Journal* **282**, 1757–8.
Folkow B. and Neil E. (1971). *Circulation*, p. 344. Oxford University Press, Oxford.

Ledingham J.G. and Rajagopalan B. (1979). Cerebral complications in the treatment of accelerated hypertension. *Quarterly Journal of Medicine* **48**, 25–41.

Pickering G.W. (1968). *High Blood Pressure*, p. 451. Churchill, London.

Strandgaard S., Olesen J., Skinhoj E. and Lassen N.A. (1973) Autoregulation of brain circulation in severe arterial hypertension. *British Medical Journal* **1**, 507–510.

Woods J.W. and Blythe W.B. (1967). Management of malignant hypertension complicated by renal insufficiency. *New England Journal of Medicine* **277**, 57–61.

8 · Pulmonary Embolism

D. F. TREACHER

Prophylaxis

In any disease, identifying those patients at risk and taking measures to reduce that risk as far as possible is a vital consideration. This is particularly important where the initial event is often unheralded and a significant number of those affected may die before effective treatment can be instituted (Macintyre and Ruckley 1974). It is estimated that 20,000 people die from pulmonary embolism (PE) in the UK every year.

Numerous studies have confirmed a close correlation between deep venous thrombosis of the legs (DVT) and pulmonary emboli (Hume *et al.* 1970, International Multicentre Trial 1975). Therefore, it has been argued that any measure that will reduce the incidence of DVT will also reduce the incidence of pulmonary emboli and many trials concerning DVT prophylaxis have supported this thesis. However, it should not be assumed that any measure failing to prevent DVT will be similarly ineffective in preventing pulmonary emboli. For example, Kline *et al.* (1975) demonstrated that although dextran 70 did not significantly reduce the incidence of DVT, it did appear to be effective in preventing pulmonary embolism. Conditions associated with an increased risk of developing a DVT and pulmonary embolus include:

1. Following surgery—risk depending on nature of surgery and length of pre- and postoperative immobilization.
2. Previous thrombo-embolism.
3. Underlying malignancy.
4. Traumatic injuries involving pelvis and legs.
5. Major burns.
6. Medical conditions associated with immobilization: myocardial infarction, congestive heart failure, 'stroke', chronic illness.
7. Obesity.
8. Varicose veins.
9. Age—over forty years old.
10. Pregnancy and puerperium.
11. Oestrogen-containing drugs, contraceptive pill (but still disputed—Macrae 1980).
12. Polycythaemia.
13. Antithrombin III deficiency.
14. Blood group A.

Since about one third of all patients develop small calf thrombi post-operatively, it is not surprising that most of the studies evaluating methods of prophylaxis have been performed on surgical patients. From these studies, surgical patients may be categorized according to their risk of developing DVT or PE into:
(a) 'High' risk—examplified by the fat, elderly patient with a recent history of thrombo-embolism, or who is undergoing major surgery for advanced malignant disease.
(b) 'Moderate' risk—typically obese patients over the age of forty, undergoing abdominal or thoracic surgery, with a history of varicose veins or heart disease, and who also develop a postoperative complication.
(c) 'Low' risk—under the age of forty with no relevant past history and undergoing minor surgery (Table 8.1).

Table 8.1. The risks of developing DVT and PE in postsurgical patients (Hirsch 1981)

Category of risk	DVT %	PE %	Fatal PE %
High	30–40	6–12	1–2
Moderate	10–40	2–8	0.1–0.7
Low	< 3	< 1	< 0.01

Measures shown to be effective in preventing DVT and pulmonary embolus are:
(i) Subcutaneous heparin: 5000 u b.d. or t.d.s.
(ii) Oral anticoagulants, preferably starting pre-operatively.
(iii) Dextran 70:500 ml pre-operatively and then daily for 2–5 days.
(iv) External pneumatic compression (EPC)—starting pre-operatively and continuing until the patient is mobile.

There is conflicting evidence about the efficacy of physical methods other than EPC (e.g. elastic compression stockings, electrical calf muscle stimulation, pedalling devices), and 'anti-platelet' drugs such as aspirin. These forms of prophylaxis await further evaluation.

It cannot be assumed that measures effective in one situation will be effective in another. For example, subcutaneous heparin fails to protect patients undergoing open bladder and prostate surgery and may produce excessive bleeding (Rosenberg et al. 1975). Although an estimated 80 per cent reduction in pulmonary emboli would occur if the more effective forms of prophylaxis (heparin and oral anticoagulants) were widely used peri-operatively, it would be unreasonable to subject everyone to the risks of such prophylaxis for the benefit of the few (about 1 per cent) who will suffer a significant pulmonary embolus. The choice of treatment must be influenced by the risks of bleeding complications in the individual patient and by situations where even minor bleeding is unacceptable, e.g. neurosurgery and ophthalmic surgery.

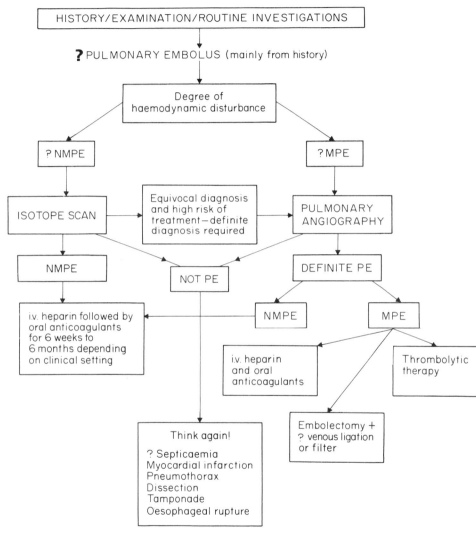

Fig. 8.1. Flow diagram for diagnosis and management in pulmonary embolism.

Successful prophylaxis requires both the identification of those particularly at risk and the selection of the most appropriate treatment. Although in many cases the hard evidence to make such a decision is lacking, the consensus opinion at present would be to treat 'high risk' patients with subcutaneous heparin (5000 u t.d.s.), oral anticoagulants or even with a heparin infusion if there is a very high risk. 'Moderate risk' patients should be treated with subcutan tous heparin (5000 u b.d.), dextran 70 or EPC. Finally, 'low risk' patients should be treated by EPC or nothing unless complications arise.

Where a definite risk of DVT developing exists, it is not acceptable to await clinical evidence before starting treatment since less than half of DVTs are detectable clinically. It is a widely held belief that the 'silent leg' is often the more deadly.

It should be remembered that early mobilization is successful in reducing thrombo-embolic events and is both cheap and free from major complications. Other common-sense measures such as advising the patient to avoid both faulty posture and the wearing of constrictive clothing around the upper legs should not be forgotten. In addition, patients should be encouraged to exercise their calf muscles while in bed.

The management of established DVT is obviously of great importance in the prevention of pulmonary emboli; this has been reviewed in detail by Buckler and Douglas (1982).

Diagnosis and management

Every clinician will recognize the syndrome of sudden pleuritic chest pain associated with dyspnoea and cough with haemoptysis. However, pulmonary emboli present with widely differing clinical pictures which explains why the diagnosis is often difficult and in many cases is only made in the postmortem room. A summary of the diagnosis and management is given in Figure 8.1.

The various clinical patterns produced can usefully be divided into five syndromes on the basis of the size of the embolus and resulting degree of obstruction to the pulmonary vascular bed (greater or less than 50 per cent), the time for which the embolus has been present, and the gross clinical picture produced.

Clinical syndromes of pulmonary thrombo-embolism

A. Silent.
B. Sudden death.

C. Acute non-massive pulmonary embolus (NMPE).
   < 50 per cent occlusion and present for < 48 hours.
D. Acute massive pulmonary embolus (MPE).
   > 50 per cent occlusion and present for < 48 hours.
E. Chronic thromboembolic disease
   progressive occlusion over months or years.

A. Silent

Various postmortem studies have shown that pulmonary emboli occur without producing any clinical signs or symptoms (Moser *et al.* 1981). This may
simply reflect either the interruption of a natural process where small
thrombi are filtered and then disposed of by fibrinolytic mechanisms, or an
imbalance between thrombosis and fibrinolysis occurring generally in the
body as an agonal event. Further study of this group may yield important
clues concerning the control of the thrombotic and fibrinolytic processes in
the body.

B. Sudden death

Acute massive pulmonary embolism is a common cause of sudden death
(Gorham 1961; Macintyre and Ruckley 1974). However, it is difficult to
assess the real extent of the problem since it is probable that in many cases
the true diagnosis is never made. For example, how often is pulmonary
embolism the cause of death in patients with known cardiopulmonary
disease, whose sudden death has been attributed to their pre-existing
disease?

In this group the aim must be prevention. This requires identification of
those at risk, improved recognition of earlier warning events and the more
widespread application of effective prophylactic measures.

C and D. Acute non-massive and acute massive pulmonary embolism

Bell *et al.* (1977) analysed the various symptoms, signs and associated
conditions in a series of 327 patients with either massive or non-massive
acute pulmonary embolus. Their findings are shown in Table 8.2.

This analysis shows that although most patients will complain of chest
pain, dyspnoea, cough with haemoptysis and have the well-recognized
clinical findings, some patients do not. However, if a patient does not
experience chest pain or dyspnoea and is neither tachypnoeic nor has a
raised jugular venous pressure, then the diagnosis of a major pulmonary
embolus is unlikely.

Table 8.2. Frequency of symptoms and signs in acute pulmonary embolus (expressed as % of total patients)

	Massive PE	Non-massive PE	Overall
Symptoms			
Chest pain*	79	89	83
pleuritic**	67	82	74
non-pleuritic	16	13	14
Dyspnoea	85	82	84
Apprehension**	65	50	59
Cough	53	52	53
Haemoptysis*	23	40	30
Sweats	29	23	27
Syncope***	20	4	13
Signs			
Respiration > 16/min.	95	87	92
Rales	57	60	58
Loud pulmonary 2nd sound*	58	45	53
Pulse > 100/min.	48	38	44
Temperature > 37.8°C	43	42	43
Profuse sweat**	42	27	36
Gallop rhythm**	39	25	34
Phlebitis	36	26	32
Murmur	28	27	28
Oedema	23	25	24
Cyanosis***	25	9	19
Association conditions			
Immobilization	60	55	58
Current venous disease	47	42	45
Pre-existing cardio-pulmonary disease	36	40	38
Malignancy	8	5	6

(Where marked *, indicates significant difference between massive and non-massive PE: $p < 0.05$ = *, $p < 0.01$ = **, $p < 0.001$ = ***)

    In distinguishing massive from non-massive pulmonary emboli, central chest pain with postural syncope and a sensation of apprehension (often well-founded), together with profuse sweating, cyanosis and evidence of right heart strain, suggests massive embolism. Whereas, pleuritic chest pain with haemoptysis but without haemodynamic disturbance suggests non-massive embolism. However, the complete classic triad of acute pleuritic chest pain, dyspnoea and haemoptysis occurs in less than 20 per cent of these cases.

Although over 85 per cent of pulmonary emboli are multiple and usually bilateral, 30 per cent of cases have a normal chest X-ray (CXR) and more relevantly so do 15 per cent of patients with massive emboli (Wenger *et al.* 1972; Talbot *et al.* 1973). Diffuse infiltration on the CXR develops in less than half of the cases and usually represents pulmonary haemorrhage rather than true infarction. Infarction occurs in only 10 per cent of cases and usually only where there is pre-existing cardiopulmonary disease (Dalen *et al.* 1977). Pleural effusion occurs in about one third of cases, but is frequently transient and resolves rapidly unless true infarction has occurred. Increased radiolucency from impaired vascular filling, prominence of the pulmonary artery with a sharp 'cut-off', right ventricular enlargement, elevation of a hemidiaphragm and areas of plate atelectasis all occur. However, these signs are often much more obvious in retrospect!

Although more consistently found with massive pulmonary embolism (MPE), electrocardiographic (ECG) changes do occur in 85 per cent of all cases but are often non-specific and transient. The Urokinase Pulmonary Embolism Trial (1973) found T wave inversion in 40 per cent, right bundle branch block in 12 per cent, right axis deviation in 5 per cent, left axis deviation in 12 per cent and the supposedly classic SI, QIII, TIII, pattern in only 11 per cent of cases. Sinus tachycardia is a regular finding but although other rhythm disturbances are unusual, the sudden unexplained onset of atrial flutter or fibrillation should always suggest the possibility of pulmonary embolism. The main value of the ECG lies in excluding acute myocardial infarction in the collapsed patient with right heart failure. It is said that the pattern of ST elevation in leads II, III and aVF, with developing Q waves is not seen in pulmonary embolism. However, in my experience even this pattern of an apparently evolving inferior myocardial infarction may occur with MPE.

Arterial blood gases are an important initial investigation, characteristically showing a low P_aO_2 (< 10 kPa) and P_aco_2 (< 4.5 kPa). Certainly, a P_aO_2 > 10.5 kPa makes a major pulmonary embolus unlikely.

Various blood tests, including patterns of serum enzyme changes, bilirubin levels in blood and urine and levels of fibrin split products, have been studied but no discriminating test or pattern of tests has emerged. Sipes *et al.* (1978) have recently reported encouraging results in correlating plasma DNA levels with pulmonary emboli but this awaits further evaluation.

On the basis of history, examination and routine investigations, alternative diagnoses may be made or eliminated. Nevertheless, whenever the clinical suspicion of pulmonary embolism persists, a lung scan and possibly pulmonary angiography are necessary.

Acute non-massive pulmonary embolus (NMPE)

The vast majority of pulmonary emboli occurring in clinical practice fall into this category in which there is usually no major circulatory disturbance and by definition, angiography demonstrates less than 50 per cent obstruction to the pulmonary vascular bed. Such a division is arbitrary, particularly when it is realized that pre-existing cardiopulmonary disease and vasospasm may considerably modify the clinical picture produced by a given degree of mechanical obstruction. Nonetheless, the distinction is useful in providing guidelines for further investigation and treatment.

Although angiography remains the final arbiter in the diagnosis of pulmonary embolism, it is neither logistically possible nor desirable to perform an angiogram on all suspected cases. For this reason the isotope lung scan is the mainstay of diagnosis in this group of smaller, more peripherally situated emboli.

Perfusion scans performed with technetium-99 labelled albumin microspheres or macro-aggregates will identify areas of impaired lung perfusion but cannot distinguish with any certainty between pulmonary emboli and other pulmonary lesions, e.g. infiltrates, chronic obstructive airways disease or central tumours. However, in pulmonary embolism areas of abnormal perfusion are usually ventilated normally. Therefore, if a ventilation scan, usually with xenon-133, is also performed areas with abnormal perfusion but normal ventilation (ventilation-perfusion mismatch) can be identified. This is a more specific finding in pulmonary embolism. Various series have confirmed that multiple segmental mismatched defects correlate well with angiography, giving a sensitivity and specificity of about 90 per cent (McNeil 1976; Urokinase Pulmonary Embolism Trial 1973; Sharma and Sasahara 1979). In addition, these studies showed that a normal ventilation-perfusion scan virtually excludes a diagnosis of pulmonary embolus.

The conventional treatment in this group is intravenous heparin followed by oral anticoagulation. The local release of vaso-active substances (serotonin, histamine, catecholamines, prostaglandins, thromboxanes, etc.), predominantly from platelets adherent to the thrombus, causes vasospasm and constriction of small peripheral airways both by direct action and reflexly via various pulmonary receptors (Widdicombe 1973). Heparin will reverse and block certain of these effects and a bolus of 15,000 u should be given as soon as the diagnosis of pulmonary embolism is made, particularly in massive embolism, where the resulting additional obstruction may be critical.

Thereafter a constant infusion of heparin, at a rate of 1200 u per hour for an average 70 kg adult, should be started. This is preferable to intermittent boluses since less heparin is required and there are fewer bleeding complications. The simplest test for monitoring intravenous heparin therapy is the activated partial thromboplastin time, which should be prolonged to between two and three times the control value. Such monitoring is essential if bleeding problems occur or are anticipated and, if used routinely, it permits a maximum therapeutic effect to be achieved with a minimum of side effects.

Heparin and oral anticoagulants are not thrombolytic but whereas heparin directly and rapidly inhibits clotting, oral anti-coagulants act by depleting clotting factors (mainly II, VII, IX, X) and this effect occurs differentially over several days. Factor VII falls most quickly and although prolonging the prothrombin time, does not result in an adequate anti-thrombotic effect. Therefore, intravenous heparin should continue for five days after starting oral anticoagulants even though the prothrombin time may reach the desired level of about twice the control by the third day.

Opinions vary concerning how long oral anticoagulation should continue. Six weeks is a minimum period, suitable for an otherwise healthy individual in whom a predisposing risk factor had been eliminated (e.g. contraceptive pill stopped, fully mobile again after elective surgery), and treatment beyond six months is only appropriate if an unavoidable high risk persists or if repeated, well-documented emboli have occurred. When oral anticoagulation is stopped, there is no need to taper the dose, since a rebound hypercoagulable state does not occur (Michaels 1971). The risks of oral anticoagulation can be minimized by careful dosage control, thorough instruction of the patient and an awareness by both patient and doctor of the danger of drug interaction.

Oakley (1977) pointed out that two-thirds of those ultimately dying from pulmonary embolism have had previous warning emboli. Furthermore some series indicate that over one-third of patients have a second potentially lethal embolus (Browse and Solan 1969). Therefore, it is important to diagnose and treat non-massive emboli. There are, in fact, no adequately designed clinical trials that demonstrate significant benefits from conventional treatment. Barritt and Jordan (1960) did attempt a trial but abandoned it before significance was achieved when several patients died in the control group. Reaction in the profession at large would now make it virtually impossible to perform a definitive trial. Therefore, as so often happens in clinical practice, one must continue to use a treatment which is most probably effective but which has never unequivocally been proven to be so.

Acute massive pulmonary embolus (MPE)

Although a significant cause of death, as an event recognized ante mortem, massive embolism is relatively rare. Gorham (1961) reported that two-thirds of patients suffering from MPE die within two hours of the event, so that the diagnosis is often not made or even suspected before death. In the first phase of the Urokinase Pulmonary Embolism Trial (1973), it took almost two years to collect 160 patients from fourteen major centres in the United States and of these only eight had MPE with marked circulatory impairment. Therefore, it is apparent that speed in diagnosis and treatment is vital and that trials of therapy in this condition are fraught with difficulty.

When the diagnosis of MPE is suspected, a pulmonary angiogram should be performed without delay. In experienced hands it is a safe procedure. It is indicated whenever the treatment contemplated carries a high risk or if the diagnosis remains unclear after a lung scan.

Digital subtraction angiography (DSA) is a new radiological technique which may supersede conventional pulmonary angiography (Meaney *et al.* 1980). Contrast material is injected into a peripheral vein at a rate of 15 ml/sec via a pressure injector and subsequent images of the pulmonary arteries are digitized and stored. A computer then selects a suitable image before arrival of the contrast and subtracts this from subsequent contrast images. This produces subtraction images which are viewed in real time. High quality pictures of the pulmonary arteries, beyond third order branches, have been obtained in normal subjects but several injections are required to visualize each lung. Evaluation in patients with pulmonary emboli, in particular MPE, is awaited since marked respiratory movements and poor flows may considerably reduce the quality of pictures obtained. A further advantage of this technique would be that views of leg and pelvic veins could be obtained at the same time.

The hallmark of MPE is the significant circulatory disturbance produced by the mechanical obstruction and associated vasospasm. The resulting fall in cardiac output may be rapidly fatal and is central to the ensuing problems. The aim of management in the acute phase is to restore and maintain an adequate cardiac output. Bradley (1977) has described the altered relationship between right and left ventricular function curves which implies that the most appropriate manipulation of the circulation is to infuse fluid, ideally Dextran 70, until the right atrial pressure (RAP) is around +12 mmHg. This achieves a significant increase in right ventricular (RV) stroke volume and hence cardiac output by increasing RV stroke work and also by expanding the pulmonary vascular bed, thereby reducing the pulmonary vascular resistance. Although values of RAP > 12 mm Hg could be tolerated without risking pulmonary oedema, higher values do not further increase RV stroke work but do increase the likelihood of (i) tricuspid regurgitation from RV distension, (ii) abdominal pain from hepatic distension and (iii) paradoxical embolism via a patent foramen ovale. Spontaneous levels of RAP > 15 mm Hg suggest imminent RV failure with circulatory collapse and would be an indication for urgent embolectomy with, if necessary, a period on cardiopulmonary bypass to allow the RV to recover.

The initial management of a patient presenting with MPE should include:

(i) Insertion of central venous and arterial lines to monitor RAP and BP and for regular sampling of blood gases.

(ii) Intravenous heparin 15000 u as a bolus dose.

(iii) Oxygen via face mask.

(iv) Correction of acidosis.

(v) Consideration of digitalization, since fast atrial fibrillation may develop.

(vi) Avoidance of measures which reduce RAP such as diuretics, opiates, and sitting patient up in bed.

The contrast material used in angiography may produce vasodilation and reduce RAP and therefore an α-agonist such as phenylephrine should be readily available or, in severe cases, given prophylactically. Inotropic support with dopamine and artificial ventilation may become necessary. If cardiac arrest occurs, vigorous external cardiac massage may break up the embolus and propel it distally. Despite full resuscitative measures, the patient may remain very unstable and in this situation emergency embolectomy without prior angiography may be considered as a last life-saving procedure.

After confirmation of the diagnosis of MPE by angiography, the options for subsequent management are either pulmonary embolectomy with or without a venous interruption procedure or thrombolytic therapy or heparin alone.

Embolectomy is the preferred treatment if there is marked haemodynamic disturbance (systolic BP < 100 mm Hg. and RAP > 15 mm Hg), or if cardiac arrest has already occurred or if heparin alone is considered inadequate and thrombolytic therapy is either contra-indicated or has already been tried unsuccessfully. Under these circumstances, impressive results are possible but all studies emphasize the importance of having experienced personnel and preferably cardiac bypass facilities available. In addition, pre-operative angiography is essential since 'blind' embolectomy on a patient in fact suffering from one of the conditions well known to mimic MPE, particularly acute myocardial infarction or septicaemia, is disastrous.

Since the vast majority of pulmonary emboli originate in the veins of the legs or pelvis, attempts at preventing further emboli by ligation or filtering procedures would seem logical. Superficial femoral vein ligation is a relatively simple procedure, but although it secures or 'locks-in' thrombus in the superficial system, it clearly provides no protection against emboli from the deep femoral system. Common femoral vein ligation is neither particularly successful nor acceptable due to the resulting severe obstruction to venous drainage. Various operations to ligate, plicate or clip the inferior vena cava (IVC) as well as attempts at non-surgical interruption by umbrella filter

(Mobin-Uddin *et al.* 1971) or balloon catheter have all been tried but found to have substantial morbidity (DeMeester *et al.* 1967). Complete interruption often produces significant lower body oedema and venous ulceration of the legs. Even successful plication still allows smaller emboli to pass and complete obstruction may occur later (Wolfe and Sabiston 1980). The various filter devices may themselves embolize or become infected and none of these procedures ensures protection against further MPE since thrombus may propagate either on the balloon or filter or at the site of operation on the IVC (Wingend *et al.* 1978).

All series show that second massive pulmonary emboli are very rare. Therefore, on current evidence the only venous interruption procedures that can easily be justified are superficial femoral vein ligation, if venography shows that the deep system is clear of thrombus, or the temporary transvenous placement of one of the new filter devices (Kim–Ray–Greenfield) which are much less thrombogenic.

The role of thrombolytic therapy in MPE is difficult to assess since no trial has yet demonstrated improved survival compared to intravenous heparin therapy alone. The Urokinase Pulmonary Embolism Trial (1973) was a prospective, randomized multicentre trial which compared intravenous heparin therapy alone with a twelve hour infusion of urokinase followed by heparin. Assessment by lung scanning, angiography, haemodynamic measurements and overall outcome showed that although urokinase produced significant angiographic and haemodynamic improvement after twenty-four hours, by one week there was no difference between the groups for any of these criteria. A subsequent trial showed similar results following a twenty-four hour infusion of urokinase or streptokinase. Although intuitively one feels that more rapid clearance both of the pulmonary vascular bed and the source of further emboli should be beneficial, at present the only unequivocal benefit from thrombolytic therapy is a much lower incidence of chronic venous disease of the legs. Prevention of late pulmonary hypertension and recurrent emboli is disputed since several studies have shown that provided there was no pre-existing cardio-respiratory disease, the long-term prognosis in MPE is very good and the likelihood of a recurrent, clinically significant embolus is small (Miller 1972; Paraskos *et al.* 1973).

Most clinicians accept that thrombolytic therapy has a role in the patient in whom the haemodynamic disturbance produced and the fear of further emboli make heparin alone seem inadequate, but for whom embolectomy is unacceptable or unavailable. However, there are some contra-indications to thrombolytic therapy:

Absolute
1. Serious injury or surgery within ten days.

2. Active internal bleeding.
3. Vascular or ophthalmic surgery within two months.
4. Cerebrovascular accident or neurosurgery within three months.

Relative
1. Recent history of peptic ulcer or gastro-intestinal bleeding.
2. Arterial hypertension with systolic BP > 200 mmHg or diastolic BP > 105 mmHG
3. Bleeding diasthesis.
4. Pregnancy, purpureum or menstruation.
5. Diabetic haemorrhagic retinopathy.
6. Risk of dislodgement of left atrial thrombus.

Once instituted thrombolytic therapy should continue for at least twelve hours with monitoring of the pulmonary artery pressure via the catheter used to perform the angiogram. Failure of thrombolytic therapy due to uncontrollable bleeding, severe drug reaction or a deterioration in the patient's condition is an indication for embolectomy. If this is unavailable locally, transfer to a regional centre may be considered after instituting the initial management and an intravenous heparin infusion.

Both thrombolytic therapy and embolectomy should be followed by an intravenous heparin infusion for at least five days and oral anticoagulation for a minimum of three months.

E. Chronic thrombo-embolic disease (CTE)

The pathophysiology of this condition is poorly understood. It probably bears little relation to acute pulmonary embolic disease since it is unusual either for it to develop after acute pulmonary embolism or for patients with established CTE to give any past history of acute pulmonary emboli. Furthermore, at post-mortem examination there is often no evidence of any venous thrombosis in the pelvis or legs of these patients. It would seem more likely that there is a fundamental abnormality either in the pulmonary vasculature or in the thrombotic or fibrinolytic mechanisms. Perhaps, either *in situ* thrombosis occurs or repeated small, subclinical emboli organize rather than resolve.

Patients usually present with a long history of exertional dyspnoea or syncope but occasionally they present with recurrent episodes of pleuritic chest pain with haemoptysis. The physical signs are those of severe pulmonary hypertension resulting from the long-standing major obstruction of the pulmonary arteries. Although oral anticoagulants occasionally produce some improvement, at present there is no effective treatment and the majority die within a few years of diagnosis.

Conclusion

For the future, prevention must be the aim. Hopefully, from an improved understanding of the thrombotic and fibrinolytic processes, there will emerge screening tests to detect those at particular risk and also more effective yet safer forms of prophylaxis and treatment. Meanwhile, the more widespread application of existing prophylactic measures and, where these fail, the institution of rapid diagnosis and treatment should help to combat the problems posed by pulmonary embolism.

Further reading

Barritt D.W. and Jordan S.C. (1960) Anticoagulant drugs in the treatment of pulmonary embolism *Lancet* **1**, 1309–1313.

Bell W.R., Simon T.L. and DeMets D.L. (1977) The clinical features of submassive and massive pulmonary emboli. *American Journal of Medicine* **62**, 355.

Bradley R.D. (1977) *Studies in Acute Heart Failure.* pp. 58–67. Edward Arnold, London.

Browse N.L. and Solan M.J. (1969) The prevention of recurrent pulmonary embolism. *British Journal of Surgery* **56**, 753.

Buckler P. and Douglas A.S. (1982) Prevention and management of deep venous thrombosis. *Medicine International* **1**, 840–843.

Dalen J.E., Haffajee C.I., Alpert J.S., Howe J.P., Ockene I.S. and Paraskos J.A. (1977) Pulmonary embolism, pulmonary haemorrhage and pulmonary infarction. *New England Journal of Medicine* **296**, 1431.

De Meester T.R., Rutherford R.B., Blazek J.V. and Zuidema G.D. (1967) Plication of the inferior vena cava for thrombo-embolism. *Surgery* **62**, 56.

Gorham L.W. (1961) A study of pulmonary embolism. *Archives of Internal Medicine* **108**, 8 & 189.

Hirsch J. (1981) Prevention of deep venous thrombosis. *British Journal of Hospital Medicine* **26**, 2.

International Multicentre Trial (1975) Prevention of fatal post-operative pulmonary embolism by low doses of heparin. *Lancet* **2**, 45.

Kline A., Hughes L.E., Campbell H., Williams A., Zlosnick J. and Leach K.G. (1975) Dextran 70 in prophylaxis of thrombo-embolic disease after surgery. *British Medical Journal* **2**, 109.

Macintyre I.M.C. and Ruckley C.V. (1974) Pulmonary embolism—a clinical and autopsy study. *Scottish Medical Journal* **19**, 20.

McNeil B.J. (1976) A diagnostic strategy using ventilation-perfusion studies in patients suspect to pulmonary embolism. *Journal of Nuclear Medicine* **17**, 613.

Macrae K.D. (1980) Thrombosis and oral contraception. *British Journal of Hospital Medicine* **24**, 5.

Meaney T.F., Weinstein M.A., Buonocore E., Pavlicek W., Borkowski G.P., Gallagher J.H., Sufka B. and MacIntyre W.F. (1980) Digital Subtraction Angiography of the Human Cardiovascular System. *American Journal of Radiology* **135**, 1153.

Michaels L. (1971) Incidence of thrombo-embolism after stopping anticoagulant therapy. *Journal of American Medical Association* **215**, 595.

Miller G.A.H. (1972) The diagnosis and management of massive pulmonary embolism. *British Journal of Surgery* **59**, 837.

Mobin–Uddin K., Trinkle J.K. and Bryant L.R. (1971) Present status of the inferior vena cava umbrella filter. *Surgery* **70**, 914.

Moser K.M., Le Moine J.R., Nachtwey F.J. and Spragg R.G. (1981) Deep venous thrombosis and pulmonary embolism. *Journal of the American Medical Association* **246**, 1422.

Oakley C. (1977) Aute pulmonary embolism. *British Journal of Hospital Medicine* **18**, 15.

Paraskos J.A., Adelstein S.J., Smith R.E., Rickman R.D., Grossman W., Dexten L. and Dalen J.E. (1973) Late prognosis of acute pulmonary embolism. *New England Journal of Medicine* **289**, 55.

Rosenberg I.L., Evans M. and Pollock A.V. (1975) Prophylaxis of postoperative leg vein thrombosis by low dose subcutaneous heparin or peri-operative calf muscle stimulation. *British Medical Journal* **1**, 649.

Sharma G.V.R.K. and Sasahara A.A. (1979) Diagnosis and treatment of pulmonary embolism. *Medical clinics of North America* **63**, 239.

Sipes J.N., Suratt P.M., Teates C.D., Barada F.A., Davis J.S. and Tegtmeyer C.J. (1978) A prospective study of plasma DNA in the diagnosis of pulmonary embolism. *American Review of Respiratory Diseases* **118**, 475–478.

Talbot S., Worthington B.S. and Roebuck E.J. (1973) Radiographic signs of pulmonary embolism and infarction. *Thorax* **28**, 198.

Urokinase Pulmonary Embolism Trial (1973) National Cooperative Study. *Circulation* **47**, Supplement 2, 1–108.

Vessey M.P. (1973) Epidemiology of venous thrombosis in Poller L. (ed). *Recent Advances in Thrombosis* Churchill Livingstone. 4, p. 59.

Wenger N.K., Stein P.D. and Wilis P.W. (1972) Massive acute pulmonary embolism: the deceivingly non-specific manifestions. *Journal of American Medical Association* **220**, 843.

Widdicombe J.G. (1973) Reflex mechanisms in pulmonary thrombo-embolism. Moses K. M. and Stein M. (eds). *Pulmonary Thrombo-embolism* pp. 178–186. Chicago, Year Book Medical Publishers.

Wigend M., Bernhand V.M., Maddison F. and Towne J.B. (1978) Comparison of caval filters in the management of venous thrombo-embolism. *Archives of Surgery* **113**, 1204.

Wolfe W.G. and Sabiston D.C. (1980) Surgical management of pulmonary embolism *Major problems in Clinical Surgery* **25**, 117.

9 · Shock

J. A. R. SMITH

The very use of the word 'shock' encourages the assumption of a common disease process. As recently as 1941, Grant and Reeves explained that this was not valid. They recommended the introduction of several alternative terms to explain better the pathophysiological processes involved and to indicate the treatment required. Their detailed recommendations failed but the principles they advocated hold good today. Thus, a wide variety of processes produce a common effect at cellular level—shock is the state in which there is impaired supply of nutrients and oxygen at cellular level.

Effects of hypoxia on the microcirculation

Once blood reaches the capillary bed, the precise distribution of oxygenated blood is subject to local control. Areas in need of oxygen dilate and constrict again once that need is supplied. Where oxygen supply is reduced, increasing areas of the capillary circulation dilate, the eventual result being stagnant hypoxia and anoxia.

Cellular hypoxia

Normal cell function depends on aerobic metabolism, the elaboration of ATP stores for energy, the maintenance of sub-cellular membrane integrity, the preservation of fluid and electrolyte balance across the cell membrane by the energy requiring Na/K pump and the provision of the optimal pH for cell enzyme function.

Where the supply of oxygen is reduced, capability for conversion to anaerobic methods of metabolism does exist but has a number of serious side effects:

1. There is a build-up of lactic acid within the cell, resulting in local acidosis. This in turn interferes with enzyme function and thus with cellular activity. The release of acid metabolites from the cell results in an increasing metabolic acidosis.

2. There is a reduction in ATP available for intracellular and membrane sited energy requiring processes. At sub-cellular level, this means serious interference with vital functions but more significant is the effect on the 'sodium pump.' Reduced efficiency results in the ingress of sodium and therefore of water into the cell, with leakage of potassium into the extra-

cellular space. The alteration of osmotic relationships within the cell further impedes cellular function.

3. These effects combine to result in disruption of sub-cellular organelles with release of potentially toxic enzymes and lysosomal hydrolases, which in turn produce further sub-cellular digestion, cellular destruction and the release of cellular enzymes outside the normally protective containing membranes.

4. The toxins released are themselves digestive but also have some vaso-active properties further embarrassing the microcirculation.

5. The hypoxic reticulo-endothelial cells are unable to detoxify the increased quantities of endotoxin absorbed from the hypoxic gastro-intestinal tract. Many actions for endotoxin are claimed but the most significant is the activation of complement by the alternate pathway. Such inappropriate activation produces problems of coagulation and haemostasis, of pulmonary gas exchange and of circulatory control.

6. Certain more specific toxins have been investigated. These are believed to be produced from the hypoxic pancreatic cells and include myocardial depressant factor and reticulo-endothelial depressant factor. However, their role in severe shock is not yet entirely clear.

Clinical picture

The classical clinical presentation is of a patient in a state of collapse with cold clammy skin. Tachycardia, hypotension, tachypnoea and low urine output complete the picture. However, in the early stages of shock due to sepsis *(vide infra)* certain important differences must be recognized. Such patients are flushed and bright eyed with warm skin. The pulse is usually bounding and systolic pressure is either normal or only slightly reduced. Respiratory rate is slightly increased. If urine output is monitored, hourly flow is reduced as is arterial oxygen tension. However, because of the different clinical picture, this diagnosis will be missed if a high index of suspicion is not maintained in patients at risk—namely, emergency surgery, especially on the bowel; faecal contamination; biliary obstruction or urinary infection; immunosuppressed patients; those with serious medical illnesses.

Cardiogenic shock

Any cause of 'pump failure' may produce a shock state. Thus, acute myocardial infarction, congestive cardiac failure, cardiac tamponade, all will result in impaired peripheral perfusion.

Furthermore, certain authorities believe that in most cases of advanced or refractory shock from any primary cause, a myocardial depressant factor is elaborated from the hypoxic pancreas. This toxin is claimed to be contributory to the high mortality in advanced shock (Lefer *et al.* 1967; Ledingham *et al.* 1971).

Hypovolaemic shock

Loss of blood volume due to haemorrhage or due to loss of plasma, such as in severe pancreatitis, or widespread burn injury, is readily recognizable. More serious is the hypovolaemia which results from excessive losses of fluids and electrolytes in burns or in such disorders as gastro-enteritis or cholera. The former is particularly dangerous in paediatric practice. Of equal importance is the combination of haemorrhage and severe trauma where significant loss of blood into soft tissues secondary to major bone injury may be overlooked or underestimated.

Anaphylactoid shock

The widespread release of histamine and related compounds in response to immediate hypersensitivity reaction results in serious vasodilation. Thus, although absolute blood volume remains unchanged, at least in the early stages, the increase in available blood space results in a functional hypovolaemia, i.e. peripheral perfusion is impaired.

Vasovagal shock

It is questionable whether true shock ever results from a vasovagal episode. In response to fear or acute stress, vasodilation results in impaired cerebral flow. The resulting collapse of the patient ensures brain and heart reach the same horizontal levels and adequate flow is restored.

Septic shock

A number of factors appear to be involved in which sepsis results in impaired cellular perfusion.

    1. Toxic vasodilation results in a relative hypovolaemia, probably in response to an acute inflammatory response or to bacterial toxins.

    2. Endotoxins, resulting from gram-negative bacterial breakdown in particular, have a number of important effects which themselves contribute to the changes seen. Perhaps most important of all is the inappropriate activation of complement by the alternate pathway. This step results in widespread phenomena including disseminated intravascular coagulation, bleeding tendency and lung changes. In addition to deposits of fibrin in pulmonary capillaries, there are changes in alveolar cells resulting in an increase in membrane thickness and in reduced production of surfactant,

causing alveolar collapse. Furthermore, endotoxin may contribute to capillary vasodilation and compound the hypoxic stagnation.

3. Arterio-venous shunting—sepsis appears to cause peripheral arterio-venous shunts for reasons not immediately clear. This will impair microcirculatory supply of oxygen but more seriously there may be significant shunting in the pulmonary circulation when central oxygenation is further embarrassed.

Treatment of shock

In addition to the principles to be discussed, it is vital to remember the absolute necessity to include treatment of the primary cause as part of the overall therapy. Thus, control of haemorrhage, drainage of any septic focus etc., must be achieved. However, it must also be remembered that any patient in severe shock shows reduced resistance to infection, impaired tolerance of large infusions of fluid and increased risk of acute renal failure. Thus, aggressive therapy must be combined with careful monitoring of response and of tolerance of the therapy used.

Anaphylactoid shock

Only anaphylactoid shock can be regarded as specific when considering therapy. Intravenous hydrocortisone, 200 mg stat, may be given together with intravenous noradrenaline, 100 μg, which can be repeated up to 400 μg, if necessary. Adrenaline (0.5–1.0 ml of 1:1000) may be given intra-muscularly as an alternative to noradrenaline. 10 mg of chlorpheniramine maleate may also be given intravenously. In all cases, it is absolutely essential to investigate the cause and to avoid re-exposure.

General principles

1. *Volume infusion*

Maintenance of circulatory volume is an essential part of the therapy of shock but the volume and type of fluid used must be carefully monitored.

Thus, in addition to monitoring pulse and blood pressure, all patients in severe shock require measurement of hourly urinary output and of central venous pressure. This is particularly important in the elderly, the patient with a history of cardiac disease or where recent myocardial infarction is suspected. Even in this group of patients, it is usually valuable to assess the effects on the CVP of a trial load of 500 ml of fluid and to institute early cardiac support in those patients whose CVP rises further in response to fluid.

In general, it is important to maintain the CVP between eight and twelve cm H_2O, remembering that if assisted ventilation is required, higher levels of CVP will be necessary. Hourly urine output of over 40 ml is the aim and there is little point in prescribing diuretics of any sort to stimulate urine output until an adequate CVP has been achieved. By the same token, avoidance of excessive infusion is essential and should be achieved before the clinical evidence of congestive cardiac failure is in evidence.

The fluid of choice for volume maintenance has long been debated. Where blood or plasma has been lost in quantity, these should be replaced. However, the dangers of using stored blood and the impaired delivery of oxygen must be remembered. In addition to the biochemical and coagulation defects which may result, the fall in red cell 2–3 diphosphoglycerate in storage increases the affinity of haemoglobin for oxygen, i.e. shifts the oxyhaemoglobin dissociation curve to the LEFT.

It must be remembered that acidosis tends to move the curve to the RIGHT and thus TOTAL correction of acidosis by the infusion of bicarbonate cannot be recommended. It is clear that provided the haematocrit is above thirty (i.e. Hb above 10 g) the healthy myocardium can compensate for a degree of haemodilution to maintain tissue oxygenation. Moreover, the consequent reduction in whole blood viscosity may be beneficial to microcirculatory flow.

In the absence of plasma losses, i.e. burns or pancreatitis, there is no specific preference for plasma over Haemaccel.

There is no place for the use of crystalloid solutions alone, as these may induce pulmonary overload. Similarly, the use of colloidal solutions alone is not indicated and a mixture of both crystalloid and colloid is to be recommended (Smith & Norman 1982). Experimental evidence is in favour of ratios 2:1 colloid to crystalloid, but in clinical practice wider variation of requirement will be found. At the present time, the polygelatin solution Haemaccel is the colloidal agent of choice and has replaced the dextrans. Dextran 40 does not remain long enough in the circulation to be effective. Dextran 70 has limited shelf life, is difficult to store and is more prone to result in haemorrhage than Haemaccel. Some serious allergic reactions have been reported with Dextran 70 and minor reactions or subclinical elevation in histamine are common. The use of Dextran 70 renders cross matching of blood more difficult and washing of red cells is required after Dextran infusion. Haemaccel has the advantages of easier storage in plastic containers, fewer reactions and no antithrombotic effect. Its molecular weight is only 35,000 and thus its retention in the circulation and hence its colloidal effect appears to depend on its molecular shape rather than weight. Hydroxyethyl starch has been used on the Continent. It is an effective plasma expander (Smith & Norman 1982) but serious allergic reactions have been reported. Furthermore, the higher molecular weight fractions of this solution are ingested by the reticulo-endothelial system (RES) and this may interfere with RES function in severe shock.

It has been suggested that in the presence of severe widespread capillary permeability, colloidal solutions leaking to the extra vascular spaces will be more harmful than crystalloid. Such severe changes are seldom seen in clinical reality and attention should be directed to the preservation of capillary integrity and early institution of treatment before such changes occur.

2. *Respiratory support*

In view of the problems of oxygen delivery to the cell, all patients in shock will require oxygen supplements by mask at the very least. There is an increasing tendency to proceed to assisted ventilation whenever oxygen by mask is insufficient to maintain an arterial oxygen tension of 65 mmHg. Where more sophisticated monitoring is possible, an alveolar-arterial oxygen difference of greater than 200 mmHg is considered an indication for ventilation.

In addition to the effect on oxygen supply, it is suggested that ventilation may also reduce the risk of pulmonary fluid overload. However, the benefits of ventilation must be weighed against the increased risk of infection in such patients, particularly remembering the opportunist fungal and viral infections.

3. *Cardiovascular support*

Clearly, in cardiogenic shock, cardiovascular support is of prime importance. However, in all cases of shock, prognosis has been linked to myocardial dysrrhythmia (Ledingham 1975) and thus similar cardiac support may be required.

(a) Antiarrhythmic drugs

The patient with atrial fibrillation will require full digitalization. In addition, patients with a persistent tachycardia despite volume replacement often benefit from digitalization. Other arrhythmias are managed as described in Chapter 5

(b) Vasodilation

Experimentally α-blockade has been shown of value provided the agent is given before the shock insult. The degree of effect on the compromised circulation is so severe that there is no place for such therapy in clinical practice. More gentle vasodilation can be achieved by the use of small doses of intravenous chlorpromazine, e.g. 2–5 mg iv.

(c) Dopamine and dobutamine

Dopamine is a potent inotropic agent. It causes an increase in stroke volume by both releasing noradrenaline from nerve endings and by a direct action on adrenergic myocardial receptors. At dosages of 3–10 μg/kg/min, it acts as an inotropic cardiac stimulant with the additional benefit of splanchnic and in particular, renal vasodilatation. At higher doses, it may cause excessive vasoconstriction, ventricular arrhythmias and an increase in pulmonary capillary wedge pressure.

Dobutamine acts directly on adrenergic receptors without releasing endogenous noradrenaline. It causes an increase in cardiac output and stroke volume with a fall in capillary wedge pressure. However, it may cause a reduction in systemic arterial resistance and a small fall in arterial blood pressure in patients with low output cardiac failure. It has been suggested that dopamine is the drug of choice in septic shock (Regnier *et al.* 1979) and that dobutamine should be used in cardiogenic shock (Francis *et al.* 1982). However, it may be preferable to utilize the benefits of the two drugs combined (Richard *et al.* 1983).

(d) Diuretics

Judicious use of diuretic therapy may be necessary to avoid congestive cardiac failure and to maintain renal function and urine output. However, it must be emphasized that these should only be used once an adequate circulatory blood volume has been ensured. Where the CVP is at a therapeutic level or above, and urine output is impaired, especially where there is other evidence of incipient renal failure, a solitary bolus of frusemide intravenously in a dose of 125 mg may be sufficient to encourage restoration of renal function. However, there is little evidence to support the infusion of further volume such as mannitol as an osmotic diuretic.

4. *Renal support*

In addition to the measures of ensuring adequate blood volume and of maintaining renal function, there is a move to the early institution of dialysis when there is clear evidence of falling urine output associated with rising urea, potassium and creatinine.

Treatment of sepsis

Both in patients in shock due to sepsis and in those whose susceptibility to infection is increased by the effects of severe shock, antibiotic therapy is indicated. Blood and other appropriate cultures must be taken prior to therapy. At the present time, a combination of gentamicin (80 mg iv t.i.d.), penicillin (1 g 6 hourly) and metronidazole (500 mg t.i.d.) is the regimen of choice when the infecting organism is not known. Where renal function is impaired, the dose of gentamicin must be adjusted according to standard tables relative to the blood urea concentration.

However, alternative agents providing an adequate spectrum with fewer side effects are increasingly available. The newest generations include latamoxef disodium (Moxalactam) or ticarcillin which have good *in vitro* spectra, sound theoretical advantages but little clinical support at the present time. They are claimed to have satisfactory activity against bacteroides but most clinicians would combine them with metronidazole or one of its newer competitors, e.g. fasigyn. An important part of overall management is the thorough drainage and bacteriological investigation of any collection of pus.

Additional agents

A variety of agents such as aprotinin (Trasylol) or prostaglandins have been recommended for the treatment of severe shock but none have been supported in extensive clinical or experimental studies. The one agent which remains controversial but widely used is glucocorticoid in pharmacological dosage. This agent is particularly valuable in early septic shock, late severe shock states and cardiogenic shock. There is clear experimental evidence that the earlier the adminstration, the more likely the success (Smith & Norman 1979) and that it must be used as part of an overall therapeutic regimen (Hinshaw *et al.* 1980; Smith 1983). Only one clinical study is suitably controlled and that reported in favour of steroid therapy (Schumer 1976).

The agent of choice is methylprednisolone sodium succinate 30 mg/kg body weight intravenously. No more than three doses at six to eight hourly intervals should be given. With this regimen there is no evidence of serious side effects due to the steroids and no evidence that larger dosage or more prolonged course is any more effective. Steroid should be administered as early as possible and only as part of the overall therapeutic regimen.

The mode of action of methylprednisolone has been extensively investigated. Most recent evidence is in favour of an action to minimize the inappropriate activation of complement. However, additional factors include stabilization of cellular and subcellular membranes and prevention of alveolar cell damage.

Further reading

Francis G., Sharma B. and Hodges M. (1982) Comparative haemodynamic effects of dopamine and dobutamine in patients with acute cardiogenic circulatory collapse. *American Heart Journal* **103**, 995–1000.

Grant R.T. and Reeves E.B. (1941) Clinical observations on air raid casualties. *British Medical Journal* **21**, 293–97 and 329–332.

Grant R.T. and Reeves E.B. (1941) Observations of the general effects of injury in man. *Medical Research Council Special Report Series No.* **227** H.M.S.O., London.

Lefer A.M., Cowgill R., Marshall F.F., Hall L.M. and Brand E.D. (1967) Characterization of a myocardial depressant factor present in haemorrhagic shock. *American Journal of Physiology* **213**, 492–498.

Ledingham I. McA., Heimbach D.M., Hutton I., McArdle C.S. (1971) Cardiac function in haemorrhagic shock. *British Journal of Surgery* **58**, 868–869.

Smith J.A.R. and Norman J.N. (1982) The fluid of choice for resuscitation of severe shock. *British Journal of Surgery* **69**, 702–705.

Ledingham I.McA. (1975) Septic shock. *British Journal of Surgery* **62**, 777–780.

Smith J.A.R. and Norman J.N. (1979) The use of glucocorticosteroids in refractory shock. *Surgery, Gynaecology and Obstetrics* **149**, 369–373.

Hinshaw L.B., Archer L.T., Beller-Todd B.K., Coalson J.J., Fluomoy D.J., Passey R., Benjamin B. and White G.L. (1980) Survival of primates in E coli septic shock following steroid/antibiotic therapy. *Journal of Surgical Research* **28**, 151–170.

Regnier B., Satran D.,Carlet J. and Teisseire B. (1979) Comparative haemodynamic effects of dopamine and dobutamine in septic shock. *Intensive Care Medicine* **5**, 115–120.

Richard C., Ricome J., Rimailho A., Bottineau G. and Auzepy P. Combined haemodynamic effects of dopamine and dobutamine in cardiogenic shock. *Circulation* **67**, 620–626.

Smith J.A.R. (1983) A review of the use of steroids in shock. *Journal of the Royal College of Surgeons of Edinburgh.* **28**, 214–218.

Schumer W. (1976) Steroids in the treatment of clinical septic shock. *Annals of Surgery* **184**, 333–341.

10 · Aortic Dissection

N. A. BOON

Aortic dissection occurs when a tear in the intima allows a column of blood, driven by the force of the arterial pressure, to enter the aortic wall. This destroys the media and strips the intima from the adventitia to produce what may be described as a dissecting haematoma spreading along and around the aorta. The condition is also known as a dissecting aneurysm of the aorta, although this term is losing favour.

Pathology

It is not clear whether the primary event is a tear in the intima with secondary dissection in the media or haemorrhage within a diseased media followed by disruption of the intima. There are reports of cases occurring without identifiable intimal tears although this is generally regarded as the primary event. In up to ten per cent of cases there may be multiple intimal tears.

Aortic dissection is almost invariably associated with a variety of histological changes in the aortic media. These include cystic medial necrosis or mucoid degeneration of the media, medionecrosis, elastin fragmentation and fibrosis. At one time these features were thought to represent a specific intrinsic defect of the media intimately involved in the pathogenesis of aortic dissection. However, Schlatmann and Becker (1977a) have shown that these changes are often found in normal aortas and appear to be part of the normal ageing process. They suggested that this pattern represents the result of repeated injury and repair and would therefore be expected to occur at an earlier age in the presence of a connective tissue disorder such as Marfan's Syndrome. Careful light microscopy studies have shown that there appears to be no qualitative difference between the aortic media of patients with aortic dissection and suitable controls (Schlatmann and Becker 1977b; Hasleton and Leonard 1979; Leonard and Hastleton 1979). So there seems to be no specific underlying defect, although degeneration of the aortic media probably does play an important part in the pathogenesis of aortic dissection.

Associated conditions

There is a strong association between arterial hypertension and aortic dissection, particularly distal aortic dissection. Up to eighty per cent of patients with an acute dissection have evidence of pre-existing arterial hypertension, and more than half will be hypertensive at the time of presentation.

The association between aortic dissection and Marfan's Syndrome is well recognized. There are also recognized associations between the condition and co-arctation of the aorta, bicuspid aortic valve, floppy mitral valve, giant cell arteritis involving the aorta and hypothyroidism. There is a curious association between pregnancy and aortic dissection, when it tends to occur in the last trimester and is often but not always associated with hypertension (Hirst *et al.* 1958).

Classification

The vast majority of aortic dissections begin either within two or three centimetres of the aortic valve or in the descending thoracic aorta just beyond the origin of the left subclavian artery. Occasionally, dissection may begin in the aortic arch or the abdominal aorta and individual arteries, particularly the coronary and carotid arteries, may also be the site for isolated dissection.

De Bakey *et al.* (1965) classified aortic dissection into three types (Fig. 10.1). Types one and two both begin in the ascending aorta; type one extends around the aortic arch, whereas type two is confined to the ascending aorta. Type three begins in the descending thoracic aorta and usually

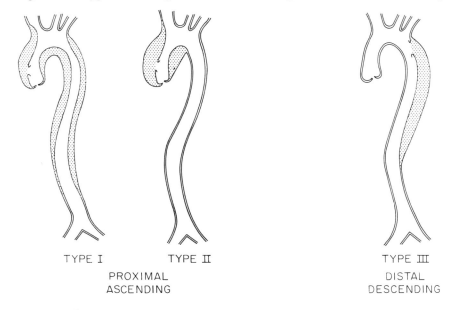

TYPE I   TYPE II   TYPE III
     PROXIMAL   DISTAL
     ASCENDING   DESCENDING

Fig. 10.1. Classification of aortic dissection.

extends distally but may also extend proximally. Cardiac catheterization may occasionally result in an iatrogenic retrograde dissection which has been classified as a type four dissection.

Classification into proximal or ascending versus distal or descending dissection has become the most widely used classification (Fig. 10.1) because it is simpler and has considerable clinical relevance. The incidence of proximal and distal dissections are probably similar although they have different clinical profiles and prognoses (Table 10.1). A distinction between acute and chronic aortic dissection is sometimes recognized; chronic dissection referring to patients who present at least two weeks after what is thought to be the primary event.

Table 10.1. Differing features of proximal and distal aortic dissection

1. Distal dissection tends to occur in an older age group and has a stronger association with arterial hypertension.
2. Anterior thoracic pain radiating into the neck or jaw suggests a proximal dissection whereas interscapular pain suggests a distal dissection.
3. Aortic incompetence and neurological manifestations are more common in proximal dissection.
4. Proximal dissections tend to rupture into the pericardium whereas distal dissections tend to rupture into the left pleural cavity.
5. Untreated proximal dissection has a worse prognosis than untreated distal dissection.

Clinical manifestations

Aortic dissection is more common in men and tends to occur between the ages of forty and seventy. The peak age of incidence is a little lower for patients with proximal dissection than those with distal dissection.

The diagnosis can often be made with a fair degree of certainty from the symptoms and signs alone. The vast majority of patients present with severe chest pain which is often described as 'ripping' or 'tearing'. The onset of pain is sudden and unlike the pain of myocardial infarction, tends to be most severe at the outset; it is often accompanied by vasovagal features and syncope may occur. The pain may migrate as the dissection progresses. Pain in the anterior chest radiating into the neck or jaw suggests a proximal lesion whereas pain between the shoulder blades is more common with a distal dissection.

The other features of aortic dissection depend on the subsequent course of the dissecting haematoma. It may occlude the origin of any of the branches of the aorta or rupture into either the pericardium or pleural space or re-enter into the aorta.

Proximal dissections tend to rupture into the pericardium which may produce tamponade characterized by hypotension, tachycardia, pulsus paradoxus, and a high venous pressure with a sharp Y descent. Distal dissections tend to rupture into the left pleural cavity which usually results in circulatory collapse. Rupture is the most common mode of death.

Acute aortic incompetence occurs in at least fifty per cent of patients with proximal dissection and may be due to distortion of the aortic valve ring or destruction of the supporting annulus. Aortic incompetence will be accompanied by an early diastolic murmur audible at the left sternal edge and a systolic flow murmur, but the peripheral signs of aortic incompetence are often absent when the lesion is acute. Left ventricular failure often supervenes.

Myocardial infarction due to occlusion of the coronary arteries occurs in one or two per cent of cases. Involvement of one of the carotid arteries associated with a weak or absent pulse in the neck and an appropriate neurological deficit is quite common. The renal arteries and mesenteric arteries may also be involved and occasionally the blood supply to the spinal cord is drastically reduced resulting in paraplegia. Occlusion of the brachio-cephalic vessels in proximal dissections and the iliac vessels in distal dissec-tions is common and may produce a vascular bruit, absent pulses and ischaemic pain. If the blood supply to the arms is affected it may be difficult to record the blood pressure accurately. Therefore, it is important to take the blood pressure in both arms and the legs if necessary.

Horner's syndrome due to compression of the superior cervical sympa-thetic ganglion and vocal cord paralysis with hoarseness due to pressure on the left recurrent laryngeal nerve have also been reported.

Diagnosis

In approximately fifty per cent of cases the ECG shows evidence of left ventricular hypertrophy, presumably due to pre-existing hypertension, but its main value is in excluding acute myocardial infarction.

In the majority of patients, the chest X-ray shows some widening of the aortic contour and may also show a localized bulge. If the aortic knuckle is calcified there may be a wide separation between the calcified intima and the adventitia which is virtually pathognomonic of aortic dissection. It is quite common to see a small left pleural effusion which is often due to a non-specific exudative reaction rather than rupture into the left pleural space. Occasionally the chest X-ray may be entirely normal.

Echocardiography cannot exclude an aortic dissection. However, it may help to establish the diagnosis in cases of proximal dissection and may also demonstrate the presence of blood in the pericardium.

Although most dissections can be visualized by CT scanning, aortography is still the definite investigation. When the diagnosis is not in doubt aortography should be carried out as soon as possible in order to confirm the diagnosis, define the entry site and extent of the dissection, and demonstrate the circulation to the vital organs. Coronary arteriography can be carried out at the same time if necessary. On the other hand, when the diagnosis is in doubt a CT scan is useful when deciding whether or not to proceed to aortography.

Management

As soon as the diagnosis is suspected, the patient should be admitted to an intensive care unit and given appropriate analgesia such as diamorphine 5–10 mg intravenously (iv) with prochlorperazine 12.5 mg iv. The heart rate, blood pressure, central venous pressure, urine output and ECG should be monitored carefully and the peripheral pulses should be checked frequently. Ideally, the blood pressure should be monitored directly from a peripheral arterial line sited in a limb whose arterial supply has not been affected. A dynamic display often provides useful information and a constant read-out is a great help in the management of hypotensive episodes.

The principal aim of treatment is to prevent the dissecting haematoma spreading or rupturing, thereby avoiding any of the major complications. The dissection will only extend when the force of the arterial pressure exceeds the forces binding the layers of the aorta together. The character of the pulse wave is a crucial factor in this equation. The maximum rate of rise of the arterial pressure (dp/dt_{max}) which is related to the velocity of left ventricular contraction (dv/dt) is probably the most important factor (Prokop 1970). The absolute level of pressure and the heart rate are also important considerations so treatment should be designed to lower the systolic blood pressure, pulse pressure, dv/dt and the heart rate.

As soon as possible, the blood pressure should be lowered using an intravenous infusion of the vasodilator sodium nitroprusside (100 mg in 500 ml of 5% dextrose). The infusion should be started at a rate of one μg/kg/minute and increased, up to a maximum of 800 μg/minute until the systolic blood pressure is around 100 mm of mercury or as low as possible without impairing cerebral or renal perfusion. The duration of action of this drug is short which makes it relatively easy to control the blood pressure from minute to minute. Sodium nitroprusside is light-sensitive so the infusion set should be wrapped in aluminium foil.

Treatment with a vasodilator alone is likely to produce a reflex increase in sympathetic nervous activity resulting in an undesirable increase in the heart rate and dv/dt. Unrelieved pain will have the same effect, so it is important to ensure adequate pain relief and to start the patient on simultaneous intravenous β-blockade. One way of achieving this is to give small doses (1.0–2.0 mg of intravenous metoprolol) every five to ten minutes until the heart rate falls to between sixty and seventy beats per minute, followed by small maintenance doses every four hours. When practical the patient can be changed to oral therapy.

The blood transfusion service should be notified and the case discussed with a cardiovascular surgeon. As soon as the blood pressure has been reduced and the patient seems stable, aortography should be carried out.

Definitive treatment

The definitive treatment may be medical or surgical. Medical therapy should consist of a six week period of restricted activity, β-blockade and strict control of the blood pressure. By this time the false lumen will have thrombosed but it is vital to keep the blood pressure as low as possible in order to minimize the risks of a second episode.

Surgical treatment involves repair or resection of the aorta with or without aortic valve replacement. Full cardiopulmonary bypass is needed to repair a proximal dissection. Such operations may be very difficult because the aorta is often friable and difficult to suture. Operative mortality obviously depends upon the age and general condition of the patient but is around fifteen to twenty per cent. Paraplegia due to ischaemic damage is an unusual but recognized complication of surgery.

Surgical treatment should always be accompanied by intensive medical therapy in the short and long-term.

The early and late results of surgical treatment are very much better than those of medical treatment in patients with proximal dissection. In patients with distal dissection the early results of medical and surgical treatment are very similar. There is a suggestion, however, that patients with distal dissection treated surgically have a slightly better long-term prognosis (Applebaum *et al.* 1976). Therefore, it seems reasonable to recommend early

Table 10.2. Scheme for management

Immediate management
1. Admit to intensive care. Monitor heart rate, blood pressure (arterial line, if possible), central venous pressure, urine output and ECG.
2. Ensure adequate pain relief. Intravenous diamorphine.
3. Reduce systolic blood pressure to around 100 mm mercury with intravenous nitroprusside and simultaneous β-blockade.
4. Aortography when stable.

Further management
1. Early surgery combined with intensive medical therapy for patients with proximal dissection or complicated distal dissection.
2. Medical therapy alone for patients with uncomplicated distal dissection and other patients not suitable for major surgery.
3. Long term follow-up and control of blood pressure is essential.

---

surgery in all cases of proximal dissection and in those cases of distal dissection who develop a major complication such as occlusion of a renal or femoral artery. Medical therapy is recommended for the remaining cases of distal dissection. Some centres recommend elective surgery after a period of six weeks intensive medical treatment in patients with uncomplicated distal dissection because they believe this offers the best long term outlook but this must be balanced against an appreciable operative mortality. Unfortunately, there are no controlled trials to clarify this dilemma.

A scheme for the management of acute aortic dissection is set out in Table 10.2. There is no doubt that the prognosis has improved considerably with the advent of effective surgical and medical therapy and the overall one year mortality is now in the region of thirty per cent.

Further reading

Applebaum A., Karp R.B. and Kirklin J.W. (1976) Ascending versus descending aortic dissections. *Annals of Surgery* **183**, 296–300.

De Bakey M.E., Henley W.S., Cooley D.A., Morris G.C., Crawford E.S. and Beall A.C. (1965) Surgical management of dissecting aneurysms of the aorta. *Journal of Thoracic and Cardiovascular Surgery* **49**, 130–149.

Hasleton P.S. and Leonard J.C. (1979) Dissecting aortic aneurysms: a clinico-pathological study. II. Histopathology of the aorta. *Quarterly Journal of Medicine*, **48**, 63–76.

Hirst A.E., John V.J. and Kime S.W. (1958) Dissecting aneurysm of the aorta: a review of 505 cases. *Medicine (Baltimore)* **37**, 217–279.

Leonard J.C. and Hasleton P.S. (1979) Dissecting aortic aneurysms: a clinico-pathological study. I. Clinical and gross pathological findings. *Quarterly Journal of Medicine* **48**, 55–63.

Prokop E.K., Palmer R.F. and Wheat M.W. (1970) Hydrodynamic forces in dissecting aneurysms. *Circulation Research* **27**, 121–127.

Schlatmann T.J.M. and Becker A.E. (1977a) Histologic changes in the normal aging aorta: implications for dissecting aortic aneurysm. *American Journal of Cardiology* **39**, 12–20.

Schlatmann T.J.M. and Becker A.E. (1977b) Pathogenesis of dissecting aneurysm of aorta. *American Journal of Cardiology* **39**, 21–26.

11 · Respiratory Failure

M. K. BENSON

The main function of the lungs is for gas exchange, maintaining arterial gas tensions for oxygen and carbon dioxide within narrow limits. Normal values for arterial oxygen tension (P_aO_2) are 11.3–13.3 kPa (85–100 mm Hg) and for arterial carbon dioxide tension (P_aCO_2) 4.8–5.9 kPa (36–44 mm Hg) with respiratory failure arbitrarily defined as a P_aO_2 of less than 8 kPa (60 mm Hg) or P_aCO_2 above 6.7 kPa* (50 mm Hg). The diagnosis of respiratory failure depends on recognition of a condition which may predispose to respiratory failure together with clinical features of hypoxaemia and hypercapnia. Confirmation and assessment of the degree of failure rests with arterial blood gas analysis (see Appendix 1).

Classification of respiratory failure

Respiratory failure can be classified into three categories which differ in terms of the underlying pathophysiology, clinical determinants and treatment.

Pure ventilatory failure results from alveolar hypoventilation. Carbon dioxide tension is raised and oxygen tension reduced to a corresponding degree.

Hypoxaemic respiratory failure results in a low oxygen tension with carbon dioxide tension being normal or low. This results from ventilation–perfusion inequalities with some areas of lung being perfused but poorly ventilated. However, total alveolar ventilation is normal and thus P_aCO_2 is not elevated.

The third group of patients has a combination of hypoxic and ventilatory failure. Arterial carbon dioxide tension is raised with oxygen tension being reduced disproportionately because of disturbed ventilation–perfusion relationships ($\dot{V}_A:\dot{Q}$).

Pure ventilatory failure

Alveolar ventilation ($\dot{V}_A$) is related to total ventilation ($\dot{V}_T$) and the amount wasted by ventilating areas of lung which are not perfused ($\dot{V}_D$) where

$$\dot{V}_A = \dot{V}_T - \dot{V}_D$$

*S.I. units alone will be used for the remainder of the chapter. For those who wish to convert 1 kPa ≈ 7.5 mm Hg.

117

When alveolar hypoventilation occurs in the presence of abnormal lungs it is usually associated with disturbed $\dot{V}_A:\dot{Q}$ relationships and will be considered subsequently. 'Pure' ventilatory failure results from a fall in total ventilation and is usually due to reduced neural drive or loss of mechanical function of the thoracic cavity.

At rest the alveolar tension for carbon dioxide ($P_A CO_2$) is determined by the alveolar ventilation. As $\dot{V}_A$ falls, $P_A CO_2$ rises which in turn results in an increase in arterial PCO_2. This increase in $P_a CO_2$ will lead to an increase in dissolved CO_2 and carbonic acid with a rise in hydrogen ion concentration H^+ since

$$CO_2 + H_2O \rightleftharpoons H_2CO_3 \rightleftharpoons H^+ + GCO_3$$

In the *acute* situation the relationship between $P_a CO_2$ and $[H^+]$ is represented graphically in Figure 11.1. For an increase in $P_a CO_2$ of 1 kPa, $[H^+]$ will rise by approximately 5.1 mmol 1^{-1}. Although $[HCO_3{}^-]$ will also rise, the

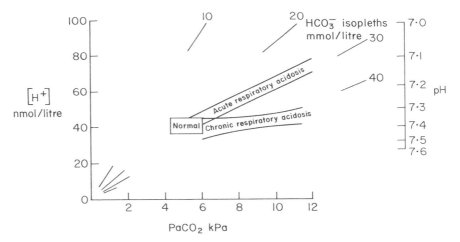

Fig. 11.1. Acid base diagram showing the relationship between arterial acidity (H^+ activity) and $P_a CO_2$. A fan of isopleths for bicarbonate values radiates from the origin.

acute changes are relatively small. *Chronic* CO_2 retention leads to renal compensation with retention of bicarbonate which is thus disproportionately high, and a return of $[H^+]$ towards normal. Knowledge of the relationship between $P_a CO_2$, $[H^+]$ and $[HCO_3{}^-]$ is of considerable clinical importance since information can be derived as to whether the changes are acute and hence potentially reversible, or chronic and possibly irreversible. In the majority of clinical situations in which there is pure ventilatory failure, the changes are relatively acute.

There is a reciprocal relationship between alveolar carbon dioxide and alveolar oxygen tension which is defined by the equation:

$$\text{Alveolar } PO_2 = \text{inspired } PO_2 - \frac{\text{alveolar } PCO_2}{R}$$

where R is the ratio of carbon dioxide eliminated/oxygen uptake (normally equals 0.8). Since alveolar and arterial PCO_2 are equal, substituting normal values we have

$$\text{Alveolar } PO_2 = 20 - \frac{5.3}{0.8} = 13.3 \text{ kPa}$$

If alveolar ventilation falls and the P_ACO_2 doubles

$$\text{Alveolar } PO_2 = 20 - \frac{10.6}{0.8} = 6.7 \text{ kPa}$$

Clinical features

The main clinical disorders in which 'pure' ventilatory failure can occur are listed in Table 11.1. They can be divided into four main groups namely: depression of the respiratory centre, neuromuscular disorders, mechanical dysfunction of the chest wall and acute large airway occlusion. In such a heterogeneous group, the clinical manifestations of respiratory failure will

Table 11.1. Clinical disorders resulting in ventilatory failure

Depression of respiratory centre	Anaesthetics/sedatives/opiates
	Head injury
	Subarachnoid haemorrhage
	Encephalitis
	'Central' sleep apnoea
Neuromuscular disorders	Cervical cord transection
	Poliomyelitis
	Acute polyneuritis
	Myaesthenia gravis
	Tetanus
Deranged chest wall mechanics	Flail chest
	Tension pneumothorax
	Gross obesity
	Kyphoscoliosis
Large airway obstruction	Inhaled foreign body
	Angioneurotic oedema
	'Obstructive' sleep apnoea

be masked by the underlying disorder. Thus following a drug overdose resulting in respiratory depression, the patient is likely to be unconscious with shallow and infrequent respiration. In contrast, patients with acute upper airway obstruction will be distressed and tachypnoeic with excess respiratory effort but inadequate ventilation. Central cyanosis will obviously reflect arterial hypoxia but severe hypercapnia will also be present before it becomes clinically obvious.

In view of the difficulty of clinical assessment, in situations where ventilatory failure is likely to occur, careful objective monitoring is necessary. Minute ventilation is the product of respiratory rate and tidal volume. Whilst the rate can be easily counted, clinical assessment of the tidal volume is unreliable. The Wright respirometer provides a simple and reliable measurement of the minute volume especially in patients who are unconscious. In neuromuscular disorders the vital capacity reflects the adequacy of respiratory reserve. These non-invasive techniques will need supplementing with arterial blood gas analysis.

Management

In a limited number of situations, rapid correction of the primary disorder reverses the respiratory failure. A foreign body may be displaced using the Heimlich manoeuvre whereby sudden pressure is applied to the abdomen. A tension pneumothorax can also be rapidly treated by insertion of a needle or catheter into the pleura. In an acute emergency when faced with a moribund patient who is making infrequent or inadequate respiratory effort, the basic principle applies of ensuring airway patency and maintaining ventilation artificially. The administration of increased concentrations of inspired oxygen will reduce the degree of hypoxaemia but will not by itself correct the hypercapnia and respiratory acidosis.

Other than sudden cardio-respiratory arrest, the commonest cause of ventilatory failure is drug overdosage. Opiates are powerful respiratory depressants and their effect can be specifically reversed by naloxone 100–200 micrograms administered intravenously and repeated if necessary. Among the hypnotics and sedatives, barbiturates are most likely to produce severe respiratory depression. The respiratory complications arise partly from this respiratory depression but also from the aspiration of secretions from the oropharynx. Initial management should concentrate on maintaining the airway by nursing in the lateral position, regular turning and frequent aspiration of the pharynx. Oxygen at a concentration of 40 per cent should be given by face mask. In patients who are deeply comatose with absent gag and cough reflexes, a cuffed endotracheal tube should be inserted. This not only prevents aspiration but facilitates physiotherapy with intermittent manual hyperventilation to prevent atelectasis. The decision to initiate mechanical ventilation will depend on the clinical picture, the arterial P_{CO_2} and the presence of secondary pulmonary complications. A P_aCO_2 above 8 kPa is unusual even if the minute ventilation is severely depressed, mainly because of a reduced metabolic rate. Ventilation is more likely to be needed in patients who have taken a long acting sedative, those with pre-existing lung disease and those who have aspirated.

Similar considerations will also apply to patients with neuromuscular disorders. An ineffective cough leads to retention of secretions. Aspiration is a particular problem in patients who have a bulbar or pseudo-bulbar palsy. In general, respiratory problems can be anticipated if the vital capacity falls to about one third of its predicted value. The decision to undertake tracheostomy and assisted ventilation will be modified by knowledge of the natural history of the underlying condition. Tracheostomy is preferable to endotracheal intubation since it can be maintained indefinitely. A cuffed tracheostomy tube can be used to protect the airway, aspirate secretions and if necessary apply intermittent positive pressure ventilation. It also reduces the anatomical dead space. Some patients with neuromuscular disorders maintain adequate gas exchange when awake, but hypoventilate when asleep. Augmented ventilation can be achieved using a cuirass ventilator during sleep.

It is not within the scope of this chapter to discuss the various types of ventilators and the practical problems associated with their use. However, mechanical ventilation in patients with ventilatory failure is relatively easy. High inflation pressures are unnecessary since the lungs are essentially normal and similarly high levels of inspired oxygen are not needed to maintain adequate arterial oxygenation.

Hypoxaemic respiratory failure

Hypoxaemic respiratory failure occurs in patients in whom there is some degree of right to left shunting of blood. This may be through a true anatomical shunt, but more commonly is due to perfusion of areas of lung which are poorly ventilated. If other areas of the lung are well or over ventilated, the net effect in terms of arterial gases will be hypoxaemia with a normal or low arterial P_{CO_2}.

The physiological mechanism whereby this occurs can be explained by the difference in dissociation curves for carbon dioxide and oxygen. There is an approximate linear relationship between P_aCO_2 and content such that areas of lung with high $\dot{V}_A:\dot{Q}$ ratios can correct for the hypercapnia present in areas with low $\dot{V}_A:\dot{Q}$ ratios. Hypoxaemia results from the 'shunting' of blood through poorly ventilated areas of lung. Well ventilated alveoli will have an increased P_AO_2 but because of the shape of the oxygen dissociation curve, this will have little effect in terms of oxygen saturation.

The hypoxaemia can only be corrected if oxygenation of poorly ventilated alveoli is improved by increasing the inspired oxygen concentration.

Clinical features

Central cyanosis is the cardinal sign of arterial hypoxaemia and can generally be recognized if arterial oxygen saturation is below 90 per cent (P_aO_2 8kPa). Severe cerebral hypoxia results in confusion and restless agitation progressing to stupor and coma. Minute ventilation is invariably increased and the patient is tachypnoeic. The increased drive to respiration results partly from the hypoxaemia but also from the reflex mechanism originating in the lung and airways.

The main clinical disorders in which hypoxaemic respiratory failure occurs are listed in Table 11.2. Acute interstitial and alveolar oedema usually results from left ventricular failure with an elevated pulmonary venous pressure. Patients with adult respiratory distress syndrome or 'shock lung' also have pulmonary oedema due to abnormal pulmonary capillary permeability. There are a number of potential pulmonary insults which may initiate this event although the precise mechanism has yet to be defined (see chapter 14).

Table 11.2. Clinical disorders resulting in hypoxaemic respiratory failure

Acute	Pulmonary oedema
	Pneumonia
	Asthma
	Pulmonary emboli
Chronic	Pulmonary fibrosis
	Chronic airway obstruction (see text)
	Pulmonary a-v shunts

Some patients with chronic airway obstruction (chronic bronchitis and emphysema) become hypoxaemic but are able to maintain a normal P_aCO_2. Other patients however are unable to maintain adequate alveolar ventilation and hence become hypercapnic, (combined hypoxaemic and ventilatory failure).

In the majority of patients with acute asthma, pulmonary oedema, pneumonia and pulmonary emboli, alveolar ventilation is usually increased with hypocapnia. However in extremis, hypercapnia may develop as a pre-terminal event. This may in part result from a fall in total ventilation due to increasing exhaustion of the respiratory muscles.

Management

Management of patients with hypoxaemic respiratory failure includes treatment of the underlying condition, correction of the hypoxaemia and, if possible relief of symptoms.

Specific measures directed at the primary pathology will include antibiotics, bronchodilators and diuretics. Although in most instances it is possible to make a definitive diagnosis on clinical grounds, it may on occasions be difficult to distinguish between cardiac failure, acute asthma or infective bronchitis and bronchopneumonia. A chest radiograph, electrocardiograph, white blood count and sputum examination should give further guidance and in some instances a right heart catheter with measurement of pulmonary wedge pressure will help to determine the underlying pathophysiology. However, since this is not always available, it may be necessary to institute 'blunderbuss' treatment to include all three possibilities in the acutely ill patient.

Hypoxaemia will be present to a greater or lesser extent in all the above conditions. This fact is often overlooked particularly when it is not clinically obvious but it should be remembered that oxygen requirements will be increased in febrile conditions and that oxygen delivery to the tissues is dependent on adequate haemoglobin and a normal cardiac output. Since there is no contra-indication to the administration of oxygen this can be given in relatively high concentration (40–60 per cent). The only situation in which lower concentrations are indicated is the co-existance of *chronic* lung disease and hypercapnia ($P_aCO_2 \uparrow$, $[HCO_3^-] \uparrow$).

Symptomatic relief of extreme dyspnoea can be achieved by the use of opiates and in certain disorders, eg. acute pulmonary oedema, it forms a standard part of treatment. It may also help in other conditions but its use always carries the risk of precipitating hypercapnia needing artificial ventilation.

The indications for artificial ventilation depend primarily on the severity of the respiratory failure but will be modified by the nature of the underlying disorder. Any patient admitted comatose due to severe hypoxia represents an acute emergency and will need immediate intubation and ventilation. Patients who are conscious but unable to maintain adequate arterial oxygenation despite high concentrations (60 per cent) of inspired oxygen may also require ventilation. An arterial PO_2 of below 6 kPa is potentially life-threatening so that unless a rapid improvement in the underlying condition is anticipated, ventilation should be considered. A practical problem, frequently encountered, results from the agitation and confusion in patients with severe hypoxia in that they will not tolerate using an oxygen mask. Sedation may enable additional oxygen to be administered *provided the patient can be ventilated if this fails*. A third indication for ventilation is increasing exhaustion. This can be difficult to quantitate clinically, but is partly related to the duration of the respiratory distress. The patient feels tired and the respiratory rate may fall as the respiratory muscles tire. The best objective indicator is an elevated arterial PCO_2 and in any patient with asthma, pulmonary oedema or a primary pneumonia, indicates a need for assisted ventilation. Respiratory stimulants are not appropriate for this group of patients.

When ventilating patients with asthma, two practical problems should be borne in mind. Firstly, endotracheal intubation is potentially hazardous since the patient will become hypoxic after only a brief period of apnoea. In addition, the insertion of the tube may provoke bronchospasm and except in an emergency, intubation should be performed by a competent anaesthetist. The ventilator used must be capable of producing high inflation pressures in the range of 7–10 kPa and have flexible controls in order to achieve the most appropriate pattern of ventilation in each patient. In general, it is better to use a relatively slow respiratory rate, expiration being prolonged.

In any patient with severe hypoxic respiratory failure, correction of the hypoxaemia may be difficult despite assisted ventilation. It will require high inspired concentrations of oxygen although prolonged administration of concentrations above 60 per cent should be avoided if at all possible since they are likely to cause further lung damage. The use of positive end-expiratory pressure improves arterial PO_2 by increasing functional residual capacity but has the disadvantage of reducing cardiac output. If oxygenation is difficult it is better to aim for a 'safe' rather than normal P_aO_2. The practical problems involved in the ventilation of patients with 'shock lung' are discussed in chapter 14.

Combined ventilatory and hypoxaemic respiratory failure

Patients in this category combine the pathophysiological abnormalities of the previous two groups. Ventilation perfusion abnormalities result in arterial hypoxaemia but additionally there are insufficient well ventilated alveoli to maintain a normal P_aCO_2.

Clinical features

'Combined' respiratory failure may occur as an end stage of any of the causes of hypoxaemic failure. However, it is most frequently seen in patients who have chronic airflow limitation (chronic bronchitis and emphysema). There is usually a long history of breathlessness on exertion and many such patients are chronically hypoxaemic and hypercapnic. It thus requires a relatively minor additional pulmonary insult to produce a sudden and life-threatening deterioration in gas exchange. Most frequently this results from a respiratory tract infection but it may also occur postoperatively or following inappropriate use of hypnotics or sedatives.

The clinical features are essentially those of the underlying lung disease. The patient is likely to be dyspnoeic and tachypnoeic although this does not reflect adequate alveolar ventilation because of the increased dead space. Hypercapnia may result in vasodilation with a warm periphery, bounding pulse, headaches and occasionally papilloedema. A coarse flapping tremor may also be present although these signs are unreliable and correlate poorly with blood gas tensions. The best clinical indicator of severe hypercapnia is increasing drowsiness although unconsciousness is rare. In contrast, cerebral hypoxia results in restlessness and agitation before progressing to coma. Since many patients have severe hypoxaemia and hypercapnia, clinical signs may be unreliable and make blood gas analysis essential.

In any patient with respiratory failure it is essential to obtain information as to the chronicity and severity of the underlying disease, since this will influence management and prognosis. There is obviously less potential for treatment in a patient who is a chronic respiratory cripple than in a patient with a severe infection superimposed on relatively mild chronic disease. If previous lung function or arterial gases are not available a clear history should be obtained of the patient's exercise capabilities during the weeks leading up to admission.

Management

The main aims of management are the treatment of infection, improving lung function and relieving dangerous hypoxaemia. It may include the administration of antibiotics, bronchodilators, additional inspired oxygen and respiratory stimulants as well as vigorous physiotherapy to assist expectoration. If these measures fail, assisted ventilation will have to be considered.

In a patient with acute on chronic bronchitis who has respiratory failure but who is nevertheless alert and orientated, the initial measures will consist of antibiotics, bronchodilators and physiotherapy. Most common infecting organisms are *Haemophilus influenzae* or *Strep. pneumonia* both of which should be sensitive to Ampicillin or its derivatives.

Bronchodilators in the form of a beta-stimulant, e.g. salbutamol (ventolin) or an anticholinergic, e.g. ipratropium bromide (atrovent) may produce a small increase in ventilatory capacity with some relief of dyspnoea. If given as a nebulized solution they may have the additional benefit of preventing excess drying of the bronchial mucosa and aiding expectoration. Intravenous aminophylline (250–500 mg) given as a slow injection or infusion has a bronchodilator action. It also acts as a mild respiratory stimulant and in animal studies has been shown to increase the power in fatiguing respiratory muscles.

Although the usefulness of physiotherapy has been questioned, expectoration should be encouraged in any patient with excess sputum production. In its simplest form the patient should undertake forced expirations following inhalation to total lung capacity. Some form of regular stimulation is especially important in patients who are drowsy and unco-operative.

The need for additional inspired oxygen will depend primarily on the arterial PO_2. Whilst somewhat arbitrary, a level greater than 7 kPa is relatively safe and does not require correction whereas below 6 kPa is dangerous. Complete correction of the hypoxaemia is unnecessary and likely to lead to increasing hypercapnia. The aim is therefore to administer relatively low concentrations of oxygen usually twenty-four or twenty-eight per cent to achieve a safe level of arterial oxygenation. A modest increase in P_aCO_2 is acceptable provided it does not lead to increasing drowsiness. Intermittent use of oxygen is dangerous in a severely hypoxic patient and once started should be given continuously until there is overall clinical improvement.

Respiratory stimulants have a limited therapeutic role in patients who are drowsy with severe hypercapnia ($P_aCO_2 > 10$ kPa). They can be regarded as buying time in order to treat the underlying condition. Doxapram (dopram) is the drug of choice and is given as an intravenous infusion. The dose can be titrated against the clinical state and arterial PCO_2.

If despite the above measures, the patient fails to improve and remains dangerously hypoxaemic and hypercapnic, ventilation will have to be considered. The major determinant for the use of assisted ventilation is the potential for recovery. If the underlying condition is likely to respond to treatment ventilation can be undertaken readily. If however the pattern is one of chronic and progressive respiratory failure with little potential for improvement, ventilation is inappropriate since if started it may be impossible to wean the patient off the ventilator.

Appendix 1

Arterial blood gas analysis

A number of methods exist for assessment of arterial blood gases. Mixed venous PCO_2 can be measured using the re-breathing technique of Campbell and Howell. Arterial oxygen saturation can be monitored using an ear oximeter. Recently, skin electrodes have been developed which can measure arterial gas tensions transcutaneously. Although all these methods are non-invasive they have practical limitations and analysis of an arterial blood sample is currently the method of choice.

The best sites for direct arterial puncture are the radial or brachial arteries. A small amount of local anaesthetic (1 per cent lignocaine) should be injected subcutaneously prior to arterial puncture. Ideally, the blood should be collected into a heparinized glass syringe since, unlike plastic, this is impermeable to gas diffusion. In practice, glass syringes are difficult to obtain and provided there is no long delay between collection and analysis, plastic syringes are acceptable. A 23G needle is used and should be advanced at an angle of 30° to the skin. When using glass syringes, the blood should enter the syringe under its own pressure, thus confirming it is arterial. Plastic syringes are at a disadvantage in this respect but pulsation can be seen in the tubing of a 'butterfly' needle. It is essential that the dead space of syringe and needle should be filled with heparin (5000 units/ml). Most modern arterial gas analysers require only micro-samples of blood although generally between 2–5 ml are aspirated. When the needle is removed, firm pressure should be applied to the puncture site for several minutes. The needle should be removed from the syringe, any gas bubbles present expelled and the syringe capped. The syringe should be rotated to ensure adequate mixing. If there is likely to be more than a few minutes delay before analysis, the syringe should be placed in ice. This reduces the metabolism of white blood cells.

Most modern gas analysers are fully automated and are relatively easy to use. Even so the operator should be familiar with the machine since mistakes are inconvenient and potentially costly to rectify.

Appendix 2

Oxygen administration

It is not unusual to see an oxygen mask (usually a Ventimask) dangling ineffectively beside a patient. This usually indicates a lack of thought as to whether the patient needs additional oxygen and if so what is the most appropriate way of administering it. The main factor determining the type of delivery system is whether oxygen is needed in high or low concentration. Other considerations relate to patient comfort and ease of use.

Oxygen masks can be divided into two main groups depending on their mode of action. Fixed performance devices operate on the Venturi principle. A jet of oxygen entrains air from holes around the oxygen inlet to produce a concentration which is constant and is independent of the patient's rate and depth of breathing. Variable performance devices supply a flow of oxygen which is less than the patient's minute volume. The volume of air added and thus the inspired concentration of oxygen is determined by the relationship between oxygen flow rate and the patient's ventilation. For any given flow rate as ventilation increases so oxygen concentration falls. The majority of masks operate on this principle.

The *Ventimask* is a fixed performance device available in five models giving concentrations of 24, 28, 35, 40 and 60 per cent oxygen. The lower concentrations of 24 and 28 per cent are especially useful in patients at risk of CO_2 narcosis. These concentrations are achieved at recommended flow rates of 2 and 4 l/min respectively and are within 1 per cent of predicted. With the entrained air there is a high total flow and minimal rebreathing. The 60 per cent mask requires a flow of 15 l/min of oxygen and although precise control is less necessary at this level there is considerable merit in knowing the exact concentration of oxygen being delivered.

The Ventimask is slightly heavier than most others and less comfortable to use. Like other masks operating on the Venturi principle some patients find it noisy. If it is held in the hand, performance is affected by obstruction of the air inlet thus giving a higher oxygen concentration. In common with all other masks it interferes with activities such as eating, talking and expectoration.

The *Edinburgh mask, M.C. mask* and *Hudson 'See-Thru' mask* are all examples of variable performance devices. The inspired concentration varies with the flow rate. These masks are less suitable for patients requiring low concentrations of oxygen although the Edinburgh mask has been safely used in patients with carbon dioxide retention. Oxygen flow rates of 1 or 2 l/min should achieve concentrations of less than 30 per cent whilst 'high' concentrations in the region of 40–60 per cent will require oxygen flows of 10–15 l/min.

Nasal cannulae are modern versions of the Tudor-Edwards' spectacles and deliver oxygen through twin tubes into the anterior nares. There are a number of different versions which differ in detail only. The ideal requirements are that the prongs should not project too far into the nose, the ends should be rounded to avoid mucosal irritation and oxygen is best delivered diffusely through a series of outlets rather than as a fine jet. For patient comfort and convenience, nasal cannulae are preferable to face masks although at high flow rates there may be some nasal irritation. The fractional concentration of oxygen varies with flow but flows of 1 or 2 l/min are safe in patients requiring low concentrations.

Further reading

Cotes J.E. (1979) *Lung Function*. 4th ed. Blackwell Scientific Publications, Oxford.
Cumming G. and Semple, S.J. (1980) *Disorders of the Respiratory System*. 2nd ed. pp 100–153. Blackwell Scientific Publications, Oxford.

Lane D.J.S, (1976) Respiratory failure. In Lane, D.J., (ed) *Respiratory Disease.* pp 286–314. William Heinemann Medical Books Ltd, London.

Sykes M.K., McNicol M.W. and Campbell E.J.M. (1976) *Respiratory Failure.* 2nd ed. Blackwell Scientific Publications, Oxford.

12 · Acute Severe Asthma

D. J. SHALE

Despite effective therapy and ready access to intensive therapy units, acute severe asthma remains a significant cause of death in young adults. There are about 1500 deaths per annum in the United Kingdom (Leading Article, *British Medical Journal* 1978). Surveys of community and hospital asthma deaths suggest that they could be avoided if patients, general practitioners and hospital doctors had a better appreciation of the severity of such attacks. Part of the failure to appreciate the severity of an attack of asthma is due to the difficulties posed by the definition of various forms of asthma (Luksza 1982). Terms such as status asthmaticus, continuous symptomatic asthma or chronic severe asthma, based on a failure of response to more than average treatment (Clark 1983), are of little value and lead to confusion. Luksza (1982) has proposed that acute severe asthma is associated with primary cardiovascular disturbance and as such should be separated from entities such as gradually deteriorating airways obstruction where circulatory features are absent. Acute severe asthma may occasionally occur against a background of relatively normal respiratory function, but usually there is evidence of gradually deteriorating airways obstruction for days or weeks before this (Bellamy & Collins 1979; Davis *et al.* 1980; Arnold *et al.* 1983).

Assessment of the patient with acute asthma

Acute asthma and its severity is recognized from the history and a number of reliable and easily elicited signs. The necessary history can be obtained in minutes from the patient or relatives, if need be. The required details are given in Table 12.1. Observation usually reveals the patient to be distressed, but his condition may vary from severe dyspnoea to coma. Conscious patients typically sit bracing the shoulders back with their hands on their knees or the bed side. In addition, use of accessory respiratory muscles, costal recession, over-inflation of the chest, cyanosis, tachypnoea and wheezy breathing will be noted. On examination of the patient, attention should be paid to signs known to indicate the severity of the asthma attack. These signs are confined to the cardiorespiratory system and can be rapidly checked. Tachycardia is a reliable sign of severity, which is indicated by a rate of 120 beats per minute or more, or a continuously increasing heart rate. Bradycardia is a grave sign in acute asthma and indicates extreme hypoxia. Immediate treatment is demanded as bradycardia in this setting often

Table 12.1. Essential aspects of history to be obtained from the patient or relatives

1. A past history of asthma.
2. Severity of previous acute episodes e.g. hospital admissions, ventilated or not.
3. Duration of present symptoms, both the immediate and those preceeding, and any precipitating factors.
4. Usual maintainance therapy.
5. Medication given during the present episode. Note especially parenteral methylxanthines and β_2 agonists, e.g. Ask how many puffs taken on day of admission.
6. Fluid loss, e.g. vomiting and fluid intake.

heralds cardiac asystole. Hypotension and pulsus paradoxus also indicate severity. The pulsus paradoxus of asthma is an accentuation of the normal respiratory effect on blood pressure by the large intra-thoracic pressure swings. A finding greater than 10–15 mm Hg of paradox is considered significant. On auscultation of the chest the expiratory phase will be prolonged and the classical high pitched expiratory rhonchi associated with asthma will be heard at some stage. However, in the majority of patients inspiratory and expiratory rhonchi will be heard. As the severity of airways obstruction increases, so will airflow limitation causing the chest to become quieter. Hence, a silent chest is a sign of extremely severe asthma and indicates a life-threatening state. Various grading schemes have been described, e.g. Whiston grading, which allow severity to be expressed in a series of grades based on clinical findings (Davis *et al.* 1980). These are said to reduce time spent on investigation, but in the author's experience the detailed questioning required for accurate grading is equally time consuming. The time spent assessing the patient is a matter of judgement and should be dictated by the condition of the patient.

Table 12.2 gives an outline of suggested helpful investigations. In any one case they may not all be necessary. In most cases arterial blood gas analysis and the peak expiratory flow rate (PEFR) will be required. The

Table 12.2. Suggested useful investigations in acute asthma

1. Full blood count including eosinophils.
2. Sputum – eosinophils
        – culture and bacterial sensitivities.
3. Peak expiratory flow rate or spirometry.
4. Arterial blood gas analysis.
5. Blood electrolytes and urea.
6. Chest radiograph.
7. ECG
8. Blood for viral titres.

PEFR can be obtained in seconds and is easily performed by an assisting nurse. The PEFR is a further guide to severity which is indicated by a reading of less than 120 litres/minute. Arterial blood for gas analysis should be obtained by radial or brachial artery puncture, but excessive time should not be spent obtaining arterial blood if the patient's overall condition is poor. Venous blood samples can be withdrawn at the time of insertion of an intravenous cannula. Sputum can be obtained after the patient's condition has stabilized. A chest radiograph should also wait until the patient's condition allows, unless there are good indications of a pneumothorax, which is the main finding on X-ray that would alter the management to be outlined. Generally the yield from chest radiography in asthma is poor. An electrocardiogram is not usually necessary, but should one be obtained it is important to understand its interpretation. In severe asthma an acute p pulmonale may be seen with a dominant R wave and T wave inversion in V_2–V_3 chest leads. These changes resolve on treatment of the asthma.

Management of the patient with acute asthma

On completion of the assessment of the patient an intravenous cannula should be inserted.

Bronchodilators

These should be given intravenously and by inhalation in most cases. Intravenous aminophylline or β_2 agonist (e.g. salbutamol or terbutaline) should be used. Aminophylline must be given in sufficient quantity to obtain a therapeutically effective blood level of 10–20 μg/ml. This represents an optimum therapeutic level. Levels greater than 20 μg/ml are associated with increasing incidence of toxic effects (Trembath *et al.* 1979). In most patients a level in the region of 10–20 μg/ml can be obtained by giving 5.6 mg/kg by slow intravenous injection (i.e. 250–500 mg given over ten minutes). This acts as a loading dose and should be continued with an infusion of 0.5 mg/kg body weight/hour. An approximation for a 70 kg patient is 500 mg aminophylline in 500 ml normal saline given over sixteen hours. Ideally, blood levels of aminophylline should be monitored, but this is rarely possible. Careful dosage as outlined will give adequate blood levels in a majority of patients, with few failures due to underdosage or toxic effects from overdosage. For patients already on treatment with xanthine bronchodilators the loading dose should be omitted and the infusion, if required, given at the same dosage as above. Salbutamol can be given by intravenous injection or infusion. An intravenous injection of 200 μg can be given over a five minute period or it can be infused at 5 μg per minute rising to 10 or 15 μg per minute if required. A useful regime is salbutamol 5 mg in 500 ml normal saline infused at a rate of 30 ml per hour. Johnson *et al.* (1978) and Evans *et al.* (1980) reported no advantage for salbutamol over aminophylline in acute severe asthma, and for most physicians aminophylline remains the drug of first choice. Salbutamol can be given in addition to aminophylline via a nebulizer or by intermittent positive pressure breathing (IPPB) via a Bennett or Bird machine. For adults 5 or 10 mg should be given in normal saline in a concentration of 0.5 per cent and nebulized with 35 or 40 per cent oxygen. This can be given by nursing staff immediately treatment is instituted and can be repeated four hourly. Salbutamol delivered by nebulizer has been shown to be as effective as IPPB (Campbell *et al.* 1978), which itself is as effective as the intravenously administered drug (Bloomfield *et al.* 1979).

Ward *et al.* (1981) have reported that ipratropium bromide, an anticholinergic bronchodilator, is as effective as salbutamol (10 mg) when given by nebulizer at a dose of 500 μg. A mixture of salbutamol (at doses outlined above) and ipratropium bromide (100 μg, i.e. 0.4 ml of 0.025 per cent nebulizer solution) given by nebulizer is becoming a popular mode of inhaled bronchodilator therapy in acute severe asthma.

Corticosteroids

There is continuing controversy regarding the use of corticosteroids in acute severe asthma. Luksza (1982) recently suggested that the main threat to life in severe asthma is the associated cardiovascular disturbance. This primary cardiovascular disturbance would be unaffected by corticosteroids. Following this argument Luksza (1982a) has recently reported on the treatment, with and without corticosteroids, of ninety patients with acute severe asthma. He reported no difference between the groups in their rates of recovery as measured by PEFR and heart rate changes. These findings again raise questions about the use of corticosteroids in the acute setting. The evidence for the use of corticosteroids is based on the Medical Research Council report of 1956 and is open to criticism. However, hydrocortisone is generally considered essential in acute severe asthma and as the controversy remains unresolved the following regime is still applicable. The severest cases should receive hydrocortisone hemisuccinate 200 mg intravenously and then six hourly for at least twenty-four hours. For less severe cases and after improvement on parenteral treatment, oral prednisolone is commenced at a dose of 40–60 mg per day, which can then be reduced as recovery occurs.

Oxygen

Prompt treatment with oxygen is essential to reverse the hypoxia associated with an episode of severe asthma. Correction is important as a hypoxic myocardium is more prone to arrhythmias and particularly following arrhythmogenic agents, e.g. aminophylline and β_2 agonists, given early in the treatment of asthma. If the $P_a CO_2$ is known to be elevated or for any reason considered likely to be, then 28 per cent humidified oxygen can be given via a Venturi mask (e.g. ventimask) or nasal catheter (2 to 4 litres per minute). A normal or low $P_a CO_2$ allows freedom to give higher concentrations of oxygen, i.e. 35 or 40 per cent. However, care should be exercised because $P_a CO_2$ may rise in older patients with elements of chronic bronchitis in addition to their asthma.

Antibiotics

If the asthmatic episode was precipitated by or complicated by infection then antibiotics should be given. Purulent sputum and a raised white blood cell count can be taken as an indication of infection and treatment started whilst awaiting results of sputum culture. Amoxycillin 250 mg t.i.d. or erythromycin 250 mg q.i.d., if penicillin allergic, are appropriate initial choices.

Dehydration

In severe asthma, extra fluid loss occurs and the ability to replace fluid by drinking is limited. Fluid can be replaced by a regime of normal saline (1 litre) and 10 per cent dextrose (2 litres) per twenty-four hours. This regime is suitable for most adults, but care is needed in older patients to avoid fluid overload. Potassium chloride 4 grams per twenty-four hours (53 mmol) should be included in this regime. In addition to fluid losses hypokalaemia may be induced by hydrocortisone and salbutamol therapy.

Bronchial secretions

Respiratory tract secretions are usually viscous and retained. Sputum plugging of airways is a prominent feature in the lungs of patients dying of severe asthma. Expectoration can be improved by physiotherapy, inhalation of nebulized saline and rehydration. Mucolytics are of no proven value in severe asthma and may increase the volume of secretions to the disadvantage of the patient. Rarely, bronchoscopic lavage is needed to remove tenacious secretions.

Acidosis

This arises as a primary respiratory acidosis due to CO_2 retention or as a secondary metabolic acidosis due to hypoxic metabolism. Severe acidosis is rarely a problem in adults. If blood pH falls to 7.0 or less sodium bicarbonate (1.4 per cent isotonic or 8.4 per cent hypertonic) at a dose of 2–4 mmol/kg can be infused over 30–60 minutes.

Once treatment is instituted it is essential to monitor its effectiveness. Pulse rate and PEFR are useful measurements which can easily be made at the bedside by nursing staff. The heart rate should be recorded regularly, half hourly, during the initial phase of recovery and then less frequently as the patient's condition improves. The PEFR should be checked before and after each dose of nebulized salbutamol throughout the recovery period, which should include the transition from emergency treatment to maintainance therapy. Arterial blood gas analysis should be repeated if there is a poor clinical response to treatment, evidence of CO_2 retention or continued hypoxia despite treatment. It should be remembered that there is no direct correlation between clinical condition and the degree of hypoxia or CO_2 retention. Medical and nursing staff must remember that asthmatic patients can deteriorate rapidly and that asthmatic deaths in hospital have been associated with inadequate treatment and monitoring.

Assisted ventilation

The aim of intermittent partial pressure ventilation (IPPV) is to support life until severe airways obstruction is reversed. It has the advantages of improving gas exchange and haemodynamics and allows safe drug-induced sleep. Fortunately, only a small number of asthmatics need ventilatory support. These subjects form two groups, but the indications for ventilation are the same (table 12.3). Some patients will be admitted to hospital in a moribund state and require immediate ventilation. The other group of patients are those who fail to respond to treatment, as described above, and become increasingly fatigued and develop respiratory failure. Intermittent partial pressure ventilation requires the expertise and extra care of an intensive care unit. Asthmatic patients can be difficult to ventilate due to their raised airways resistance. In view of this a low tidal flow is used, e.g.

Table 12.3. Indications for endotracheal intubation and assisted ventilation in acute severe asthma

$P_aO_2 < 6.5$ kPa and falling.
$P_aCO_2 > 6.5$ kPa and increasing.
Arterial pH < 7.2 and falling

Hypotension–systolic blood pressure less than 90 mm Hg.
Intolerable respiratory distress.
Cardiorespiratory arrest.

6–7 ml/kg, as large tidal volumes will further increase the over-inflation of the lungs. A low breath frequency, e.g. twelve breaths per minute, is used to allow time for adequate airflow during expiration. This will rapidly reverse hypoxaemia but may not increase alveolar ventilation and hence reduce P_aCO_2. This situation can be improved by bronchial lavage which should only be used in the setting of an intensive care unit. Lavage will remove mucous plugs improving ventilation and airways resistance and reduce the period of IPPV needed. During mechanical IPPV the tidal volume can be increased gradually as the airways resistance falls. As ventilation is improved the P_aCO_2 will fall and this should produce a normal or low P_aCO_2 over 24–48 hours. Usually IPPV is necessary for 48–72 hours and the patient can be easily removed from the ventilator. During this, standard treatment is continued and the patient converted to maintenance therapy when appropriate.

Conversion to maintenance therapy should be based on the condition of the patient and improvements in PEFR. It may be possible to convert to oral prednisolone and slow release aminophylline between twenty-four and seventy-two hours after admission in patients not requiring ventilation. The author usually continues nebulized salbutamol whilst the need for oral slow release aminophylline or β_2 agonist is assessed and oral steroid doses are reduced. Changes should always be monitored clinically and with PEFR measurements. If the asthma deteriorates after changes in therapy then the rate of change should be modified using PEFR measurements as a guide. This approach allows morning dipping to be controlled and the right balance of maintainance therapy to be obtained. Inhaled corticosteroids (beclomethasone, betamethasone or budesonide) should be started when oral prednisolone is at 10 mg/day. This phase of recovery is an ideal time to ensure that the patient and his relatives understand his disorder and its implications. Details of therapy should be explained, particularly the role of bronchodilators versus that of prophylactic treatments like sodium chromoglycate and inhaled corticosteroids. The patient's ability to effectively use inhalers should be checked and new patients should be taught their proper use. It is of great importance to explain to the patient when medical help should be sought; e.g. bronchospasm occurring in the setting of a respiratory infection, increasing nocturnal disturbance whilst normal therapy is maintained and increasing bronchospasm unresponsive to bronchodilators in any setting. A small number of 'brittle' asthmatics should be able to refer themselves to specialized units and their relatives instructed in the basics of cardiorespiratory resuscitation. Some of this group may also need a supply of injectable bronchodilator (e.g. adrenalin, terbutaline or salbutamol) at home and they and their relatives should be instructed in its use.

Even with the use of measures described, there are still deaths due to asthma and little evidence that they are reducing nationally. As noted already, some deaths could be avoided if patients and their doctors were more aware of the severity of an asthma attack. An awareness of the development of acute asthma is important in this respect. A few patients will experience sudden deterioration of their asthma and may rapidly die before treatment can be given. However, most patients will probably have a phase of gradual deterioration preceding the severe episode. Bellamy & Collins (1979) reviewed forty-four patients and found a mean period of five weeks deterioration before the severe episode and Davis *et al.* (1980) noted deteriorating asthma for at least fourteen days before the severe episode. If Luksza (1982) is correct, this prodromal phase of deterioration is the time when vigorous use of corticosteroids would be most effective. Judicious use of steroids at this time may halt further deterioration to severe asthma when they may be of little direct value (Luksza 1982a). In surveys of deaths occurring in and out of hospital, Cochrane & Clark (1975), Macdonald *et al.* (1976), Macdonald *et al.* (1976a), Bateman & Clark (1979), Ormerod & Stableforth (1980) and the BTA (1982) found that under-use of corticosteroids, inadequate initial assessment and failure to objectively and regularly monitor the effects of treatment were probable extra contributory factors.

Clearly, careful attention to diagnosis, assessment of severity and adequate treatment including ventilation when required will help to reduce those avoidable asthma deaths. Further, it is essential that patients are told about their asthma, their medication and about the indicators of deterioration of their asthma. The value of this approach has been reported by Davis *et al.* (1980) who carefully educated their asthmatic patients and provided easy access to medical advice. In their three hundred patients over a ten year period there was one death and only two patients required ventilation as they had vigorously dealt with asthma at an early stage of deterioration. It is possible that this type of preventative care of the asthmatic patient will reduce the incidence of acute severe asthma and therefore asthma deaths.

Further reading

Arnold A.G., Lane D.J. and Zapata E. (1983) Current therapeutic practice in the management of acute severe asthma. *British Journal of Diseases of the Chest* 77, 123–135.

Bateman J.R.M. and Clarke S.W. (1979) Sudden death in asthma. *Thorax* 34, 40–44.

Bellamy D. and Collins J.V. (1979) Acute asthma in adults. *Thorax* 34, 36–39.

Bloomfield P., Carmichael J., Petrie G.R., Jewell N.P. and Crompton G.K. (1979) Comparison of salbutamol given intravenously and by intermittent positive-pressure breathing in life-threatening asthma. *British Medical Journal* 1, 848–850.

British Thoracic Association, BTA (1982). Death from asthma in two regions of England. *British Medical Journal* 285, 1251–1255.

Campbell I.A., Hill A., Middleton H., Momen M. and Prescott R.J. (1978) Intermittent positive-pressure breathing. *British Medical Journal* 1, 1186.

Clark T.J.H. (1983) Acute severe asthma. In Clark T.J.H. and Godfrey S. (eds) *Asthma,* pp. 393–414. Chapman and Hall, London.

Cochrane G.M. and Clark T.J.H. (1975) A survey of asthma mortality in patients between ages 35 and 64 in Greater London hospitals in 1971. *Thorax* **30**, 300–305.

Davis B., Gett P.M., and Jones E.S. (1980) A service for the adult asthmatic. *Thorax* **35**, 111–113.

Evans W.V., Monie R.D.H., Crimmins J., and Seaton A. (1980) Aminophylline, salbutamol and combined intravenous infusions in acute severe asthma. *British Journal of Diseases of the Chest* **74**, 385–389.

Johnson A.J., Spiro S.G., Pidgeon J., Bateman S. and Clarke S.W. (1978) Intravenous infusion of salbutamol in severe acute asthma. *British Medical Journal* **1**, 1013–1015.

Leading Article (1978) Management of severe acute asthma *British Medical Journal* **1**, 873–874.

Luksza A.R. (1982) A new look at adult asthma. *British Journal of Diseases of the Chest* **76**, 11–14.

Luksza A.R. (1982a) Acute severe asthma treated without steroids. *British Journal of Diseases of the Chest* **76**, 15–19.

Macdonald J.B., Seaton A. and Williams D.A. (1976) Asthma deaths in Cardiff 1963–74: 90 deaths outside hospital. *British Medical Journal* **1**, 1493–1495.

Macdonald J.B., Macdonald E.T., Seaton A. and Williams D.A. (1976a). Asthma deaths in Cardiff 1963–74: 53 deaths in hospital. *British Medical Journal* **2**, 721–723.

Medical Research Council (1956) Cortisone acetate in status asthmaticus. *Lancet* **2**, 803.

Ormerod L.P. and Stableforth D.E. (1980) Asthma mortality in Birmingham 1974–7: 53 deaths. *British Medical Journal* **1**, 687–690.

Trembath P.W., Boobis S.W. and Richens A. (1979) Theophylline: Biochemical pharmacology and pharmacokinetics. *Journal of International Medical Research* **7**, 4–15.

Ward M.J., Fenthem P.H., Roderick-Smith W.H. and Davies D. (1981) Ipratropium bromide in acute asthma. *British Medical Journal* **282**, 598–600.

13 · Pneumonia

A. G. ARNOLD

In pathological terms pneumonia is an illness in which there is an inflammatory reaction in the lower respiratory tract. The cellular exudate of neutrophils, red blood cells and macrophages in the alveolar spaces results in a non-aerated portion of lung that is relatively radio-opaque and an abnormal chest X-ray. This is most often a response to an infecting organism, usually bacterial and less commonly a virus or organism such as Mycoplasma or Coxiella. Non-infective causes are infrequent and include 'allergic' (e.g. pulmonary eosinophilia) or 'physical' causes (e.g. irritant gases, inhalation, irradiation). Neoplasia can mimic pneumonia, as in lymphangitis carcinomatosa.

Clinical classification is usually on the basis of the aetiological agent involved, or on the radiological distribution of consolidation, but is difficult because of the low specificity of either method. Not only might a certain organism such as *Streptococcus pneumoniae* (pneumococcus) cause anything from a classical lobar pneumonia to bronchopneumonia, but there may be a variability in the clinical manifestation of the disease from a fairly well patient to one who is moribund. This variability depends to some extent on host factors. Accurate classification is often a retrospective exercise and is less important than the prompt initiation of appropriate antibiotic therapy, based on clinical judgement. When assessing a patient with acute dyspnoea three important questions need to be answered before an antibiotic is chosen (Fig. 13.1):

1. Is this pneumonia? The usual symptoms are of a cough (that may or may not be productive), dyspnoea, malaise, fever and pleuritic chest pain. All or none of these symptoms may be present and the time course can vary from a few hours to several weeks. The presentation may be particularly obscure in the elderly, where pneumonia may lead to recent loss of mobility or confusion, so that a high index of suspicion is required. General features include pyrexia, tachypnoea and buccal herpes infection. A localized reduction of chest wall movement can occur, with inspiratory crackles, or bronchial breathing and whispering pectoriloquy, and possibly a pleural friction rub. Physical signs can be entirely absent. A chest X-ray will usually confirm the diagnosis and may suggest the type of pneumonia (Fig. 13.2), but it can be normal early in the illness.

2. Is there pre-existing lung disease? A distinction between primary pneumonia, when there is no pre-existing pulmonary disease, and secondary

STAGE I~Presentation.

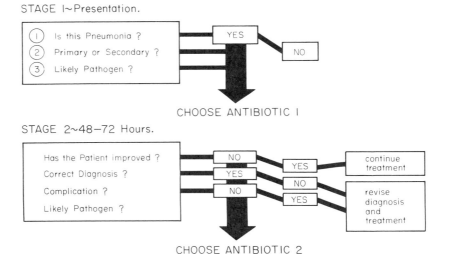

CHOOSE ANTIBIOTIC I

STAGE 2~48–72 Hours.

CHOOSE ANTIBIOTIC 2

Fig. 13.1. Flow diagram of management decisions.

pneumonia, when pulmonary conditions such as bronchiectasis or chronic obstructive lung disease already exist, is useful. Not only does this provide some guide to the likely pathogen, but it significantly affects the general management.

3. What is the most likely pathogen? The choice of initial antibiotic depends on this assessment, and since substantial bacteriological evidence only becomes available much later, the decision becomes a matter of clinical and radiological judgement. An immediate Gram stain of the sputum will sometimes suggest the likely pathogen. If a patient has a primary lobar pneumonia it is likely to be due to the pneumococcus, but if that patient has already failed to respond to ampicillin from his general practitioner the pathogen is more likely to be *Staphylococcus aureus* or *Klebsiella* species. Another example would be a young adult presenting with a relatively long history and marked constitutional symptoms, when a non-bacterial cause might be suspected. The provisional diagnosis is therefore based on the 'best fit', taking into account the usual clinical picture of each pathogen, as detailed later.

Investigations—stage I (Fig. 13.1)

(a) Non-bacterial. Chest X-ray, full blood count with differential white cell count and ESR, blood gas analysis, urea and electrolytes, first of paired sera and cold agglutinins. The second serum sample for antibody titres should be sent after ten days.

(b) Bacteriological. *Sputum culture.* Meaningful results are more likely if the doctor personally supervises the collection of a good sputum sample, rather than leaving the task to the most junior nurse, when the laboratory will often receive a sample of saliva. Ideally, the sample should be taken before antibiotics are given. If there are problems in obtaining a good sample then physiotherapy may help, as may laryngeal stimulation or the use of an intermittent positive pressure breathing (IPPB) device. Sputum should always be examined for tubercle bacilli.

Blood culture. This ought to be regarded as a routine and undertaken as early as possible without waiting for a spike of fever.

Pleural fluid culture. When arranged early in a pneumonic illness this can yield the pathogen. Repeated diagnostic aspiration is indicated if empyema is suspected.

General management

The management of severe pneumonia was considered by Harvey (1982). The following considerations are important.

1. Hydration. Insensible fluid losses are high because of pyrexia and tachypnoea. Therefore an intravenous infusion may be required.

2. Analgesia. Severe pleurisy must be countered since ventilation and expectoration are hindered. If mild analgesics are not adequate then it is entirely reasonable to use morphine, *providing* that there is no evidence of carbon dioxide retention or of chronic obstructive lung disease.

3. Oxygen. The physiological consequence of pneumonia is hypoxaemia due to ventilation/perfusion mismatch, and central cyanosis is not unusual. Initially, the area of consolidation is perfused but not ventilated. However, hypoxic vasoconstriction then leads to local redistribution of pulmonary blood flow to minimize the shunt. Increased ventilation does not improve the hypoxaemia significantly but may result in some lowering of the arterial $P\text{CO}_2$. Type I respiratory failure (without elevation of $P\text{CO}_2$) requires treatment with continuous inspired oxygen at a concentration of up to 60 per

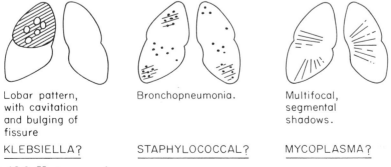

Lobar pattern, with cavitation and bulging of fissure
KLEBSIELLA?

Bronchopneumonia.

STAPHYLOCOCCAL?

Multifocal, segmental shadows.

MYCOPLASMA?

Fig. 13.2. X-ray examples.

cent, using masks such as the MC type. An elevated arterial P_{CO_2} (Type 2 respiratory failure) is seen in secondary pneumonias complicating, for example, chronic obstructive lung disease, or at a late stage of a pneumonic illness when the patient is tiring. The exhausted patient sometimes requires artificial ventilation. Type 2 respiratory failure is treated with continuous low dose oxygen (24–28 per cent) using a Ventimask, or nasal speculae delivering between one and three litres per minute; repeated blood gas estimations are required.

4. Physiotherapy.

5. Bronchodilators. These are likely to be necessary in cases of secondary pneumonia, with continued observations of an objective measure of air flow obstruction, such as peak flow rate or the forced expiratory volume in one second (FEV_1). For most patients a β_2-adrenergic bronchodilator is indicated, with delivery via a simple nebulizer.

6. Antibiotics. These should be commenced as soon as possible; for ill patients they should be given parenterally during the early stages.

Reassessment—stage 2 (Fig. 13.1)

Continual observation is required after treatment has been started. If the patient has failed to respond after 48–72 hours, by which time full bacteriological data should be available, then reassessment is indicated. Failure to respond may be because either the original diagnosis was incorrect (Table 13.1), or a complication has developed (Table 13.2), or the unidentified

Table 13.1. Differential diagnosis

1 Pulmonary emboli.
2 Bronchial neoplasm.
3 Tuberculosis.
4 Bronchopulmonary aspergillosis.
5 Foreign body.

pathogen is being treated inappropriately. The antibiotic often needs to be changed at this point and the base-line investigations repeated. The following additional investigations can help:

(a) Fibre-optic bronchoscopy. By this means lavage, suction and brush specimens can be obtained directly from the area of consolidation, with transbronchial biopsies if necessary. Bronchoscopy is particularly useful when a proximal obstructing bronchial neoplasm or foreign body is suspected. There are two problems with this technique in these circumstances. Bacterial contamination can occur as the specimen is retrieved through the suction channel, and some local anaesthetics used in the procedure may inhibit growth of the pathogen.

Table 13.2. Complications

1 Pulmonary abscess
2 Empyema
3 Pneumothorax
4 Septicaemia · meningitis · endocarditis · peritonitis · septic arthritis
5 Respiratory, circulatory or renal failure
6 DVT
7 Pleural effusion

(b) Trans-tracheal aspiration. A fine gauge needle is inserted through the cricothyroid membrane into the trachea. Local anaesthetic is not necessary. A sputum sample can be aspirated after the insertion of 2 ml of sterile saline, and is usually free of upper respiratory tract contaminants. This technique is relatively free of complications.

(c) Direct lung puncture. This is most useful when the X-rays reveal a peripheral area of consolidation. Under local anaesthesia, with X-ray screening, a fine gauge needle can be used to aspirate a few ml of fluid. There is some risk of a pneumothorax.

Bacterial pneumonias

The following examples of pneumonias are not exhaustive and exclude many of the less common types, as well as tuberculosis. More information may be obtained from Crofton and Douglas (1981).

Pneumococcal pneumonia *(Streptococcus pneumoniae)*

This is the commonest bacterial pneumonia seen in hospitals in this country (White *et al.* 1981). It can complicate influenza, or other upper respiratory tract viral illnesses. Immuno-compromised hosts (e.g. post splenectomy patients) are vulnerable but most cases occur in normal subjects. The classical symptoms are described earlier and the history is often as short as a few hours. Although the sputum is typically 'rusty' in colour it may be clearly blood-stained. In addition to the usual physical signs the spleen is occasionally palpable and jaundice can occur. A chest X-ray will characteristically show unifocal consolidation of a lobe, or part of a lobe, but other patterns occur, particularly if the pneumonia is superimposed upon chronic obstructive lung disease. Gram staining of the sputum may show Gram-positive diplococci in large numbers but this will be affected by prior use of antibiotics. A moderate neutrophil leucocytosis $(12-15,000/mm^3)$ and moderate elevation of the ESR (50–100 mm) is common. Benzylpenicillin (parenterally) is the antibiotic of choice because it is bactericidal and the pneumococci are highly susceptible. The spectrum of action is more narrow than ampicillin or amoxycillin, causing less disturbance of the normal bacterial gut flora. Nevertheless, many clinicians now use ampicillin or amoxycillin because they can be given orally and are well absorbed. amoxycillin is better absorbed than ampicillin and produces higher levels in sputum, particularly when sputum purulence clears (Stewart *et al.* 1974). It is usual to continue antibiotics for three days after the temperature has fallen, and for at least seven days.

Staphylococcal pneumonia *(Staph. aureus)*

This organism can cause either a lobar pneumonia or a bronchopneumonia. There is a marked tendency to cause tissue destruction and thin-walled abscess formation. The abscesses may rupture, especially in children, leading to pyopneumothorax. Cases are seen more frequently during influenza epidemics and are then a major cause of mortality. A patchy secondary bronchopneumonia is common, particularly amongst hospital acquired infections. Gram stains of the sputum show Gram-positive cocci in clusters. The majority of strains of staphylococci are resistant to benzyl-penicillin, due to their production of beta-lactamases, so that a penicillinase resistant penicillin like Flucloxacillin is chosen (Table 13.3). The development of a potent beta-lactamase inhibitor, clavulanic acid, has led to the introduction of a combined oral preparation with amoxycillin that may prove valuable.

Klebsiella pneumonia *(Kl. pneumoniae)*

This relatively rare pneumonia often affects the ill and the elderly, and is associated with a high mortality (20–50 per cent) and morbidity. There is a predilection for upper lobes and the typical early appearance is of a lobar consolidation with bulging down of the adjacent fissure. The consolidation may be bilateral. Chronicity is a helpful clinical pointer towards the diagnosis and cavitation and empyema tend to occur. Over many months chronic fibrocavitatory disease can develop with a risk of septic complications (e.g. meningitis). Sputum production is a prominent feature and the sputum is often blood-stained, mimicking tuberculosis. The mainstay of treatment used to be chloramphenicol or streptomycin, but they have been superseded by gentamicin and third generation cephalosporins, such as cefotaxime (Davies 1982).

Haemophilus pneumonia *(H. influenzae)*

Haemophilus is most often seen in secondary pneumonias and particularly

Table 13.3. Antibiotics.

Pathogen	1st line choice	2nd line choice
Strep. pneumoniae	Penicillin, Ampicillin	Erythromycin
Staph. aureus	Flucloxacillin	Na. fusidate+Lincomycin
Kleb. pneumoniae	Gentamicin*	Cefotaxime
H. influenzae	Ampicillin	Tetracycline
Other Gm.-ve organisms		
· aerobic–Gentamicin* (+Azlocillin for Pseudomonas)		
· anaerobic–Metronidazole		
M. pneumoniae	Tetracycline	Erythromycin
Coxiella burneti	Tetracycline	Erythromycin
Chlamydia psittaci	Tetracycline	Erythromycin
Legionella pneumophila	Erythromycin+Rifampicin	

*Gentamicin may soon be replaced by more modern aminoglycosides, such as Netilmicin (Davies 1982)

complicates bronchiectasis and chronic obstructive lung disease. The expected pattern is a bronchopneumonia, which can be part of a mixed infection, usually accompanying the pneumococcus. Gram-negative pleo-morphic cocco-bacilli are seen in the sputum. Ampicillin or amoxycillin are the drugs of first choice in the treatment of Haemophilus.

Other Gram-negative organisms

These are characteristically seen in ill hospitalized patients, often after a previous course of antibiotics. Those with urinary tract infections are especially vulnerable. The chest X-ray would be expected to show a pre-dominantly basal bronchopneumonia. Care is needed in the interpretation of sputum cultures; not infrequently, Gram-negative organisms are isolated due to contamination with oral flora or due to overgrowth related to anti-biotic therapy. Pathogenicity is suspected if the clinical condition of the patient is deteriorating, and can be confirmed by isolation from the blood or pleural fluid. *Pseudomonas* infections may follow the use of nebulizers or ventilators, since this organism thrives in moist conditions. Whereas most Gram-negative aerobic infections respond to gentamicin, azlocillin or piperacillin must be added if *Pseudomonas* infection is suspected. Ceftazidime is a recent useful alternative. Metronidazole is effective in treating anaerobic infections.

Non-bacterial pneumonias

Mycoplasma pneumonia *(M. pneumoniae)* (Alexander *et al.* 1966)

Neither a bacterium nor a virus, mycoplasmas are one of the smallest of known free living organisms. The younger age-group of patient is often involved. Characteristically, cases are seen in epidemics but about half of the cases are sporadic. Serological tests reveal that many cases go unrecognized. A recent study showed this type of pneumonia in 15 per cent of hospital cases (White *et al.* 1981). Symptomatic patients may have marked constitutional symptoms that can last several weeks, with upper respiratory tract features as well as a cough. Skin rashes, otitis media, an arthropathy, or a haemolytic anaemia may complicate the illness. Several neurological complications have been recorded that include cranial nerve palsies, aseptic meningitis and transverse myelitis. The radiological appearances are very variable. Lobar consolidation can be seen, as can an effusion, but a multifocal consolidation is more usual. The wide extent of radiological consolidation is often out of proportion to the scant physical signs found on clinical examination. Often the serum from affected patients has the ability to agglutinate human Group O red blood cells at low temperatures. These 'cold agglutinins' are seen in up to two thirds of cases, and are virtually diagnostic since they are infrequently seen in other types of infection and they may be present before specific antibodies can be detected. The diagnosis is confirmed by a rising antibody titre. Treatment is with tetracycline for between ten and fourteen days.

Q fever *(Coxiella burneti)* (Marmion and Stoker 1958)

The disease was first described in Queensland, Australia, before the causative organism was identified—hence Q, for query. Cows and sheep provide the reservoir for infection. Infected animals can excrete the organism in milk, but this is not a common route of infection unless unpasteurized milk has been consumed. Human infection usually follows contact with infected straw or hides and dust-laden air, and outbreaks have been reported in abattoir workers. There are no clinically distinctive features and the illness normally lasts up to three weeks. There is also a chronic form of infection that tends to be associated with endocarditis, abnormal liver function tests and thrombocytopenia. Diagnosis is by rising titres of complement-fixing antibodies, and treatment is with tetracycline. A typical chest X-ray appearance is of multiple segmental or sub-segmental lesions.

Ornithosis *(Chlamydia psittaci)* (Anderson and Bridgewater 1968)

This disease was initially termed psittacosis when the infection was thought to involve psittacine birds alone (e.g. parrots), but it is now appreciated that infection can follow contact with non-psittacine birds such as pigeons, budgerigars and ducks. Routine serological testing shows that mild and sub-clinical infections can occur. A history of avian contact is obtained in only about 50 per cent of cases. The bird involved need not appear to be sick since it can be a chronic carrier of the organism. Now it is accepted that infection occurs in other domestic animals (cattle, sheep, cats) and human-to-human transmission may occur. There is a spectrum of severity but patients tend to be more ill than with mycoplasma infection, and some cases are fatal. A high fever and headaches are usual. Cough need not be prominent and there is no specific pattern of radiological consolidation. Rose spots, erythema nodosum, encephalitis, or hepatosplenomegaly may complicate the picture. Again, the diagnosis is established by a rising antibody titre; tetracycline is the antibiotic of choice.

Legionnaire's disease *(Legionella pneumophila)* (Hutchinson 1981)

Recognition of this condition has only come in recent years. In part the delay has been due to the fastidious growth requirements of the organism, which is one of a group of flagellate motile Gram-negative rods. Now the organism can be cultured and serological tests have been developed. It can survive for over a year in water, at optimal temperatures, and this may be related to ingestion by amoebae. Common source outbreaks have often involved air-conditioning systems, or other water systems; infection is thought to have occurred by inhalation of an aerosol of organisms. Male patients and smokers seem to be predisposed to this illness and it also occurs in immuno-compromised hosts, where the organism assumes an opportunistic role. Legionnaire's disease should not be considered unduly rare and only 25 per cent of cases seen in this country have been infected abroad. It should be distinguished from Pontiac fever, also due to *Legionella* sp., which is a milder non-pneumonic illness.

In a typical patient the symptoms evolve over about five days as a high fever gradually develops. Most of the early symptoms are non-specific, but headache is prominent and diarrhoea is a feature in at least a third of patients. The respiratory symptoms are of a dry cough, dyspnoea and often a pleuritic pain. By the time that the patient is admitted to hospital he is likely to be very ill and confused. On examination the patient may be dehydrated and can exhibit meningism. Auscultation of the chest reveals coarse crackles, bronchial breathing, or a friction rub but on occasions minimal signs. Chest X-rays may show a diffuse bronchopneumonia but more often there is lobar consolidation of at least one area. This consolidation resolves very slowly, over two to three months, which often raises the question of an underlying bronchial neoplasm. Laboratory results show a lymphopenia, perhaps a thrombocytopenia and an elevated ESR. Hyponatraemia, elevation of the blood urea and abnormal liver function tests are clues as to the diagnosis. Demonstration of the organism by immunofluorescence has been achieved. This is beyond the scope of most hospital laboratories but is usually available in regional reference laboratories, as is serological testing. IgM specific antibody is usually detectable by the tenth day of illness, but can be greatly delayed, so that appropriate antibiotics must be given on the basis of a strong clinical suspicion. The patients are often so ill that they require early ventilatory support and intravenous fluid replacement. Erythromycin (2–4 g daily, iv) is probably the best single antibiotic, but it is wise to combine this with Rifampicin (Table 13.3). Despite intensive management the mortality rate is between 20 and 40 per cent.

Pneumonia in immuno-compromised patients

This is becoming an increasingly common problem as more patients are treated with drugs that impair the immune mechanisms and as organ transplantation occurs more often. Shadowing on the chest X-ray does not necessarily indicate pneumonia in such patients as it can be due to drugs, irradiation, pulmonary lymphoma, intrapulmonary haemorrhage or pulmonary oedema. When a pneumonia is present it is often due to the common bacterial pathogens which will respond to broad-spectrum antibiotics. Tuberculosis must enter the differential diagnosis. Full diagnostic tests should be arranged at Stage 1 (Fig. 13.1) rather than Stage 2. If there is no early response to treatment then opportunistic infections must be seriously considered. An open lung biopsy is sometimes necessary to resolve the problem. The commonest opportunistic infections are those due to *Pneumocystis carinii, Candida* sp., *Aspergillus fumigatus* and viruses such as cytomegalovirus or herpes simplex. *Pneumocystis* infections are treated with high doses of co-trimoxazole. Sometimes this treatment has to be given without confirmation of the diagnosis, which is only possible with direct examination of lung tissue or of bronchoscopic material. Systemic fungal infections are treated with amphotericin B, alone or in combination with 5-fluorocytosine. The latter can be given orally, as can ketoconazole, which is currently under evaluation. Cytomegalovirus infection often co-exists with *Pneumocystis* infection. The treatment of viral pneumonia is essentially supportive.

Non-infective pneumonias

These pneumonias are much less common than bacterial pneumonias. The presence of an excess of eosinophils in the blood or sputum should alert the clinician to the possibility of pulmonary eosinophilia. The commonest cause of this condition in Britain is bronchopulmonary aspergillosis. An asthmatic history is usual. The diagnosis is supported by the isolation of mycelial elements in the sputum, a positive immediate skin prick test, positive serum precipitins and a rapid response to steroid therapy. Simple pulmonary eosinophilia (Löffler's syndrome) causes mild symptoms, transient chest X-ray infiltrates and a slight eosinophilia. It is usually caused by drugs when seen in Britain. Chronic pulmonary eosinophilia (CEP) presents with a very ill patient, a high eosinophil count and a chest X-ray with dense peripheral areas of consolidation. There is a prompt response to steroid therapy but there is a tendency to relapse. Polyarteritis nodosa is a rare cause of pulmonary eosinophilia. The lung is involved in about one third of cases of polyarteritis and there is usually evidence of multisystem involvement.

Probably the commonest form of 'physical' pneumonia is that due to aspiration/inhalation. The presentation may be cryptic and often without gastro-intestinal symptoms. Particular clues are the presence of a nocturnal cough and multifocal areas of consolidation and fibrosis on the chest X-ray. Barium studies will demonstrate the underlying cause (e.g. achalasia). The immediate treatment is steroid therapy and prophylactic broad-spectrum antibiotics. Surgery may be necessary at a later date to correct the underlying lesion. The treatment of other forms of 'physical' pneumonia is similar, with steroid therapy and oxygen in the first instance. Occasionally antibiotics and mechanical ventilation are required.

Further reading

Alexander E.R., Fog H.M., Kenny G.E., Kronmal R.A., McMahan R., Clarke E.R., Macoll W.A. and Grayston J.T. (1966) Pneumonia due to Mycoplasma pneumoniae. *New England Journal of Medicine* **275**, 131–136.

Anderson J.P. and Bridgewater F.A.J. (1968) Ornithosis in a chest clinic practice. *British Journal of Diseases of the Chest* **62**, 155–166.

Crofton J. and Douglas A. (1981) *Respiratory Diseases*, 3rd ed. Blackwell Scientific Publications, Oxford.

Davies A.J. (1982) New antimicrobials. *British Journal of Hospital Medicine* **27**, 136–142.

Harvey J. (1982) Severe pneumonia. *British Journal of Hospital Medicine* **27**, 278–285.

Hutchinson D.N. (1981) Legionnaires Disease. *Hospital Update.*, November, 1129–1146.

Marmion B.P. and Stoker M.G.P. (1958) The epidemiology of Q fever in Great Britain: an analysis of the findings and some conclusions. *British Medical Journal* **2**, 809–816.

Stewart S.M., Anderson I.M.E., Jones G.R. and Calder M.A. (1974) Amoxycillin levels in sputum, serum and saliva. *Thorax* **29**, 110–114.

White R.J., Blainey A.D., Harrison K.J. and Clarke S.K.R. (1981) Causes of pneumonia presenting to a district general hospital. *Thorax* **36**, 566–570.

14 · Adult Respiratory Distress Syndrome (ARDS)

A. FISHER

The development and accessibility of improved resuscitative techniques during the last two decades, associated with the technical and pharmacological ability to support failing body systems in the early stages of disease, has improved the survival of critically ill patients. It is now recognized that catastrophic respiratory failure associated with pulmonary oedema of non-cardiogenic origin frequently occurs in the critically ill following a large and ever increasing number of initiating clinical disorders of both pulmonary and non-pulmonary origin. In 1967 Ashbaugh *et al.* introduced the term 'adult respiratory distress syndrome' to replace the many synonyms (such as traumatic wet lung or congestive atelectasis) previously used to describe this respiratory failure. However, this term omits reference to the many precipitating disorders listed in Table 14.1. Why such a diverse galaxy of diseases should have the lung as a common target organ and produce a syndrome of uniform clinical, radiological, physiological and pathological features is only now becoming clear as the pathogenesis of the disorder becomes better understood. A single aetiological cause is often difficult to identify and usually the syndrome is associated with multiple clinical disorders, the most common being hypovolaemic shock, sepsis, trauma and aspiration (Petty 1982).

Incidence and mortality

It is not possible to give an accurate incidence in the United Kingdom for this disorder, but extrapolating data from the Division of Lung Disease Task Force (Lung Program 1972) in the USA about 40,000 to 50,000 cases would occur annually. The mortality remains depressingly high and in most published series is between fifty and sixty per cent (Petty and Newman 1978). Failure to respond to the use of positive end expiratory pressure, the presence of sepsis or associated renal failure adversely affects the prognosis.

Clinical features

Gas exchange

Tachypnoea and hypoxaemia are the cardinal features of the syndrome when it is established but there is often a deceptively encouraging period of

12–48 hours between the initiating event and the fully developed disorder, during which the patient appears to be haemodynamically stable with no overt respiratory distress. However, it is possible that serial blood gas analysis at this time would reveal subclinical hypoxaemia in spite of a normal chest X-ray and dry lung fields on auscultation. Clinically there is no hint of the imminent disastrous deterioration in pulmonary function nor, as yet, any routine laboratory or respiratory investigation that might predict the change. As the disease becomes established, increasingly high concentrations of oxygen are required to maintain adequate oxygenation until a P_aO_2 in excess of 6.7 kPa cannot be achieved and ventilatory support becomes mandatory. The cause of this hypoxaemia is threefold:

Impaired diffusion

Thickening of the alveolar capillary septum produces a restriction in the diffusing capacity. Oxygen transfer is further impaired by a reduction in pulmonary capillary volume and an increased cardiac output decreasing the red blood cell transit time (Lamy *et al.* 1976).

Ventilation perfusion (V_A/Q) mismatch

Interstitial and peribronchial oedema produce narrowing of the small airways with less ventilation of normally perfused alveoli. This reduced but finite V/Q ratio is found particularly in the dependent lung zones.

True shunt

Alveolar atelectasis and alveolar flooding result in perfusion of completely non-ventilated lung units and up to sixty per cent of the cardiac output may be shunted without oxygenation through the lungs.

The relative contribution of each of these mechanisms is difficult to assess but the main cause of the hypoxaemia is undoubtedly true shunting of blood through the non-ventilated alveoli and the corner-stone in the management rests with reversing this defect. In the early stages of the disease, carbon dioxide is eliminated efficiently and sometimes excessively (especially if there is pain) producing a respiratory alkalosis and hypocarbia. However, during the later stages, embolization of the pulmonary microcirculation can reduce perfusion of certain lung units producing relatively high V/Q ratios, an increase in dead space volume with impaired CO_2 elimination and a respiratory acidosis. Often, at this critical stage, the acidosis is compounded by a metabolic element produced by hypoxaemia and tissue hypoperfusion.

Lung compliance

Stiff non-compliant lungs requiring increasingly high inflation pressures to maintain adequate alveolar ventilation are a consistent finding and the resulting high intrathoracic pressures can lead to complications such as pneumothorax or reduced cardiac output. The main determinants of compliance are lung volumes, tissue elasticity and alveolar surface tension. All lung volumes are reduced in ARDS, and there is increased elastic recoil. However, surfactant abnormalities leading to alveolar instability and micro-atelectasis probably produce the major change in lung compliance (Petty *et al.* 1982).

Pathogenesis

One common feature in ARDS, whether the initiating cause is mediated via the circulation or the airways, is an increase in lung water caused by a disturbance in the normal fluid flux between the intravascular and extra-vascular compartments in the lungs. The factors governing transvascular fluid filtration are related in the Starling equation:

$$F = K(P_{cap} - P_{is}) - \theta(\Pi_{cap} - \Pi_{is})$$

Where F = net filtration rate, K = filtration coefficient, P_{cap} and P_{is} the capillary and interstitual hydrostatic pressures, Π_{cap} and Π_{is} the capillary and interstitial protein osmotic pressures and θ the protein reflection coefficient. Thus, fluid transfer in the lung is influenced by capillary permeability, hydrostatic pressure difference and oncotic pressure difference. Normally, the outward transcapillary hydrostatic gradient slightly exceeds the inward transcapillary oncotic pressure gradient producing a continuous flow of water and solutes removed by the lymphatics.

Lung water

Methods of estimating lung water include measurement of electrical impedence, thermal dilution techniques, nuclear imaging methods and external radioflux detection, but they are limited by complex methodology, complicated apparatus and variation in accuracy (Staub and Hogg 1980). A preliminary study using the differential absorption through an intact chest wall of two photo peaks emitted by 123 iodine albumin indicates the following values for lung water (in ml/cm^3 lung) in normal patients and patients with ARDS (Lee *et al.* 1982):

	Normal	*ARDS*
Plasma	7.5±1.5	8.1±2.4
Interstitial	7.4±1.4	16.7±3.9

The sequence in the pathogenesis of ARDS is thus:

Initiating event → increased interstitial water → over-loaded lymphatic drainage → alveolar flooding → intrapulmonary shunting → hypoxaemia. In an attempt to identify the defect producing the increased lung water which is at first confined to the interstitial compartment, the variables of Starling's equation have been investigated.

Plasma oncotic pressure and lymph drainage

Trauma and acute illness can lead to a reduction in plasma protein concentration often compounded by crystalloid infusions (Skillman *et al.* 1970). It has been suggested that this may produce interstitial and pulmonary oedema but as there is an accompanying interstitial loss of oncotically active material, the transcapillary gradient is preserved (Staub 1974). Raised intrathoracic pressures have been shown to reduce lymph flow in sheep but this is unlikely to play a primary role in the genesis of ARDS in the human.

Pulmonary capillary permeability and hydrostatic pressure (Fig. 14.1)

Although stress evoked stimulation of the sympathetic nervous system in the critically ill will produce pulmonary venoconstriction, emphasis is moving away from neurohumoral mechanisms in the pathogenesis of ARDS. Evidence is accumulating that embolization by circulating blood constituents with release of vasoactive materials produces permeability and hydrostatic changes in the pulmonary microcirculation (Ogletree and Brigham 1980).

Complement activation

Many clinical causes of ARDS, such as endotoxaemia, trauma and pulmonary infection also activate the complement cascade (Craddock *et al.* 1977). Vaso-active products (termed anaphylatoxins) of the third, fourth and fifth components can increase smooth muscle contraction, vascular permeability and histamine release. In addition, the peptide fragment C5a released via the alternate pathway is a chemo-attractant for polymorpholeucocytes (PML) producing aggregation and non-uniform embolization in the pulmonary microcirculation. Pulmonary capillary hypertension with increased transvascular filtration is produced in the exchanging vessels. However, the change in pulmonary capillary permeability following endothelial cell damage is probably more important. This is caused by the release of proteinases destroying structural proteins (such as collagen, elastin or fibronectin) and also by toxic oxygen radicals. Proteinases may also cleave fibrinogen and the Hageman factor, predisposing to intravascular coagul-

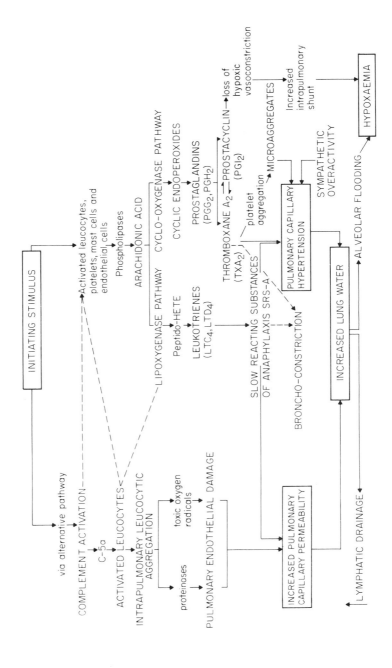

Fig. 4.1. Pathogenesis of adult respiratory distress syndrome.

Table 14.1. Disorders associated with ARDS

1.	Hypovolaemic shock	
2.	Infection	(a) Pulmonary (microbial, fungal, pneumocystis) (b) Extrapulmonary (septicaemia)
3.	Trauma	(a) Thoracic (b) Extrathoracic
4.	Embolism	(a) Fat (b) Amniotic fluid (c) Cellular aggregates

5.	Inhalation	(a) Gas (i) irritant (e.g. nitric oxide, smoke)
		          (ii) non-irritant (e.g. oxygen)
		(b) Liquid (i) gastric juice
		          (ii) fresh and salt water

6.	Haematological	(a) Disseminated intravascular coagulopathy (b) Massive blood transfusion
7.	Metabolic	(a) Diabetic ketosis (b) Uraemia
8.	Neurogenic	(a) Cerebral oedema (b) Intracranial haemorrhage
9.	Drugs	Including heroin, aspirin, propoxyphene, barbiturates
10.	Others	(a) Pancreatitis (b) High altitude

ation. Moreover, depletion of the plasma opsonin fibronectin impairs the phagocytic action of the reticolo-endothelial system leading to further embolization of the pulmonary microcirculation by platelets, PMLs and products of intravascular coagulation (Scovill *et al.* 1976). Thus PML-mediated and coagulation-mediated mechanisms produce micro-embolization, endothelial cell damage and permeability changes in the pulmonary circulation in ARDS, while release of vaso-active substances such as histamine, serotonin and prostaglandins further influence permeability and pulmonary vascular resistance.

Arachidonic acid metabolism

The products of arachidonic acid metabolism have a remarkable spectrum of biological activity and there is direct and indirect evidence linking these products with pulmonary dysfunction. Following release from cell membrane phospholipids in the lung by activated platelets, mast-cells, leucocytes and complement dependent mechanisms, arachidonic acid is metabolized by two pathways producing two functionally active groups of substances, the prostaglandins (PG) and the leukotrienes (LT).

The cyclo-oxygenase pathway converts arachidonic acid to the labile endoperoxidases, prostaglandins PG G_2 and PG H_2 which are further metabolized into a host of vaso-active products, the most important being prostacyclin (PGI_2) and thromboxane (TXA_2). Present studies indicate that PGI_2 has the capacity to dilate the constricted pulmonary vascular bed, prevent intrapulmonary platelet aggregation and dilate narrowed airways. Thromboxane elicits severe pulmonary hypertension by directly constricting the vascular bed and mechanically obstructing the microcirculation with platelet aggregates. A disturbance in the normally balanced metabolism of arachidonic acid in favour of TXA_2 production, increases pulmonary capillary hydrostatic pressure and disrupts the Starling equilibrium (Hyman *et al.* 1980). Increased prostacyclin production may increase intrapulmonary shunting and hypoxaemia by preventing the normal hypoxic pulmonary vasoconstriction (Gerber *et al.* 1980).

The alternative lipoxygenase pathway of arachidonic acid metabolism produces several groups of metabolites, depending on the source of the lipoxygenase enzyme (Valone *et al.* 1980). Leucocytes possess the enzyme responsible for producing 5-hydroperoxyeicosa tetranoic acid (5, HPETE) which is the precursor of a family of peptido-HETEs termed leucotrienes. Not only are these extremely powerful vasoconstrictors (Dahen *et al.* 1980), but two (LTC4 and LTD4) are the main constituents of the slow-reacting substance of anaphylaxis (SRS-A) which has been shown to increase capillary permeability in peripheral vascular beds.

The pathogenesis of ARDS is thus extremely complex and in parts speculative. It involves the interaction of immune, coagulation and biochemical responses and, although end stage manifestations are similar with differing aetiologies, the pathological pathway may vary according to the specific aetiology. A schematic representation of the pathogenesis is given in Fig. 14.1.

Diagnosis and management (Tables 14.2 and 14.3)

Early supportive and pharmacological therapy favourably influence the prognosis in ARDS (Schmidt *et al.* 1976). However, prediction of patients at risk is difficult. The indices of pulmonary gas exchange and pulmonary compliance are not sufficiently sensitive to detect early interstitial oedema. They become abnormal only when alveolar flooding occurs. Changes in lung volumes, particularly FRC, and closing volumes do occur earlier but are not applicable to bedside monitoring. Although it is not yet known if early pulmonary capillary permeability changes are gradual or abrupt, non-invasive methods of measuring lung water using, for example, radioisotope-labelled albumin, may prove useful in screening patients. Perhaps the most promising means of identifying incipient ARDS is by C5a assays, high levels of which have been positively associated with the development of ARDS (Hammerschmidt *et al.* 1980).

Table 14.2. Diagnosis

Clinical	
	Hypoxaemia
	Tachypnoea
	Recognized initiating event
Physiological	
	$P_aO_2 < 6.7$ kPa with $FIO_2 > 0.6$
	Reduced overall compliance (< 30 ml/cm)
	Increased shunt fraction (Qs/Qt > 15 per cent)
	Normal or increased cardiac output
Radiological	
	Diffuse bilateral pulmonary infiltrates
	Sparing of apices and costophrenic angles
	Normal cardiac size
	Pruning and beading of pulmonary arterioles on balloon-occluded segmental pulmonary angiogram
Exclusions	
	Left ventricular failure
	Chronic pulmonary disease

The diagnosis (Table 14.2) is made partly by clinical, radiological and blood gas findings. Tachypnoea, hypoxaemia and similar X-ray changes make the differentiation from cardiogenic pulmonary oedema difficult. However, ARDS should be suspected if acute respiratory failure ($P_aO_2 < 6.7$ kPa breathing 60 per cent O_2) occurs in association with one of the precipitating causes listed in Table 14.1, and if the circulation is hyper-dynamic with normal or only slightly raised pulmonary capillary wedge and central venous pressures. Blood gas analysis may often reveal evidence of hypoxaemia and increased intrapulmonary shunting before the classical X-ray appearance of ARDS develops.

The aim of the management of patients with ARDS is to support all body systems until the integrity of the alveolar-capillary membrane is restored.

Table 14.3. Management of ARDS

Respiratory	
	Oxygen uptake
	Intermittent positive pressure ventilation
	Positive end expiratory pressure
	Membrane oxygenation
	High frequency ventilation
	Low frequency ventilation and CO_2 removal
	Oxygen delivery
	Maintain oxygen content
	Maintain cardiac output
	Oxygen availability
	Maintain normal dissociation curve
	Oxygen demand
	Control with analgesia and sedation
Fluid balance	
	Maintain normovolaemia
	Monitor pulmonary capillary wedge pressure
	Oncotic pressure
	Osmolarity
Antibiotics	
	Daily screening
Corticosteroids	
	Early administration
Parenteral Feeding	
	Preserve nitrogen balance

Maintenance of oxygenation

Intermittent positive pressure ventilation

Only in mild cases can a P_aO_2 of > 6.7 kPa be sustained using controlled oxygen-enriched air delivered by a face mask. Endotracheal intubation and mechanical ventilation is usually necessary. A volume pre-set ventilator delivering a large tidal volume (10–15 ml/kg), with a slow inspiratory phase and prolonged expiratory pause produces the most efficient gas exchange.

If satisfactory oxygenation cannot be achieved with a non-toxic (< 0.5 per cent) fractional inspired oxygen concentration (FIO_2), other methods of improving gas exchange must be sought.

Positive end expiratory pressure (PEEP)

There is evidence that PEEP can exert a prophylactic as well as a therapeutic role in the management of ARDS. The effect is to decrease intrapulmonary shunting by recruitment and opening up of lung units previously unavailable for gas exchange and to enhance further oxygenation by increasing FRC (Ashbaugh and Petty 1973). The compliance of the lung may also be improved by the increase in lung volume and by surfactant conservation (Wyszogrodski *et al.* 1975). However, the benefits are limited by cardiac output changes and the dangers of barotrauma, such as pneumothorax, pneumomediastinum and surgical emphysema. Although positive end expiratory pressures between 5 and 10 cm H_2O are unlikely to lower cardiac output, more precise information of oxygen transport can be obtained by either thermodilation cardiac output measurements or assessment of mixed venous oxygen content ($C\bar{v}O_2$) changes. Assuming a fixed oxygen uptake, a fall in $C\bar{v}O_2$ would indicate a reduction in oxygen delivery attributable to a decreased cardiac output. Another practical method of obtaining optimum PEEP is to correlate pulmonary compliance and oxygen delivery (Suter *et al.* 1975). Incremental increases (3 cm H_2O) in PEEP are made until no further improvement in static compliance (tidal volume/peak inspiratory pressure-PEEP) is obtained. 'Super' levels of PEEP in excess of twenty-five cm of water with inotropic support of the heart have been advocated but the obvious dangers impose limitations on its use.

Tracheostomy

The use of large volume/low pressure cuffed endotracheal or nasotracheal tubes with scrupulous aseptic technique during suctioning considerably lessens the incidence of tracheal stenosis and post-extubation degluttition problems. Thus, early tracheostomy is reserved for patients with flail segments following chest trauma and patients in whom efficient suctioning and tracheal toilet is impossible through an endotracheal tube.

Asynchronous independent lung ventilation (AILV)

This technique attempts to obtain optimum respiratory function from each lung independently (Hillman and Barber 1980). Each limb of the double lumen endobronchial tube is connected to a separate ventilator, thus allowing ventilatory indices, respiratory gas concentrations and positive end-expiratory pressure to be varied independently.

Occasionally, the ARDS predominantly affects one lung. Conventional IPPV in these patients may preferentially inflate the more compliant lung with the risk of causing a pneumothorax and PEEP may divert blood from the better to the more diseased lung, thus increasing the V/Q mismatch. By selectively delivering a calculated tidal volume to each lung, more effective distribution of ventilation can be obtained. Furthermore, by delivering a low FIO_2 to preserve pulmonary vasoconstriction and raising the mean intra-alveolar pressure with PEEP, blood may be diverted from the diseased lung with improved perfusion of the better lung.

Although the concept of AILV is attractive, in practice it demands a high degree of nursing care to preserve accurate tube placement and the duration is limited by the risk of trauma to the bronchial tree.

High frequency ventilation (HFV)

It is now well established that satisfactory gas exchange can be maintained by high frequency ventilation using volumes considerably less than the 'dead space' (Bohn *et al.* 1980). A broad division can be made into high frequency jet ventilation at frequencies of 1–10 Hz and high frequency oscillation at frequencies up to 40 Hz. The physical principles applied to explain this physiologically surprising phenomenon invoke the enhancement of convection and accelerated diffusion of gas molecules but have yet to be fully explained (Slutsky *et al.* 1980). Specially designed ventilators with negligible compressible volumes delivering pulses of oxygen enriched air (at frequencies ranging from 1–40 Hz) achieve adequate alveolar ventilation and arterial oxygenation at low intratracheal and transpulmonary pressures with reflex inhibition of spontaneous respiratory drive. The risks of barotrauma are thus lessened and both pulmonary and systemic circulations are unaffected. However, in clinical use, the place of HFV in the management of ARDS has yet to be established and the assessment of variables such as pressure, pressure flow amplitude, waveform and frequency is limited by measurement technology.

Membrane gas exchange

Advances in extracorporeal oxygenation for open heart surgery led to the hope that, by diverting a proportion of the cardiac output through a membrane oxygenator, the lungs of patients with ARDS would have time to recover while oxygenation and perfusion of the vital organs was maintained. However, the results of a prospective multi-centre trial of extracorporeal membrane oxygenation (ECMO) were disappointing (Zapol and Snider 1980). Recently more attention has been paid to low frequency ventilation with CO_2 removal (Gattinoni *et al.* 1980). This method utilizes a large area membrane lung with low blood flow (1–1.5 l/min) to remove CO_2, maintain normocapnia and reduce respiratory drive. Transpulmonary oxygen uptake is maintained by the use of a carinal catheter delivering 200–300 ml of oxygen per minute. The low intra-alveolar tension, low ventilatory rate (3/min) and low inflation pressures avoid the adverse iatrogenic effects of conventional IPPV. Further experience is required before the place of LFV with CO_2 R in the respiratory management of ARDS is established.

Augmentation of oxygen availability

The availability of oxygen to the tissues is influenced not only by the arterial content but also by the cardiac output and the position of the dissociation curve. To obtain optimum oxygen transport, anaemia should be corrected by transfused filtered fresh blood and the cardiac output augmented by inotropic support. Oxygen availability at the tissue level is improved if leftward shifts of the oxyhaemoglobin dissociation curve produced by decreases in 2,3-DPG and alkalosis, are avoided. The role of hypothermia is controversial. It increases dissolved oxygen and reduces oxygen uptake but the reduction may reflect the leftward shift of the oxyhaemoglobin dissociation curve and hence a decreased availability rather than a decreased demand.

Weaning from ventilators

During conventional IPPV with PEEP, the FIO_2 is lowered in stages as the patient's gas exchange improves until it is less than 0.5. PEEP can then be reduced in increments of 2–4 cm of water according to satisfactory blood gas analysis. At this stage in the patient's recovery, intermittent mandatory ventilation (IMV) may be introduced. This divides the work load of ventilation between the patient and the ventilator by reducing, in a controlled manner, the number of ventilator cycles. Spontaneous breathing increasingly takes over to maintain oxygenation until ventilatory support is unnecessary. An alternative method of weaning patients from ventilators is to substitute short periods of spontaneous ventilation starting with five minutes every hour and gradually increasing their duration according to the patient's progress.

Oxygen toxicity

It is paradoxical that oxygen therapy, although fundamental in the management of ARDS, carries the risk of tissue damage. This toxicity was first suggested by Smith in 1899 but it was not until 1970 that it was conclusively demonstrated in man by Barber. It is the alveolar oxygen tension (P_AO_2) and not the arterial oxygen tension (P_aO_2) that is responsible for the toxicity but the precise FIO_2 at which this occurs depends on a large number of variables, such as duration of exposure, previous exposure, age, weight and endocrine status of the patient (Deneke and Fanburg 1980). Thus a maximum safe FIO_2 cannot be accurately predicted but oxygen concentrations of less than 0.5 can be tolerated for extended periods without deleterious effects. Investigations also suggest that 100 per cent oxygen is safe at sea level for between twenty-four and forty-eight hours, although tracheitis might develop within six hours. In the long term, the harmful effects of oxygen concentrations above 0.5 are time related.

The mechanism of oxygen toxicity is specific cell damage caused by free oxygen radicals (superoxide radical, hydrogen peroxide, hydroxyl radical and singlet excited oxygen) overwhelming the normal anti-oxidant defence mechanisms, such as superoxide dimutase, producing enzyme inactivation and nucleic acid damage (Deneke and Fanburg 1980). Although a time-related fibrogenic effect of high inspired oxygen concentrations has been demonstrated, total resolution is possible if the initial damage is not overwhelming.

Corticosteroids

Despite many retrospective and prospective clinical trials, controversy continues to surround the use of high dose corticosteroids in the prevention and management of septic shock and ARDS (Ledingham and McArdle 1978). However, a recent comprehensive review of the literature suggests that early use is indicated (Nicholson 1982). Their demonstrated ability to stabilize lysosomal membranes, depress lysosomal enzyme release, restore reticulo-endothelial function and clear 'myocardial depressant substance' are all potentially favourable. Moreover, the evidence that some cases of ARDS may result from complement-induced pulmonary leucostasis and the accompanying endothelial cell damage provoked by oxygen radicals has suggested another mechanism. High dose corticosteroids (30 mg/kg methyl-prednisolone six hourly for forty-eight hours) inhibit C5a activation, leuco-cytic aggregation and superoxide production, thus protecting the capillary endothelium.

Antibiotics

The role of infection in the aetiology and prognosis of ARDS cannot be over-emphasized. Nearly all patients dying of ARDS have either a pulmonary or extrapulmonary focus of infection. A recent ultra-structure analysis of the alveolar capillary barrier in patients dying of trauma or shock revealed that most of the pulmonary capillary lesions appeared to be the consequence of systemic or local pulmonary infection. Strict aseptic suctioning techniques must be adopted and sterility of ventilators ensured. Intensive efforts must be made to identify micro-organisms by daily monitoring of tracheobronchial secretions and blood cultures, early identification allowing the appropriate antibiotic regime to be adopted. Until culture and sensitivity results are available, broad spectrum coverage should be extended to most patients.

Fluid management

The pathogenesis of ARDS has a direct bearing on the fluid management of the critically ill patient, particularly in the early resuscitative phase. The hydrostatic, oncotic and permeability determinants of the starting equilibrium all influence the amount and type of fluid used.

There is unanimous opinion that the initial therapeutic goal must be restoration of circulating blood volume to prevent the possible development of ARDS and acute tubular necrosis, but the type of fluid recommended is controversial. The dilemma exists because it is not known at which stage in the genesis of ARDS the pulmonary capillary leak occurs, nor if it is a sudden or gradual process. The clinical significance is whether early infused colloid solutions remain within the pulmonary vascular bed with improved plasma volume, or leak into the interstitium abolishing the transcapillary oncotic gradient (Weaver *et al.* 1978). When the pulmonary capillary leak becomes established, even large molecules pass into the interstitium and the protein content of tracheobronchial aspirates may approach that of plasma (Brigham 1979). Several prospective randomized studies have demonstrated significant advantages in administering colloid solutions to critically ill patients (Boutros *et al.* 1979; Jelenko *et al.* 1979). Therefore, it would seem reasonable to correct a low plasma oncotic pressure particularly as pulmonary oedema can be produced at normal or low left atrial pressures in the presence of hypo-albuminaemia. The choice of 25 per cent albumin, 5 per cent plasma protein fraction, single donor plasma or large molecule synthetic solutions such as dextrans, Haemaccel or hydroxyethyl starches, depends on many factors, such as speed of availability, anaphylaxis, cost and compatibility with subsequent blood cross-match. The ability of Dextran 70 to decrease fibrinolysis inhibition particularly following trauma (Modig and Saldeen 1981) indicates a potential place in the preventive management of the ARDS and filtered fresh whole blood has obvious advantages in terms of oxygen carriage but is not always readily available. The volume of fluid infused is also critical. The avoidance of fluid overload while maintaining efficient pulmonary and systemic perfusion demands careful monitoring. Central venous pressure measurements do not accurately reflect pulmonary capillary hydrostatic pressures or pulmonary perfusion (Beck *et al.* 1975). A flow directed Swan–Ganz balloon catheter measuring the pulmonary wedge pressure (PCWP) is of great benefit in assessing the haemodynamic status of the patient but if levels of PEEP greater than 10 mm Hg are used, the measured wedge pressure may over-estimate the left atrial pressure. By maintaining a PCWP within the range of 8–12 mm Hg a guide to the rate and volume of infused fluid is obtained while sequential measurements of plasma oncotic pressure and haematocrit will enable the type of fluid to be more precisely selected. The use of restricted fluid intake and diuretic therapy to induce hypovolaemia and lower PCWP is open to question as impaired oxygenation and organ perfusion may adversely effect the final outcome. The interdependence of biventricular function must be remembered. Right ventricular failure, secondary to increased pulmonary vascular resistance, will restrict left ventricular forward flow and may also produce left ventricular compression by a leftward shift of the interventricular septum.

In such instances, the pharmacological reduction of the pulmonary vascular resistance with vasoactive drugs such as glyceryl trinitrate or prostacyclin might be considered, but the loss of protective hypoxic pulmonary vasoconstriction can increase V/Q mismatch with a decrease in P_aO_2. More recently it has been suggested (Richardson *et al.* 1984) that ultra filtration is more efficient than diuresis in treating pulmonary oedema and, by controlling pulmonary hypertension with prostacyclin infusion, adequate cardiac output can be maintained in spite of diminished blood volume.

Implications of pathogenesis in therapy

The better understanding of the pathogenesis of ARDS suggests various therapeutic methods in the management.

The depletion of plasma fibronectin by proteinases can be overcome by infusing agents such as Damazol with known anti-proteinase activity, or a fibronectin-rich cryoprecipitate. Beta-amino-propionitrile (an inhibitor of collagen cross-linking) and structural analogues of proline have been used successfully in animals as anti-fibrotic agents to decrease collagen deposition, although their role in man has yet to be assessed.

Aspirin and non-steroidal anti-inflammatory drugs block the conversion of arachidonic acid to both the vasoconstrictor TXA_2 and the vasodilator PGI_2 and also tend to shift the metabolism to the leukotriene pathway. Corticosteroids, on the other hand, inhibit cyclo-oxygenase and lipoxygenase pathways by selectively stabilizing cell membranes and preventing the release of arachidonic acid.

Pulmonary capillary hypertension may be treated with drugs such as sodium nitroprusside or ketanserin (an anti-serotonin agent) but the use of imidazoles to inhibit TXA_2 production is still unproven.

Outcome

The fate of patients surviving ARDS has received considerable attention (Yahav *et al.* 1978). There is a high and unchanging mortality usually associated with severe interstitial and intra-alveolar fibrosis. The early fibrotic response, possibly due to acutely impaired pulmonary endothelial and epithelial cells failing to inhibit fibroblasts is reversible (Simpson *et al.*

1978). Improvement in lung function can occur for up to six months and, although minor impairment of gas exchange is common, only one-third of survivors have a permanent reduction in vital capacity or restriction in air flow (Elliott *et al.* 1981). The quality of life of survivors thus justifies the demanding and expensive care necessary in their management.

Further reading

Ashbaugh D.G., Bigelow D.B., Petty T.L. and Levine B.E. (1967) Acute respiratory distress in adults. *Lancet* **11**, 319–323.

Ashbaugh D.G. and Petty T.L. (1973) Positive end expiratory pressure: physiology, indications and contra-indications. *Journal of Thoracic and Cardiovascular Surgery* **65**, 165–70.

Baek S.M., Makabali G.C., Bryan-Brown C.W., Kusek J.M. and Shoemaker W.C. (1975) Plasma expansion in surgical patients with high central venous pressure (CVP); the relationship of blood volume to haematocrit, CVP, pulmonary wedge pressure and cardiorespiratory changes. *Surgery* **78**, 304–315.

Barber R.E., Lee J. and Hamilton W.K. (1970) Oxygen toxicity in man; a prospective study in patients with brain damage. *New England Journal of Medicine* **283**, 1478–84.

Bohn D.J., Miyasaka K., Marchak B.E., Thompson W.K., Froese A.B. and Bryan A.C. (1980) Ventilation by high frequency oscillation. *Journal of Applied Physiology* **48**, 710–716.

Boutros A.R., Ruess R., Oslon L., Hoyt J.L. and Baker W.H. (1979) Comparison of hemodynamic, pulmonary and renal effects of use of three types of fluids after major surgical procedures on the abdominal aorta. *Critical Care Medicine* **7**, 9–13.

Brigham K. (1979) Pulmonary oedema—cardiac and non-cardiac. *American Journal of Surgery* **138**, 361–367.

Craddock P.R., Fehr J., Brigham K.L., Kronenberg R.S. and Jacob H.S. (1977) Complement and leukocyte—mediated pulmonary dysfunction in hemodialysis. *New England Journal of Medicine* **296**, 769–774.

Deneke S.M. and Fanburg B.L. (1980) Normobaric oxygen toxicity of the lung. *New England Journal of Medicine* **303**, 76–86.

Dahén S.E., Hedqvist P., Hammarström S. and Samuelsson B. (1980) Leukotrienes are potent constrictors of human bronchi. *Nature* **288**, 484–486.

Elliott C.G., Morris A.H. and Cengiz M. (1981) Pulmonary function and exercise gas exchange in survivors of adult respiratory distress syndrome. *American Review of Respiratory Disease* **123**, 492–55.

Gattinoni L., Agostoni A., Presenti A., Pelizzola A., Rossi G.P., Langer M., Vesconi S., Uziel L., Fox U., Longoni F., Kolobow T. and Damia G. (1980) Treatment of acute respiratory failure with low frequency positive–pressure ventilation and extracorporeal CO_2 removal. *Lancet* **11**, 292–294.

Gerber J., Voelkel N., Nies A., McMurty I. and Reeves J. (1980) Moderation of hypoxic vasoconstriction by infused arachidonic acid: role of PGI_2. *Journal of Applied Physiology* **49**, 107–112.

Hammerschmidt D.E., Weaver L.J., Hudson L.D., Craddock P.R. and Jacob H.S. (1980) Association of complement activation and elevated plasma—C5a with adult respiratory distress syndrome. Pathophysiologic relevance and possible prognostic value. *Lancet* **1**, 947–949.

Hillman K.M. and Barber J.D. (1980) Asynchronous independent lung ventilation (AILV). *Critical Care Medicine* **8**, 390–395.

Hyman A.L., Spannhake E.W. and Kadowitz P.J. (1980) Divergent responses to arachidonic acid in the feline pulmonary vascular bed. *American Journal of Physiology* **239**, H40–H46.

Jacob H.S., Craddock P.R., Hammerschmidt D.E. and Moldon C.F. (1980) Complement-induced granulocyte aggregation: an unexpected mechanism of disease. *New England Journal of Medicine* **302**, 789–794.

Jelenko C. III, Williams J.B., Sheeler M.L., Callaway B.D., Fackler V.K., Albers C.A. and Barger A.A. (1979) Studies in shock and resuscitation, 1: use of a hypertonic, albumin-containing fluid demand regime (HALFD) in resuscitation. A physiologically appropriate method. *Critical Care Medicine* **7**, 157–167.

Lamy M., Fallat R.J., Koeniger E., Dietrich H.-P., Ratliff J.L., Everhart R.C., Tucker H.J. and Hill J.D. (1976) Pathology and mechanisms of hypoxemia in adult respiratory distress syndrome. *American Review of Respiratory Disease* **114**, 267–284.

Ledingham I.M. and McArdle C.S. (1978) Prospective study of the treatment of septic shock. *Lancet* **1**, 1194–1197.

Lee G. de J., Chapel H., Husseim A., Kanazawa M., Loyd J. and Scott M. (1982) Pulmonary oedema due to increased lung capillary permeability. *Quarterly Journal of Medicine* **51**, 502.

Lung Program, National Heart and Lung Institute. *Respiratory diseases: task force on problems, research approaches, needs.* Washington D.C.: Government Printing Office, 1972, 171. (DHEW Publication no. (NIH) 73–432.)

Modig J. and Saldeen T. (1981) Some aspects of the etiology and treatment of adult respiratory distress syndrome. *Critical Care Medicine* **9**, 148.

Nicholson D.P. (1982) Glucocorticoids in the treatment of shock and the adult respiratory distress syndrome. *Clinics in Chest Medicine* **3**, 121–132.

Ogletree M. and Brigham K. (1980) Arachidonate increases pulmonary vascular resistance without changing lung vascular permeability in unanaesthetized sheep. *Journal of Applied Physiology* **48**, 581–586.

Petty T.L. (1982) Adult respiratory distress syndrome: Definition and historical perspective. *Clinics in Chest Medicine* **3**, 3–7.

Petty T.L. and Newman J.N. (1978) Adult respiratory distress syndrome. *Western Journal of Medicine* **128**, 399–407.

Petty T.L., Silvers G.W. and Paul G.W. (1982) Further surfactant observations in the respiratory distress syndrome. *American Review of Respiratory Disease.*

Richardson A., Wells F.C. and Branthwaite M.A. (1984) Use of prostacyclin and ultrafiltration in adult respiratory distress syndrome. *Intensive Care Medicine* **10**, 107–109.

Schmidt G.B., O'Neill W.W., Kit B.K., Hwang K.K., Bennet E.J. and Bombeck C.T. (1976) Continuous positive airway pressure in the prophylaxis of the adult respiratory distress syndrome. *Surgery, Gynecology and Obstetrics* **143**, 613–618.

Scovill W.A., Saba T.M., Kaplan J.E., Bernard H. and Powers S. Jr. (1976) Deficits in reticulo-endothelial humoral control mechanisms in patients after trauma. *Journal of Trauma* **16**, 898–904.

Shoemaker W.C., Appel P., Czer L.S.C., Bland R., Schwarz S. and Hopkins J. (1980) Pathogenesis of respiratory failure (ARDS) after hemorrhage and trauma. *Critical Care Medicine* **8**, 504–512.

Simpson D.L., Goodman M., Spector S.L. and Petty T.L. (1978) Long-term follow-up and bronchial reactivity in survivors of the adult respiratory distress syndrome. *American Review of Respiratory Disease* **117**, 449–454.

Skillman J.J., Parikh B.M. and Tanenbaum B.J. (1970) Pulmonary arteriovenous admixture: improvement with albumin and diuresis. *American Journal of Surgery* **119**, 440–447.

Slutsky A.S., Drazen J.M., Ingram R.H. Jr., Kamm R.D., Shapiro A.H., Fredberg J.J., Loring S.H. and Lehr J. (1980) Effective pulmonary ventilation with small volume oscillations at high frequency. *Science* **209**, 609–611.

Smith J.L. (1899) The pathological effects due to increase of oxygen tension in the air breathed. *Journal of Physiology* **24**, 19–35.

Staub N.C. and Hogg J.C. (1980) Conference report of a workshop on the measurement of lung water. *Critical Care Medicine* **8**, 752–759.

Staub N.C. (1974) 'State of the Art' review: Pathogenesis of pulmonary edema. *American Review of Respiratory Disease* **109**, 358–372.

Suter P.M., Fairly H.B. and Isenberg M.D. (1975) Optimum end-expiratory pressure in patients with acute pulmonary failure. *New England Journal of Medicine* **292**, 284–289.

Valone F.H., Franklin M., Sun F.F. and Goetal E.J. (1980) Alveolar macrophage lipoxygenase products of arachidonic acid: Isolation and recognition as the predominant constituents of the neutrophil chemotactic activity elaborated by alveolar macrophages. *Cellular Immunology* **54**, 390–401.

Weaver D.W., Legerwood A.M., Lucas C.E., Higgins R., Bouwman D.L. and Johnson S.D. (1978) Pulmonary effects of albumin in resuscitation for severe hypovolaemic shock. *Archives of Surgery* **113**, 387–391.

Wyszogrodski I., Kyei-Aboagye K., Taeusch H.W. Jr. and Avery M.E. (1975) Surfactant inactivation by hyperventilation: conservation by end-expiratory pressure. *Journal of Applied Physiology* **38**, 461–466.

Yahav J., Lieberman P. and Molho M. (1978) Pulmonary function following the adult respiratory distress syndrome. *Chest* **74**, 247–250.

Zapol W.M. and Snider M.T. (1980) Editorial: Membrane lungs for acute respiratory failure: current status. *American Review of Respiratory Disease* **121**, 907–909.

15 · Pneumothorax

T. W. EVANS

The term pneumothorax defines a condition in which air is present outside the lung tissue but within the pleural cavity and is one of the commonest respiratory emergencies encountered in the accident room of any general hospital. As the clinical consequences of this problem may be catastrophic, the importance of early diagnosis and appropriate management cannot be over-estimated. This can only occur if a high level of diagnostic suspicion is maintained, arising from an appreciation of the wide variety of pulmonary disease that may be complicated by pneumothorax.

Classification

The terminology used in textbooks to classify pneumothorax is frequently vague and imprecise. The importance of an organized approach to the subject must be emphasized. Traditionally the terms 'spontaneous' and 'tension' have been used to classify pneumothorax. Unfortunately, there has been frequent misuse of the former division to include all pneumothoraces

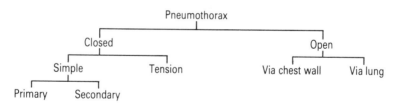

Fig. 15.1. Classification of pneumothorax (from: Thompson D.T. (1981). Pneumothorax reconsidered. *South African Medical Journal* **59**, 377–381). Definition of terms:

1. Open pneumothorax: Open communication between the pleural space and the exterior
2. Closed pneumothorax: Communication through which air has entered the pleural space is closed off
3. Tension pneumothorax: The hole in the lung or chest wall is covered by a flap of tissue that acts as a ball valve allowing air to enter the pleural space during expiration causing a progressive rise in intrapleural pressure
4. Simple pneumothorax: A closed pneumothorax with no tension changes which may complicate pre-existing lung pathology (secondary), or occur apparently spontaneously (primary)

not of the tension type. This is misleading, as in a large proportion of cases underlying pathology can be found, and the only truly 'spontaneous' pneumothorax occurs in a defined group of patients discussed in more detail below. This disparity of terms has led to a new classification by Thompson (1981) which divides closed pneumothoraces into 'tension' and 'simple' types. The latter category is further sub-divided into primary and secondary pneumothoraces according to the presence or absence of underlying lung pathology. This classification, illustrated in Fig. 15.1, not only provides an excellent framework for considering, or discussing, aetiology but also accords tension pneumothorax a leading and separate category. This is more than justified in view of the serious clinical consequences that may accrue from its going unrecognized.

Pathophysiology and functional disturbance

Within the thoracic cavity the lung occupies more than twice the volume that it would if exposed to the atmosphere. This tendency to collapse is just balanced by the tendency of the chest wall to recoil in the opposite direction. The chest wall: lung interface is lined by a double thickness of moist pleura which permits easy movement of the lungs on the chest wall but resists a separation of the two. There is consequently a negative pressure in this potential space which varies in health between -2.5 mm Hg and -6.0 mm Hg with quiet respiration. When air is admitted to the pleural space through either a rupture in the lung or a hole in the chest wall the lung on the affected side collapses as the intrapleural pressure approaches atmospheric pressure. If the communication between the pleural space and the exterior remains open (open pneumothorax) either directly via the chest wall or via the alveolar spaces and bronchial tree, more air will move in and out of the pleural space with respiration. If the hole is large enough, resistance to the movement of air into the intact lung is greater than the resistance to air flow into the pleural space. Ventilation of the intact lung then falls, the mediastinum moves towards the unaffected side and hypoxia and respiratory distress ensue. If, on the other hand, the hole through which air enters the pleural space seals off (closed pneumothorax) air continues to enter the intact lung rather than the pleural space and unless the pneumothorax is very large, or the patient already suffers from underlying lung pathology, it does not cause as much respiratory distress. In the development of tension pneumothorax, a flap of tissue over the hole in the lung or chest wall acts as a flutter valve, permitting air to enter during inspiration, but preventing its escape during expiration. The pressure in the pleural space progressively rises leading to mediastinal shift and compression of both the great veins and the opposite lung. Eventually, venous return to the heart is impeded and circulatory collapse results.

The functional disturbances caused by pneumothorax consequently depend upon its size and type. The immediate result of collapse of one lung is to cause a gross ventilation perfusion imbalance with secondary venous to arterial shunting. In the healthy adult even complete collapse of one lung may cause only mild arterial hypoxaemia and exertional dyspnoea (Cran and Rumball 1967). This is reflected in a reduction of lung volumes and a decrease in carbon monoxide transfer, caused by the aforementioned shunting. Even this may be mild in degree if the pneumothorax is closed off, when ventilation and later perfusion are equally reduced. If the pneumothorax is of the open or tension types, which grow progressively

Table 15.1. Aetiology of pneumothorax

A. *Closed pneumothorax*
   1. Simple: (a) *Primary or idiopathic*
            (b) *Secondary: focal lung lesions*
                   tuberculosis
                   carcinoma of bronchus, and rarely other
                       intrathoracic structures
                   cysts—congenital
                       —parasitic
                   pulmonary infarction
                   lung abscess
                   eosinophilic granuloma of lung
                   tuberous sclerosis

                   generalized lung lesions
                   obstructive airways disease—reversible
                                       —irreversible
                   generalized pulmonary emphysema
                   occupational lung disease
                   diffuse fibrosing alveolitis
                   inherited connective tissue disease
                       (Marfans syndrome)
                   non-inherited connective tissue (Ehlers
                     Donlas
                   syndrome)
                   sarcoidosis
                   cystic fibrosis
                   corticosteroid therapy
   2. Tension: this may result from any of the causes listed above
B. *Open pneumothorax*
   1. Via chest wall: direct injury
                : compression injury
                : secondary to elective invasive procedures
   2. Via lung   : during positive pressure ventilation
                 : secondary to barotrauma
                : all causes listed under closed pneumothorax

---

larger, hypoxic vasoconstriction in the vascular bed of the affected lung causes diversion of blood to the unaffected lung, reducing the venous to arterial shunting. However, progressive mediastinal movement caused by the increasing intrapleural pressure in the affected hemithorax causes obstruction of the great vessels with hypoxia, activation of pulmonary deflation receptors with more marked respiratory distress, and circulatory compromise. Naturally, the effects of all types of pneumothorax are increased if there is already underlying lung pathology.

Aetiology

Table 15.1 illustrates the number and variety of clinical conditions that may be complicated by pneumothorax. Only those categories that may catch the junior clinician unawares, or that are topics of interest in postgraduate examinations will be considered here.

Direct and compression injuries to the chest wall including those resulting from closed chest cardiac massage, are major causes of pneumothorax and may be associated with intrapleural bleeding (haemopneumothorax), a complication considered in more detail below. The patient who has needed vigorous resuscitation or the road traffic accident victim with apparently minor chest injuries who gradually develop signs of respiratory compromise should be considered to have a pneumothorax until proved otherwise.

That percutaneous diagnostic procedures such as pleural and lung biopsies can result in pneumothorax is self evident and a postoperative chest X-ray should always be performed. Less obvious and more difficult to detect is pneumothorax occurring during positive pressure ventilation. This hazard is becoming increasingly recognized; Steir (1974) found that 14 per cent of all pneumothoraces in one hospital occurred during mechanical ventilation. Pneumothorax after transbronchial biopsy is uncommon, occurring in less than 5 per cent of cases (Collins 1982).

By definition, primary pneumothorax occurs when there is no demonstrable pulmonary abnormality either clinical or radiological to explain the condition. These apparently healthy individuals are usually twenty to thirty years of age, male and often of asthenic build. Lichter and Gwynne (1971) studied twenty such patients with recurrent pneumothorax requiring thoracotomy and found characteristic apical scars on the surface of the lung, with bullae and cysts adjacent to the scar in some cases. In fact, such lesions had first been described by Kjaergaard in 1932 but were then attributed to healed tuberculosis. Wedge resection of these areas revealed varying histology including gross disorganization by fibrosis, atelectasis and cyst formation. Focal emphysema, non-specific chronic inflammation, endarteritis and alveolar and bronchiolar proliferation were also described but no evidence of tuberculosis was found. Theories of the aetiology of these lesions have included congenital defects (Brock 1948) local ischaemia (Withers *et al.* 1946) and repeated trauma caused by friction against the chest wall or a sharp inner border of the first rib during coughing or deep breathing (Stephenson 1976). Whatever the cause, these patients clearly form a group apart. In view of the operative findings described, this type of pneumothorax may not fully justify the title 'primary' although the true incidence of such lesions cannot be established in patients not requiring operative intervention. It should be emphasized that the rate of recurrence of pneumothorax in this group is high and that approximately 20 per cent of these patients will develop a second pneumothorax after incurring a first. However, the chances are said to be progressively reduced after two years have elapsed (Cran and Rumball 1967).

Finally, the importance of recognizing pneumothorax in patients with pre-existing lung pathology, especially those with chronic reversible and irreversible airways disease must not be underestimated. In terms of final outcome the exclusion of this complication is paramount and should be considered before other problems such as infections or exacerbations of cardiac failure.

Clinical features (Table 15.2)

The classical symptoms of pneumothorax, namely acute dyspnoea and associated pleuritic chest pain are less frequently encountered in practice than most textbooks suggest. In addition, both symptoms and signs are modified by the pre-existing respiratory status of the patient and the size and type of pneumothorax. Consequently, in a survey of fit young air force personnel with primary pneumothorax, Cran and Rumball (1967) found that more than 10 per cent of the cases were completely asymptomatic and were detected only on routine chest radiography. Furthermore, only eighteen of the 994 patients studied were totally incapacitated by the occurrence. Breathlessness without wheeze is the main symptom of an uncomplicated large pneumothorax in an individual with previously healthy lungs. Pain, when it occurs, is due to stretching of the parietal pleura and is usually localized to the lateral part of the chest although it may radiate to the shoulder or epigastrium. Some patients experience dull, central chest pain exacerbated by an associated unproductive cough or even complain of a clicking sensation in the chest. The clinical history may be less characteristic in a patient with pre-existing chronic obstructive airways disease because the complaint may be of increased wheeze as well as breathlessness. Similarly, pneumothorax can be responsible for the sudden worsening of asthmatic symptoms and must be excluded in all cases of acute asthma. Generally speaking the more severe the pre-existing lung disease the more

Table 15.2. Clinical features of pneumothorax

The symptoms and signs indicated below may occur alone or in combination:

A. *Symptoms*
  i.   None
  ii. Dyspnoea of sudden onset
  iii. Marked increase in dyspnoea in those with pre-existing lung disease
  iv. Pleuritic chest pain
  v.   Increased wheeze may occur in those with obstructive airflow limitation

B. *Signs*
  i.   None
  ii.   Tachypnoea and sweating
  iii. Cyanosis
  iv.   Decreased movement of hemithorax on affected side
  v.   Increasing expansion of hemithorax on affected side (tension pneumothorax)
  vi.   Mediastinal shift to unaffected side (progression in tension pneumothorax)
  vii. Decreased or absent tactile vocal fremitus
  viii. Increased percussion note
  ix.   Diminished or absent breath sounds

Note:
  Tension pneumothorax: Symptoms and signs are progressive in intensity

  Open pneumothorax via chest wall: Sucking wound in chest present

---

compromised the patient will be by even the smallest pneumothorax. An open pneumothorax, for example with a bronchopleural fistula, presents with similar symptoms only more intensely. In tension pneumothorax these symptoms are both profoundly increased and progressive. Cyanosis and shock ensue because of the prevention of adequate venous return.

The signs of pneumothorax rarely develop with less than 30 per cent collapse. Consequently a patient with pre-existing lung disease may be severely distressed with 25 per cent unilateral pneumothorax but with no detectable clinical signs. When present, the signs include diminished expansion on the side of the lesion, often with a loss of thoracic contour. The trachea is deviated to the opposite side and the apex beat may be shifted. Tactile vocal fremitus is diminished or absent with hyper-resonant percussion note. The breath sounds are decreased in volume or absent and may be associated with tinkling crepitations if fluid is present (see complications). Exotic signs like the 'coin test' are rarely present and are of no practical importance. In tension pneumothorax these physical signs are obvious and progressive. In such circumstances the release of intrathoracic pressure is vital and time must not be wasted obtaining a radiograph.

Investigations

The most important investigation in the detection of pneumothorax is obviously the chest radiograph. The emphasis should however be on detection, for the X-ray confirmation of a clinically obvious tension pneumothorax prior to management is unjustifiable. However, with this notable exception the chest radiograph is vital, not only to confirm a dubious clinical diagnosis but to establish the possibility of underlying lung pathology.

A pneumothorax is recognized radiographically by the presence of a clear zone with no lung markings between the chest wall and the edge of the lung. Consequently the condition can only be diagnosed with certainty when the edge of the lung is clearly seen. The use of films taken in inspiration and expiration will enhance this possibility. When the patient breathes out the lung will decrease in size but the volume of air in the pleural space remains constant. The pneumothorax therefore appears larger on expiration than inspiration. Chest films taken in the supine position may not reveal a pneumothorax, a factor of considerable importance in the ventilated patient. The free pleural air tends to collect anteriorly as the heavier lung falls backwards and collapse is prevented by positive pressure. A free lung margin cannot be observed until the diaphragm is depressed by which time a considerable amount of air will have entered the pleural space. Mediastinal shift occurs to the unaffected side for reasons already given. The diaphragm on the side of the lesion is usually depressed, and small pleural effusions are common. Larger volumes of fluid, especially with air–fluid levels, should suggest the possibility of haemopneumothorax, especially if trauma is involved. Subcutaneous and mediastinal air are frequent accompaniments to pneumothorax and unless extensive (see complications) are of little significance.

In patients with emphysema, the radiological distinction between a pneumothorax and large emphysematous cyst is frequently difficult to make and the two may, of course, coexist. Comparison with previous X-ray films is often helpful, and in doubtful cases the diagnosis may be confirmed by the insertion of a 21 gauge needle attached to a large syringe half filled with saline into the second intercostal space. The patient should be placed at 45° to allow free air to collect anteriorly and superiorly, and instructed to hold his breath. Gentle aspiration will produce a continuous stream of bubbles in the case of. pneumothorax, whereas if intact lung is entered only a few bubbles will be extracted before lung tissue occludes the needle. If doubt remains, and the patient is in extremis, the author would advocate the insertion of an intercostal drain, for the procedure may be life-saving in patients with a pneumothorax complicating emphysema. However if a large bullous is inadvertently entered, a bronchopleural fistula may be created but this can be dealt with in the manner described below.

The pain and dyspnoea of pneumothorax can usually be distinguished from that attributable to myocardial infarction on the grounds of history and clinical examination alone, but an electrocardiogram is nevertheless an essential investigation to exclude the latter. However, extensive ECG changes can occur with a pneumothorax including inverted T waves in the chest leads and QRS complexes of diminished amplitude (Walston 1974). Nevertheless, Q waves and the changes of acute myocardial infarction are not seen and the aforementioned changes resolve on sitting up (Copeland 1970). These artefacts are thought to result from the longitudinal rotation of the heart that may occur especially with left-sided pneumothorax, as well as changes in electrical conductivity caused by retrosternal air.

Arterial blood gas analysis in the patient with pneumothorax and no previous history of chest disease is probably not justified, especially as in such cases hypoxaemia ensues only when the ratio of lung to pleural space is less than 75 per cent (Norris *et al.* 1968). The decision regarding the insertion of a chest drain is better made on the basis of radiographic changes and the degree of clinical compromise observed at the bedside.

Management

Management of pneumothorax is aimed at re-expanding the lung, preventing recurrence and restoring the patient to normal activity as soon as possible. The wide variety of conditions that may be complicated by pneumothorax and the range of symptoms encountered make decisions on active management difficult. Consequently, this section will deal with the two basic problems of when and how to instigate active management.

When to initiate active management? (Fig. 15.2)

A. *Closed pneumothorax*

Simple pneumothorax

(a) Primary. As has been indicated, the majority of patients with simple primary pneumothorax are young fit individuals who by definition have no underlying lung pathology. Provided the pneumothorax is small (less than 30%) and the patient undistressed, conservative management is indicated (Riordan 1984). As bed rest and restricted activity are all that is needed in such cases, some clinicians believe that out-patient management is permissible with repeated X-rays to assess re-expansion of the lung. Others advocate hospital admission for all cases of pneumothorax in order that active management may be immediately instigated should complications ensue. In either case, patients should be warned that as the lung re-expands

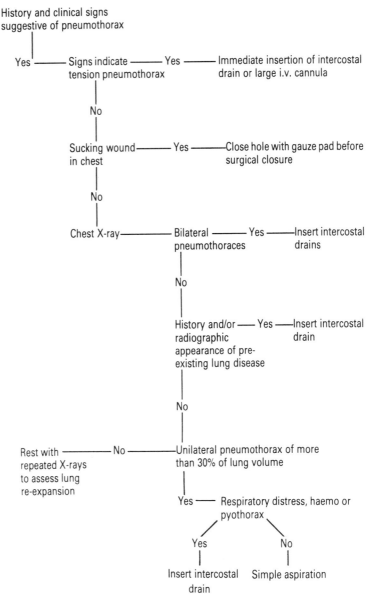

Fig. 15.2. When and how to manage pneumothorax actively.

the two layers of pleura rub together and further transient pleuritic chest pain may be encountered. Full resolution may be a slow process. Aust (1961) found that re-expansion took place over an average of sixteen days in patients treated conservatively (range 4–56 days) as opposed to only two days (range 1–5 days) in those requiring an intercostal drain. Simple aspiration (see below) is more rapid still. Although the rate of expansion can be increased by the breathing of high concentrations of oxygen (Northfield 1971) this is not always practical, and a more active approach to management may be indicated where prolonged inactivity could result in financial hardship. However, the decision to insert an intercostal drain or aspirate is more usually based on clinical assessment and radiographic estimation of the degree of lung collapse. Generally speaking, if the patient is even mildly dyspnoeic at rest and/or has a pneumothorax of 30 per cent or more active management is indicated. A useful radiographic rule of thumb states that intervention is indicated if the lung is separated from the chest wall by an air space of one-third or more of the transverse diameter of the hemithorax (Crompton 1982). Bilateral pneumothoraces must be drained.

(b) Secondary: The degree of clinical compromise induced by even a small pneumothorax in a patient with significant lung disease will necessitate the insertion of a chest drain. This is especially so where a large accumulation of pleural fluid has occurred further exacerbating respiratory distress.

Tension pneumothorax

An absolute indication for active management as soon as a diagnosis is made.

B. Open pneumothorax

Via chest wall

An absolute indication for active management as soon as the diagnosis is made.

Via lung

The presence of an open air leak between lung and pleura means that the pneumothorax will persist until the communication seals itself or is closed operatively. This means a chest drain should be inserted and managed as indicated below.

Active management of pneumothorax (Fig. 15.2)

1. Tension pneumothorax

If the patient is in extremis, any available needle or cannula inserted into any intercostal space can be life-saving. A 12 or 14 G 'Medicut' or 'Abocath' is ideal. A chest drain should then be inserted as soon as possible. Should such equipment be unavailable, Birch (1967) describes the use of a finger stall with a hole cut in the end tied over the cannula acting as a crude but effective one-way valve.

2. *Open pneumothorax via chest wall (Sucking wound)*

The hole in the chest wall must be closed as soon as possible with any available material, although a thick gauze pad or sterile dressing is ideal. Surgical closure should then be performed.

3. *Primary/secondary simple pneumothorax/open pneumothorax via lung*

Patients with a simple pneumothorax of more than 30 per cent without breathlessness, haemo or pyothorax may be treated by simple aspiration. All other patients in this category require a chest drain.

Aspiration

This technique has recently been described for the management of large (> 30 per cent) asymptomatic pneumothoraces. Air is aspirated using a 60 ml syringe, Teflon canula and three-way tap via the second intercostal space anteriorly or in the mid-axillary line laterally. A tube connected to the third arm of the three-way tap should be held in a jug of water to ensure that air is withdrawn from the intercostal space and expelled in the right direction, thus avoiding the development of a tension pneumothorax. Aspiration is stopped when resistance is felt. If more than 4 litres is withdrawn with no resistance an X-ray film should be taken. If no expansion has occurred the pneumothorax is open and a chest drain and suction will be needed (see below). Complete aspiration without recurrence was achieved in sixteen of twenty-three patients reported in two recent series (Raja and Lalor 1981; Hamilton and Archer 1983).

Insertion of an intercostal drain

The classical method of managing a pneumothorax is to insert a chest drain into the pleural cavity connected to an underwater seal drainage bottle. An alternative method of drainage, the Heimlich flutter (non-return) valve, enjoyed considerable popularity in the mid-1970s and will also be described. The traditional trocar and cannula is becoming less widely used as disposable cannulae of various types are marketed. The 'Argyle' tube is inserted directly into the pleural space using its own introducer after which it is sutured to the skin. The 'Malecot' catheter is inserted in a similar manner but incorporates a self retaining device. The traditional trocar and cannula is more clumsy in operation, involving the insertion of a rubber catheter through the cannula after which the latter is withdrawn over the tubing. However, these catheters tend to be more pliable than the disposable cannulae and have the added advantage of being more irritant to the pleura thus encouraging the formation of adhesions. Once *in situ,* these drains are connected to an underwater seal in the usual manner. The Heimlich flutter valve allowing one way drainage of air from the pleural cavity represented an attempt to reduce the inconvenience caused by these bulky underwater seals. The small rubber valve encased in perspex and weighing only 22.5 g is attached in the normal manner to an intercostal tube and then strapped lightly to the chest (Heimlich 1965). The unmistakable 'raspberry' sound as air passes through the fluttering valve indicates normal function which ceases only when lung expansion is complete. Negative pressure can however be applied to the distal end of the valve should this prove necessary. A review of the efficiency of this apparatus by Bernstein *et al.* (1973) showed that 66 per cent of patients had full expansion in one hour and 94 per cent within five days of intubation. However, a significant disadvantage occurred when the pneumothorax to be drained was associated with an effusion as fluid tended to block the valve.

The site most commonly advocated for tube insertion is the second intercostal space anteriorly. However, the cosmetic disadvantages of this site in terms of scarring together with the possibility (admittedly remote) of damaging the subclavian or internal thoracic vessels, mean that the fourth or fifth intercostal space in the mid axillary line is gradually becoming the site of choice, especially for pneumothoraces associated with effusions. Nevertheless, great care is required when inserting the cannula by this lateral approach because the vital structures in the mediastinum may be damaged if the tube is inserted with too much enthusiasm! Following skin cleansing and the insertion of an appropriate local anaesthetic a blade and surgical forceps should be used to open a track down to the parietal pleura. This dissection within the intercostal space should carry the track away from the neurovascular bundle sited under the inferior aspect of the upper rib, and permits easy insertion of the cannula in the normal way. An outrush of air indicates entry into the pleural space, and the underwater seal or valve should be connected. About 10 cm of the tube should normally be inserted and directed towards the apex, and the cannula then·sutured in place. In normal circumstances the drain should initially bubble as the patient breathes out, coughs or laughs while the lung re-expands. Subsequently the water in the seal will move up or down the drainage tubing a few centimetres as the patient breathes in or out. The seal should be placed on the floor beside the bed with Spencer Wells forceps available to clamp the tube when the patient is moved. Should this precaution be ignored and the bottle elevated above

Table 15.3. Tube troubleshooting

---

1. *Level stops swinging*

Chest X-ray

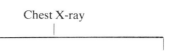

Lung re-expansion incomplete:	*Lung re-expansion complete:*
i. Tube is blocked suck blockage out with bladder syringe, if this fails inject 20 ml of sterile saline down tube	Expanded lung has blocked intrathoracic end of tube. Clamp off tube and leave for 24 hours before repeating X-ray. If no collapse, remove tube
ii. If this fails, assume tube is blocked at intrathoracic end by partially expanded lung: rotate and shorten tube change tube	

2. *Level continues to swing*

Chest X-ray

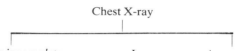

Lung re-expansion incomplete:	*Lung re-expansion complete:*
Apply suction to tube in increasing increments of 5 cm water to a maximum of 20 cm. If lung still fails to expand and tube is patent, obstruction in the bronchial tree is likely (e.g. sputum plugs, carcinoma of bronchus) and bronchoscopy should be performed	i. Clamp off tube for 24 hours and re-X-ray. If no collapse, remove tube
	ii. If lung collapses on clamping there is probably a patent air bleb on the lung surface. Apply *minimum* amount of suction needed to re-expand lung for further 48 hours and reclamp. If lung collapses, re-apply suction and consider chemical pleurodesis or operative intervention (see 'persistent air leak')

---

the level of the chest, for example on to a bedside locker, the contents will be aspirated into the pleural cavity. When the level in the drainage tube stops swinging it is likely that the lung has re-expanded and is blocking the end of the cannula although other possibilities are indicated in Table 15.3. A chest film to confirm this event should be taken and the tube clamped for forty-eight hours before re-X-raying the chest to ensure that no collapse has recurred. The tube can then be removed. The forty-eight hour period during which the tube is clamped prior to removal is the author's preference. Some clinicians prefer to leave the tube *in situ* for a longer period. A study by So and Yu (1982) divided patients with chest drains *in situ* into those who had the tube removed as soon as expansion was complete, and those who had the tube left in place for three days after this event, with the tube clamped for the final twenty-four hours. They found that although early catheter removal achieved the same overall success rate as later removal the failures in the early removal group were caused by re-collapse of the lung. However, failure of expansion was the commonest cause when the drain was left *in situ* for the full three days. In this sense early removal of the cannula seems undesirable although leaving the drain *in situ* for a prolonged period creates problems of its own including an increased chance of intra-thoracic infection.

This account represents the normal course of management of pneumothorax. Table 15.3 illustrates the other possible outcomes after drain insertion. As may be seen, the author advocates the use of suction only in certain circumstances and then applied in increasing increments as necessary up to 20 cm of water. There is no evidence that the application of suction to all cases of pneumothorax requiring drainage is beneficial in terms of speed of resolution (So and Yu 1982). In addition, too rapid lung expansion by suction may result in unilateral pulmonary oedema (Childress *et al.* 1971). However, controlled suction may be indicated for medical management of bronchopleural fistula (discussed below).

Complications

The pneumomediastinum

Pneumomediastinum and subcutaneous emphysema occur due to leakage of air via the interstitial tissues of the lung into the mediastinum and neck. Both are usually apparent on chest X-ray and are benign provided that the build up of pressure in the mediastinum is countered by a release of air into the subcutaneous tissues. If this does not happen, venous return to the heart may become compromised. Treatment with high concentrations of oxygen will rapidly alleviate this problem (Bodey 1961) although emergency mediastinotomy and thoracotomy may be necessary.

Recurrent pneumothorax

Patients who have had one primary pneumothorax have a 20 per cent chance of getting a second and this figure rises to 50 per cent in patients with chronic lung disease (Emerson 1981). Consequently most physicians consider that any patient who has had two pneumothoraces should be considered for pleurodesis or pleurectomy and that patients in the high risk categories of chronic lung disease and exposure to occupational hazards (e.g. pilots and divers) should undergo this procedure after the first.

Chemical pleurodesis is undertaken in the hope that adhesions formed between the parietal and visceral pleura will prevent recurrence. Agents used include Camphor in oil and Tetracycline, both of which can be injected into the pleural space before intubation (Goldszer *et al.* 1979). 500 mg of tetracycline in 20 ml of saline injected into the pleural cavity via the chest drain will usually initiate effective pleurodesis, especially if the patient is encouraged to lie on each side successively allowing dispersal of the fluid over the full pleural surface. However, this procedure is frequently extremely painful and full opiate analgesia must be provided before commencement. Poudrage with iodized talc is also effective. Nevertheless, thoracotomy with parietal pleurodesis is the only certain way of preventing recurrence and should be considered as the most satisfactory approach in the otherwise fit patient.

Persistant air leak (bronchopleural fistula)

This may become apparent in several ways. The lung may partially re-expand, or require suction to expand fully, and the drain continues to bubble indefinitely. Alternatively, the drain may stop bubbling but the lung persistently collapses when the drain is clamped. Thoracotomy with full examination of the pleura and surgical closure of the leak is undoubtedly the most effective means of dealing with this but many patients will be unable to withstand such surgery because of pre-existing lung pathology. Consequently, careful application of suction is required such as to permit re-expansion of the lung without enlarging the communication between the bronchial tree and pleural space. Chemical pleurodesis via the intercostal drain is then carried out in the manner described above. This procedure may need to be repeated more than once with different agents, necessitating the application of suction for several weeks before pleurodesis occurs. Careful attention to the drain site is vital to exclude infection, which may be life-threatening should the pleural space become involved.

Pyopneumothorax

A small pleural effusion is a common accompaniment to pneumothorax but the presence of a large collection should suggest the presence of pyo or haemopneumothorax. The former is common when the pneumothorax is secondary to suppurative disease such as a lung abscess or tuberculous cavity. A swinging pyrexia is accompanied by signs of an effusion in the lower part of the lung with pneumothorax above. A succussion splash may be present and chest X-ray shows a horizontal air–fluid interface. Aspiration confirms the nature of the fluid and microscopy for cell types and later culture and sensitivity should be carried out. Cytological examination for malignant cells should also be performed. Intercostal drainage and complete removal of the fluid followed by chest X-ray may reveal underlying pathology which should then be treated appropriately.

Haemopneumothorax

Bleeding into the pleural space is a common complication of traumatic pneumothorax but is otherwise rare complicating only 2–5 per cent of spontaneous pneumothoraces (Abyholm *et al.* 1973). After the initial onset of pain and shortness of breath, the patient frequently enters a latent period of comparative wellbeing and only later becomes dyspnoeic and shocked. Chest X-ray shows air and fluid in the pleural space and aspiration yields blood. The fluid (usually with haemoglobin more than 7 gm/dl) should be completely removed by aspiration and appropriate intravenous replacement should be given. Thoracotomy must be considered if the collection re-accumulates.

Conclusion

Pneumothorax is a common medical emergency and one that may have disastrous consequences for the patient. Provided a high level of diagnostic suspicion is maintained when assessing patients with any degree of respiratory compromise, the diagnosis will not be missed and management is both straightforward and satisfying.

Further reading

Abyholm F. (1975) Spontaneous pneumothorax. *Scandinavian Journal of Thoracic and Cardiovascular Surgery* **9**, 281–286.

Aust J.P. (1961) Spontaneous pneumothorax. *Postgraduate Medicine* **29**, 368.

Bernstein A., Wagaruddin M. and Shah M. (1973) Management of spontaneous pneumothorax using a Heimlich flutter valve. *Thorax* **28**, 386.

Birch C.A. (1967) *Emergencies in Medical Practice*, 8th edition, p. 164. Churchill–Livingstone, Edinburgh.

Bodey G.P. (1961) Medical mediastinal emphysema. *Annals of Internal Medicine* **54**, 46–56.

Brock R.C. (1948) Recurrent and chronic spontaneous pneumothorax. *Thorax* **3**, 88–111.

Childress M.E., Moy G. and Martha M. (1971) Unilateral pulmonary oedema resulting from treatment of spontaneous pneumothorax. *American Review of Respiratory Diseases* **104**, 119–121.

Collins J.V. (1982) Bronchoscopy. *Medicine* **I**, 21, 991–992.

Copeland R.B. (1970) E.C.G. changes suggestive of coronary artery disease in pneumothorax. Their reversibility in the upright position. *Archives of Internal Medicine* **125**, 151–153.

Cran I.R. and Rumball C.A. (1967) Study of spontaneous pneumothoraces in the Royal Air Force. *Thorax* **22**, 462–465.

Crompton K. (1982) Spontaneous pneumothorax. *Hospital Update* March, 251–262.

Emerson P. (1981) Pneumothorax and spontaneous haemopneumothorax, in Emerson, P. (Ed.) *Thoracic Medicine*, p. 649–659, Butterworths, London.

Goldszer R.C., Bennett J., Van Compen J. and Rudnitzky J. (1979) Intrapleural tetracycline for spontaneous pneumothorax. *Journal of the American Medical Association* **241**, 724–725.

Hamilton A.A.D. and Archer G.J. (1983) Treatment of pneumothorax by simple aspiration.*Thorax* **38**, 934–6.

Heimlich H.J. (1965) Heimlich flutter valve: effective replacement for drainage bottle. *Hospital Topics* **43**, 122.

Kjaergaard H. (1932) Spontaneous pneumothorax in the apparently healthy. *Acta Medica Scandinavica*, supplement 43.

Lichter I. and Gwynne J.F. (1971) Spontaneous pneumothorax in young subjects. *Thorax* **26**, 409–417.

Norris R.M., Jones J.G. and Bishop J.M. (1968) Respiratory gas exchange in patients with pneumothorax. *Thorax* **3**, 427–433.

Northfield T.C. (1971) Oxygen therapy for spontaneous pneumothorax. *British Medical Journal* **4**, 86–88.

Raja O.G. and Lalor A.J. (1981) Simple aspiration of spontaneous pneumothorax *British Journal of Diseases of the Chest* **75**, 207–8.

Riordan J.F. (1984) Management of spontaneous pneumothorax. *British Medical Journal* **289**, 71.

So Sy. and Yu D.Y.C. (1982) Catheter drainage of spontaneous pneumothorax: suction or no suction, early or late removal? *Thorax* **37**, 46–48.

Steir M. (1974) Pneumothorax complicating continuous ventilatory support. *Journal of Thoracic and Cardiovascular Surgery* **67**, 17–23.

Stephenson S.F. (1976) Spontaneous pneumothorax, the sharp rib syndrome. *Thorax* **31**, 369–372.

Thompson D.T. (1981) Pneumothorax reconsidered. *South African Medical Journal* **59**, 377–381.

Walston A. (1974) E.C.G. manifestations in spontaneous pneumothorax. *Annals of Internal Medicine* **80**, 375–379.

Withers J.N., Fishback M.E., Kiehl P.V. and Hannan J.L. (1964) Spontaneous pneumothorax. Suggested aetiology and comparison of treatment methods. *American Journal of Surgery* **108**, 772–776.

16 · Cerebrovascular Disease

R. C. D. GREENHALL

Cerebrovascular disease is common, and is a frequently cited cause of death. Clinically a 'stroke' is an acute cerebral or brain stem deficit of presumed vascular cause, either thrombo-embolic or haemorrhagic. Arbitrarily, such episodes lasting less than twenty-four hours are called transient ischaemic attacks (TIA) and those over twenty-four hours, stroke. Transient ischaemia will be considered separately from stroke in this chapter. The particular stroke from a ruptured berry aneurysm is dealt with in Chapter 19.

As defined above there is clinical presumption of the vascular cause. Clearly the first aim of management is to make a diagnosis with more certainty, as it is generally accepted that on clinical grounds alone, five to ten per cent of strokes turn out to have another diagnosis, particularly tumour. In the management of the patient who appears to have suffered a stroke there are three main problems:

(a) Is it a vascular problem?
(b) If it is, what is the type and cause?
(c) What treatment is required?

1. Is it a stroke?

A clear outline of the temporal aspects of the episode is of the utmost importance. This may be given by the patient, but where the patient is comatose or has a language disturbance, it must be obtained from a witness. In the elderly it is very easy to assume that the unconscious patient with a hemiparesis has had a stroke, perhaps failing to appreciate that the hemiparesis is old and the coma caused by something entirely different. Also, the patient with a language disturbance may be unable to communicate the fact that the dysphasia has been progressive over some weeks, and medical attention only sought because the limbs have become weak. Just as there must be caution with the facility of diagnosing stroke in the elderly because it is so common, so must there be awareness that strokes do occur in young people, although the causes may be unusual.

The deficit depends upon which part of the brain is affected and may be limb weakness, mono or hemiparesis, visual disturbance, usually hemianopic, even though the patient claims it is one eye that is affected. Certainly the retina may be involved, producing a monocular disturbance of vision either alone, or in combination with a contralateral limb disturbance with loss of feeling or use in a limb or limbs. Loss of consciousness may occur at the onset and may, or may not persist. Consciousness may also be lost after the onset.

The brain stem and cerebellum are the site of the stroke in only about ten to fifteen per cent of all strokes. Although rare, the constellation of symptoms and signs often make these syndromes easily recognizable. Thus a list of these may begin with a combination of a third nerve palsy and a contralateral hemiparesis from a cerebral peduncular lesion (Weber's syndrome) in the mid-brain and end in the medulla with the lateral medullary (Wallenberg) syndrome. The features of this are vertigo, ipsilateral trigeminal sensory symptoms, ipsilateral cerebellar incoordination, contralateral spinothalamic sensory disturbance on the trunk and limbs, ipsilateral Horner's syndrome and ipsilateral palatal and pharyngeal paresis. However, it must be remembered that the syndromes do not always have a vascular basis, for example in the younger age group the lateral medullary syndrome may be caused by demyelination.

The locked-in syndrome or de-efferented state results from more severe brain stem disturbance, usually affecting the anterior part of the pons and often the result of basilar thrombosis. In this condition the patient is quadriparetic and has bulbar disturbance, being unable to speak or swallow. However the patient is often awake and aware of what is said. Communication can be made by eye movement or eyelid closure and may allow sensory testing to be performed and often showing it to be intact. Although the prognosis for this condition is bad, the patients that do recover often remember what has been said about them on the assumption that they were unconscious. Vertigo is a common symptom of brain stem disturbance. Limb or gait ataxia may also occur in brain stem strokes, from involvement of cerebellar connections, but cerebellar infarction is unusual in view of the anastomotic vessels therein.

Cerebellar haemorrhage accounts for approximately ten per cent of intracerebral haemorrhages. Although some present with a patient deteriorating rapidly and dying within twenty-four hours, a less dramatic clinical picture is seen characterized by small but reacting pupils, lateral gaze paresis, and periodic respiration, which may progress to coma from hydrocephalus.

Awareness of past history of systemic disease, and the general examination of the patient may lead to a suspicion of neoplastic disease or a more generalized disturbance, rather than a primary neurological condition.

Recognition of clinical patterns based on a clear history and examination can increase the confidence of clinical diagnosis of a vascular event. Where doubt exists, e.g. the febrile patient, no history available and minimal focal signs, further investigation is required to try and establish an alternative diagnosis. This may include examination of the cerebrospinal fluid (CSF) when infection cannot be excluded, or neurological referral when there is the possibility of an abscess, tumour or subdural haematoma.

2. Type and cause of stroke

Pathologically, strokes can be divided into thrombo-embolic disturbances leading to infarction (CI) and haemorrhagic disease leading to cerebral haemorrhage (CH). The question is often posed as to whether it is necessary to distinguish between these. There is a clear reason to do this for epidemiological or therapeutic intervention research work. Certainly there is no reason to suppose that the treatment for CI and CH are the same. In the moribund elderly patient where the diagnosis of stroke is clear, it would be meddlesome to investigate to differentiate between these two, but in the young patient the knowledge that there is an infarct or haemorrhage can determine which further investigations are performed.

It has long been realized that it is not possible to distinguish reliably between CI and CH on clinical grounds. However, coma at the onset is a feature more in keeping with cerebral haemorrhage, as is vomiting at that time. Progressive deterioration to coma and death within hours again favours cerebral haemorrhage, whereas such deterioration in two to five days suggests cerebral infarction. This reflects the development of intracranial distortion, findings which in the past have led to the use of echoencephalography in differentiating CI and CH. The abrupt onset of the focal neurological deficit suggests an embolic problem. The finding of neck stiffness clearly favours a haemorrhagic problem. It is generally accepted that hypertension is a predisposing factor to both cerebral infarction and cerebral haemorrhage and is of no help in distinguishing between them. Other proven risk factors are heart disease, diabetes and smoking. CT scanning is now revealing how frequently enclosed cerebral haemorrhage occurs, demonstrating even further the unreliability of a bloodless CSF in distinguishing between the two.

CT scanning, can with good reliability, distinguish between infarct and haemorrhage, although the changes in cerebral infarct may not be marked in the early stages. However, it is a counsel of perfection to suggest CT scanning for all strokes in the United Kingdom. Few towns have scanners and those that have probably do not have the spare capacity.

Thrombo-embolic

Fashion varies as to whether the heart or the carotid vessels is the commoner or more important cause for thrombo-embolic stroke. Clearly this depends upon the sample used, but they are both important. The phrase 'cerebral embolus' is usually reserved for emboli from the heart, but they may arise from many other sources, in particular the origin of the internal carotid artery.

Examination of the heart together with appropriate cardiological investigation, electrocardiograph, chest X-ray and echocardiograph, may reveal a source for emboli; rheumatic valvular disease, myocardial infarction, atrial myxoma, endocarditis. Support for the heart as a source of emboli may be obtained from the existence of emboli elsewhere in the body, and certainly this would implicate with more reliability the heart as the source in the patient with isolated atrial fibrillation. Otherwise it is difficult to be certain of the relevance of isolated atrial fibrillation in the patient with a stroke.

A systolic bruit in the neck, opposite the angle of the jaw, usually indicates stenosis in the carotid arterial tree. Although most frequently the internal carotid, the external and common carotid arteries may be those involved. This bruit reasonably raises the suspicion of a source of emboli.

In both young and old patients presenting with a stroke, the possibility of an arteritic process must be considered. Examination of the whole of the cardiovascular system, especially the peripheral pulses may increase the suspicion, as may symptoms of systemic disturbance. The ESR will be of help in determining the need for further investigations, although a normal value does not preclude them. Syphilitic arteritis still occurs but very rarely.

Polycythemia is well recognized as causing thrombotic stroke and may be obvious clinically. In younger patients the stroke may result from a severe attack of migraine (complicated migraine), not only in those with the hemiplegic type of this disease. Trauma, even seemingly very trivial, may lead to damage to the neck arteries and infarction.

Haemorrhage

The chief considerations are whether the intracerebral haemorrhage is primary, or secondary to a berry aneurysm, arteriovenous malformation (AVM) or haematological disturbance. Primary haemorrhages are the commonest and AVM haemorrhages rare. It is unusual for patients with a past history of migraine and other vascular episodes to lead the clinician to a successful diagnosis of an arteriovenous malformation when they present with an intracerebral haemorrhage. It must be remembered that intracranial haemorrhage (extradural, subdural or intracerebral) is more likely in a patient with a bleeding disorder, and particularly in those taking anticoagulants.

Even though subarachnoid haemorrhage is dealt with in Chapter 19, it should be noted that blood may reach the subarachnoid space by rupture of a berry aneurysm (indeed it is extremely rare for this not to occur), or by extension from a primary intracerebral haematoma. In particular, middle cerebral artery and anterior communicating artery aneurysms may rupture into the cerebral substance, as well as the subarachnoid space. CT scanning can show the site of the haemorrhage and may increase thereby the suspicion of a berry aneurysm as the cause when in the inferofrontal, or temporosylvian areas. The use of contrast injection may show up an arteriovenous malformation.

Thus the diagnosis of the patient with a possible stroke involves a full history, from a witness if necessary, a thorough examination with especial reference to the nervous and cardiovascular systems, and the use of investigations. These may include:
Full blood count, including platelets.
Erythrocyte sedimentation rate.
Glucose, urea and electrolytes.
Syphilitic serology.
Lumbar puncture.
Chest and skull X-rays.
Electrocardiograph.
Echocardiograph.
CT scan.
Angiography.
ANF/DNA for arteritis.
Arterial biopsy.
When there is any doubt about the diagnosis, it is always reasonable to ask for an opinion from a neurologist.

Treatment

The aims of treatment are:
1. Reduction of acute mortality.
2. Reduction of morbidity.
3. Prevention of recurrence.

Acute mortality

Immediate mortality, variably stated as within about four weeks from a stroke is high. About 45 per cent of patients with undifferentiated strokes die in this period. Data obtained before CT scanning show that early mortality from cerebral infarct is lower (about 30 per cent) than that from cerebral haemorrhage (about 80 per cent). Even though CT scanning is revealing more unexpected cerebral haemorrhages, and thereby tending to reduce the mortality, it is likely that this difference is real. It is clear that the majority of patients dying in the acute phase do so in the first few days after cerebral haemorrhage, and between days two and ten, after a cerebral infarction. The commonest cause of death in this period is intracranial swelling, from the size of the haemorrhage and the reactive oedema in the surrounding brain in cases with cerebral haemorrhage. In those with cerebral infarct, it is principally the swelling of the infarct itself causing the distortion. Although the increase in intracranial volume from the haemorrhage is instantaneous, the oedema around an infarct takes longer to develop. Transtentorial downwards herniation occurs which may produce secondary brain stem haemorrhages in either situation. Disturbance of consciousness, pupil reaction, eye movements and respiration may all occur as a result. There are very few reported cases of survival from these secondary brain stem haemorrhages which are much more common than primary brain stem haemorrhage.

Gaze disturbance (an inability to look to command to the side of the hemiparesis, or to follow to that side), a severe hemiparesis and disturbance of consciousness on admission, are poor prognostic signs for survival of the acute phase. Conversely the majority of patients presenting with a normal level of consciousness survive.

Many and various methods of treatment have been suggested to reduce the acute mortality after stroke. These have mainly been aimed at reducing the swelling or increasing the cerebral perfusion. Some of these are listed in Table 16.1. By no means all of these remedies have been subjected to a reasonable trial, and only low molecular weight dextran has been shown to have an effect on this basis. However, this effect was limited to those with particularly severe ischaemic infarcts, and is not generally recommended. It is not uncommon for dexamethasone (4 mg qds) to be given, presumably on

Table 16.1. Some treatments suggested for acute ischaemic infarction

Streptokinase
Urokinase
Heparin/warfarin
Prostacyclin
Aminophylline
Papaverine
Ergot derivatives
Acetazolamide
Low molecular weight dextran
Barbiturates
Glycerol
Dexamethasone
Mannitol
Blood pressure change
Tracheostomy
$\left. \begin{array}{l} \downarrow P_{CO_2} \\ \uparrow P_{O_2} \end{array} \right\}$ inspired air
Hyperbaric oxygen
Venesection

the basis that it is reasonable to expect it to work, although it has not been proven. Intravenous mannitol (20 per cent) is also sometimes used for cerebral infarction. This mainly affects the normal brain. A rebound rise in intracranial pressure may follow, but this may perhaps be avoided by repeated administration over several days. Barbiturate anaesthesia and intensive life support measures have been suggested recently. However controlled trial work has not yet been reported and it is a technique requiring considerable resources.

The decision whether to treat intensively those with the poor prognostic signs listed above is a very difficult one, but clearly needs to be taken quickly.

The surgical treatment of acute infarction is limited, although decompression by craniotomy or temporal lobectomy on the affected side have had their proponents. Some have tried to disobliterate the internal carotid artery where this has shown to be occluded, but this again has not been proved a successful method. Evacuation of haematomas in the acute stage is also usually unrewarding, except in the case of intracerebellar haematoma where it can be life-saving.

The above discussion has been about treatment for the effect of the stroke. Clearly if the primary disorder is treatable, early intervention is appropriate. Reversal of anticoagulation is an obvious move with intra-cerebral bleeding, but may not be so appropriate in the patient on anti-coagulants with cardiac disease with a stroke. Here the differential diagnosis between cerebral infarct and cerebral haemorrhage is clearly important. In the elderly patient with a hemiparesis, tender temporal arteries and generalized malaise, with a raised ESR, immediate treatment with steroids (prednisolone 20 mg qds) is required. Many feel it mandatory to perform a temporal artery biopsy within twenty-four hours as well.

Other causes of death in the acute stage are pulmonary emboli and infection, particularly bronchopneumonia. Deep venous thrombosis in the affected lower limb is common after stroke, and some have recommended the use of low dose subcutaneous heparin (5000 units 12-hourly) until mobilization occurs. There is, however, the danger of worsening the intra-cerebral disturbance, be it cerebral haemorrhage or infarct. Although the use of prophylactic antibiotics against pneumonia has its proponents, it is probably better to encourage mobility, give chest physiotherapy and keep a careful clinical watch for the onset of a chest infection before using anti-biotics. Close attention must be paid to the urinary tract and to the skin in addition.

Morbidity

The majority of the patients who on admission have a normal conscious level will survive. These patients also require careful management and simple measures can be very helpful. Avoidance of putting the patient in a bed with a wall on his unaffected side, leaving the window on the world through the hemianopic or neglected side is not a difficult task. Stimulation and encouragement are important. Passive movements of the limbs through full range should start immediately to avoid joint disorder and contractures. Early mobilization has the advantage of reducing the risk of deep venous thrombosis. The 'painful shoulder syndrome' is very common. Passive movements and support of the limb may help in prevention. Particular care must always be exercised in moving the upper limb, as subluxation may readily occur, and if the painful shoulder is already present, intense pain be inflicted.

There is controversy as to the effectiveness of speech therapy in patients with dysphasia with strokes. A recent trial has shown that although there was no demonstrable difference between the effect of speech therapy and involvement with volunteers, both appeared to have a beneficial effect. This suggests at least that language stimulation is helpful.

Specific medical treatment has failed to produce an obvious measure to improve morbidity. Most trials of the suggested remedies for treatment of the acute stroke did not follow up long enough to shown any effect. Clearly when the natural history of a condition is one which includes possible improvement after six months, assessing the effect of a measure at six weeks is unlikely to produce a reasonable answer. Naftidrofuryl, having an effect on intracellular metabolism, given orally over twelve weeks has been claimed to lead to a reduction in neurological deficit at twelve weeks. This is clearly an interesting finding and the results of further studies are awaited. In the acute stage of stroke the blood pressure may be raised even when the patient was known to be previously normotensive. Autoregulation of the cerebral circulation may be disrupted, and the rise in systemic pressure may benefit the ischaemic area. This has to be weighed against the deleterious affects on the rest of the brain, kidneys and elsewhere. Hypotensive treatment is certainly indicated where the diagnosis is that of hypertensive encephalopathy with a focal deficit in addition.

Hypertension and cardiac disease are factors which affect the morbidity after stroke and appropriate management of these after the acute phase should be undertaken.

Prevention of recurrence

Hypertension is associated with an increased risk of recurrence of cerebral infarction. This is also probably the case with cerebral haemorrhage but there have not been enough diagnosed survivors to be able to say this.

Emboli from the heart with rheumatic valvular disease seem to come in clusters and there is some evidence that anticoagulation reduces the risk of recurrence of stroke in this condition. Although there is a risk of turning an ischaemic infarct into a haemorrhagic one if anticoagulants are used, it would seem reasonable to start them immediately rather than wait for approximately ten days for some resolution of the infarct. The small risk of misdiagnosed cerebral haemorrhage in such a patient must also be remembered.

Anticoagulants have been advocated in several other situations in cerebrovascular disease. There is some evidence of their efficiency in reducing emboli from mural thrombi after myocardial infarction. They are often used in patients with isolated atrial fibrillation, but other clinicians are hesitant and point to the problems involved with control and bleeding. However, there is no evidence that anticoagulation has a beneficial effect in the acute stage of completed cerebral infarction. It is advocated by some in 'stroke in evolution'. This clinical situation can be difficult to recognize, and even so the trials performed have not shown indisputable benefits.

Transient ischaemic attacks

These vascular events, lasting by definition for less than twenty-four hours, are presumed to be thrombo-embolic in origin. A small percentage are associated with anaemia, polycythemia, arteritis, cardiac rhythm disturbance, hypertension or hypotension. A common source for the emboli is the internal carotid artery, particularly the origin, but other parts of the arterial tree may be involved as well.

Symptoms may be of retinal, cerebral hemisphere, or brain stem origin. Thus transient blindness from one eye (amaurosis fugax), hemiparesis, hemisensory disturbance, hemivisual disturbance and dysphasia, double vision, vertigo and limb symptoms may occur. Many of these last no more than twenty minutes.

The importance of transient ischaemic attacks is that there seems to be an increased risk of cerebral infarction following them, but studies so far have shown a great disparity (5–60 per cent) in this risk. Management is usually to refer to a neurological service. Here investigation aims to exclude the causes listed above and also to exclude the rare cerebral tumour presenting this way. Investigation may include carotid angiography, the decision being influenced by the presence of retinal emboli, neck bruit, hypertension, age and general medical condition.

There is some evidence that aspirin may be effective in reducing the infarction rate after TIA and a large study is at present in progress on a multicentre basis in the United Kingdom to try to answer this unequivocally. There is, however, no conclusive evidence that anticoagulation, sulphinpyrazone or dipyridamole are effective, singly or in combination. Even if a stenotic or ulcerative lesion is found at the origin of the internal carotid artery, with no abnormality elsewhere in the arterial tree, it is not clear that endarterectomy is the appropriate treatment. Studies so far have shown that although there may be some improvement in the long term picture, this has to be balanced by the risk from the operation itself. This is also the subject of a trial at the moment.

Conclusions

Although there are no specific remedies for all patients with stroke, such patients occur commonly and must be dealt with actively. Therefore, consider alternative diagnoses and try to find the type and cause, especially in the younger patient. Identify those requiring specific management: intracerebellar haemorrhage, those on anticoagulants, those with rheumatic valvular disease, but do not neglect the others. Active management on the ward from medical, nursing, physiotherapy, speech therapy and occupational therapy staff, will improve the patient's morale and will ensure that the most is made of the natural recovery which can be expected.

Further reading

Marshall J. (1976) *The Management of Cerebrovascular Disease*. 3rd edn. Blackwell Scientific Publications, Oxford.
Ross Russell R.W. (1983) (Ed). *Vascular Disease of the Central Nervous System*. Churchill Livingstone, Edinburgh.
Warlow C.P. (1979) The young stroke. *British Journal of Hospital Medicine* 2, 252–259.
Warlow C.P. (1981) Cerebrovascular disease. *Clinics in Haematology*, Vol. 10, No. 2, 631–651.

17 · The Diagnosis and Management of 'Funny Turns'

L. D. BLUMHARDT

Transient episodes of disturbed consciousness are a common medical condition. In the UK patients often complain of 'funny turns' or 'blackouts', but a variety of phrases such as 'queer do's' or 'coming over queer' may be as close as some patients can get to describing their unfamiliar experiences. For some reason American patients have 'spells' while in Europe it is apparently common to feel 'away' or 'out of touch' as expressed by the German '*ich war veg*' and the Swedish '*jag är borta*'. Perhaps the most appropriate blend of anxiety and clinical urgency is conveyed by the old French phrase, '*le petit mort.*'

Such terms cover a wide range of events from brief episodes of 'light-headedness' to dramatic collapses with loss of consciousness. Clearly the former are more likely to be referred to a specialist clinic and the latter rushed to hospital by alarmed relatives. However, the apparent severity of the attacks does not necessarily parallel their seriousness, as relatively minor symptoms occasionally herald a potentially life-threatening condition. While undoubtedly many such episodes do not come to immediate attention, those that do should be carefully assessed. Although most attacks are 'funny' (i.e. *peculiar*) to the patient they are usually easily recognized by the physician. In the majority the problem will resolve into epilepsy versus syncope (Table 17.1). In an important minority the attacks are initially 'funny' (i.e. *undiagnosable*) to the physician and investigations then are time-consuming and expensive. Diagnosis, if achieved, is often delayed.

As the opportunity to observe a 'funny turn' seldom occurs, the GP and casualty department staff have a special responsibility to document the events and the condition of the patient soon after the attack and to interview witnesses before they are lost or memories fade. A detailed account of the episode is the most important single factor in achieving an early correct diagnosis.

Taking the history

A description of the attack must be built up in great detail. Particular attention should be paid to the events leading up to the attack, the premonitory symptoms, if any, and the circumstances of the episode itself. The patient should be allowed to give his own sequential account of the episode but most will require prompting to achieve this. It will always be necessary to

Table 17.1. Causes of transient episodes of disturbed consciousness

Syncope	'Vaso-vagal' or reflex syncope
	Acute reduction in cardiac output
	—disorders of rate and rhythm
	—mechanical obstruction to flow
	Micturition syncope
	Carotid sinus syndrome
	Cough syncope
Epilepsy	Grand mal (tonic-clonic or major seizures)
	Temporal lobe (complex partial seizures)
	Focal motor or sensory seizures
	Petit mal
	'Minor' seizures
Basilar ischaemia	Migraine
	Thrombo-embolic 'vertebro-basilar disease'
Psychiatric	Pseudoseizures ('hysterical attacks')
	Hyperventilation syndrome
	Cardiac neurosis
Miscellaneous	Transient global amnesia
	Cryptogenic drop attacks of women
	Breath-holding episodes in infants
	Reflex anoxic seizures
	Narcolepsy
	Head injury
	Acute obstruction of CSF pathways
	Metabolic (hypoglycaemia, hypocalcaemia)
	Severe vertigo
	Iatrogenic—drugs
	—pacemaker malfunction

make specific enquiries to obtain crucial information which otherwise may be forgotten, neglected, considered irrelevant or even actively suppressed. Both positive and negative answers may be of value to subsequent investigators and should be recorded. Lastly, an eye-witness account should be obtained in similar detail.

Predisposing factors

If it is the patient's first attack a search for possible precipitants should be made and the prior state of health established. Marital disorders, epilepsy, diabetes mellitus, heart disease or fainting attacks in the family history may be relevant. Is there a past history of febrile convulsions, absence attacks or fainting in childhood? Has the patient had rheumatic fever, angina, serious head injury, meningitis or encephalitis? Faints are common after recent blood loss, during convalescence or after initiation of hypotensive drugs. Is there a history of mental instability, personality disorder or other psychiatric illness? A past history of alcohol or drug abuse may suggest withdrawal seizures, while disturbed sleep, marital discord and financial problems may suggest anxiety attacks or depression.

If there have been other attacks in the past the total number or frequency and pattern, if any, of occurrence should be established. Attacks which tend to cluster or have a clear relationship to the menstrual cycle are likely to be epileptic. Episodes which occur during sleep are unlikely to be hysterical but must be distinguished from the nocturnal syncopal attacks which occur *after* rising to pass urine. Attacks with a clear relationship to food intake or drinking may be hypoglycaemic, or suggestive of the acute effect that quite small quantities of alcohol may have in precipitating seizures in some young people.

The immediate circumstances of the attack frequently provides clues. What was the patient doing? A rapid change of posture may suggest syncope. A sudden emotional shock may precipitate syncope, an anxiety attack or even a serious cardiac arrhythmia (De Boer 1952). Hysterical attacks rarely occur without an audience. Blackouts in front of television may be photosensitive epilepsy provoked by flicker, or syncope in response to an unpleasant scene. Blackouts during exercise are more likely to reflect a cardiac problem than rare forms of reflex epilepsy. The pain of migraine or venepuncture that triggers a syncope is unlikely to be forgotten but identical attacks may result from quite trivial injuries.

Premonitory symptoms

Specific enquiry should be made for the very first warning of the attack. The characteristic paraesthesiae in the fingers and around the mouth in the hyperventilating patient, the prolonged nausea, warmth and blurred vision of presyncope and the rising sensation in the epigastrium associated with temporal lobe seizures, are usually obvious enough. Palpitations or chest pain may suggest a cardiac arrhythmia, anxiety attack or neurosis. A period of confusion and sweating may precede a hypoglycaemic blackout. In many cases a clear picture of the onset can only be obtained from an eye witness.

The eye-witness account

Although powers of observation and recall vary enormously and are often inaccurate, even fragmentary information obtained from the poorest witness can be of diagnostic value. Again attention should be paid to the onset of the attack. What was noticed first? Was the onset sudden or gradual? Did the patient communicate his aura or cry out? The aura of a temporal lobe seizure and the bout of coughing which may result in a syncopal attack are frequently forgotten by the patient. Did he look strange or behave oddly? Enquiry as to whether the patient was unconscious often elicits an evasive response but it can usually be established if the patient fell to the ground and was unresponsive. The gradual slump and limpness of the victim of syncope contrasts with the sudden crash and rigidity of the seizure. Was the jaw clamped tight? What was the colour? Patients may flush during strenuous pseudoseizures while pallor is the rule in vasovagal syncope. Either may occur during temporal lobe seizures. Were there any injuries? Tongue biting is uncommon in episodes of loss of consciousness other than epilepsy but injuries may occur in syncopal and hysterical attacks. Incontinence may occur in syncope when the bladder is full. Were there any involuntary movements? Head and eyes may be driven to the contralateral side by a focal, frontal epileptic discharge, or there may be focal twitching. It may be difficult, from eye witness accounts, to distinguish the random thrashing of a pseudoseizure from rhythmic clonic epileptic movements. Either may be interpreted as 'fighting' or 'struggling'. A demonstration of the difference will often establish the correct version of events! Merely asking for 'jerking' is of little value as the slight twitches that may accompany a faint, or the trembling of an anxiety attack may be misinterpreted. Patients who clutch and grip objects during violent attacks are unlikely to be in the throes of a major convulsion.

If there was no major convulsion was the patient in touch with his surroundings? Could he respond? Was speech possible? Unresponsiveness combined with the blank stare of the child with *petit mal* or the vacant lip-smacking appearance during a temporal lobe seizure, contrast with the anxious facies of the patient with transient global amnesia who asks repeated questions. The hysteric may produce clear words or phrases in the midst of a pseudoseizure whereas the patient with epilepsy, at best, mumbles incoherently. How long did the attack last? While witnesses are notoriously bad at estimating elapsed time it is important to differentiate the very short episodes of *petit mal*, which never last more than twenty seconds, from temporal lobe seizures which are usually of several minutes duration.

Sequelae

A sore tongue or cheek, incontinence, myalgia and headache may all suggest a seizure. Rapid recovery is the rule after syncope and most 'hysterical' attacks, but post-ictal confusion, amnesia for events after an initial recovery of consciousness, and drowsiness, are features of convulsions. Complete recovery after severe convulsions may take several days. Facial flushing following cardiac asytole is usually very transient but pallor may persist long after vasovagal syncope. Polyuria may occasionally follow a paroxysmal tachyarrhythmia.

Points and problems in the diagnosis of various funny turns

Syncope and pre-syncope

'. . . the brain that dies because it fails to receive from the heart the fluid which ordinarily stimulates it.'

Xavier Bichat, Studies in Life and Death.

A critical reduction in cardiac output due to reduced cardiac filling will result in a variety of premonitory symptoms (pre-syncope or lipothymia) followed by loss of consciousness (faint or syncope, from the Greek *synkoptein*—to cut or break). The causes of syncope are listed in Table 17.2.

The premonitory symptoms include various combinations of malaise, dizziness, dimming or blurring of vision, tinnitus or fading sound, warmth and sweating ('clamminess'), increased salivation, nausea and abdominal discomfort. Faints almost invariably occur when standing up (they may occur rarely in the recumbent pregnant patient) and may be avoided by quickly lying down. Otherwise, the patient will slump to the ground unconscious and flaccid, with rolled up eyes. A 'waxy' pallor results from profound vasoconstriction in the skin. The duration of loss of consciousness is usually only five to ten seconds during which there may be flickering of the eyelids and the odd twitch of the limbs. There is then rapid recovery provided recumbency has been achieved. If the patient is unlucky enough to be held upright, as in a confined space, the anoxia may trigger a major seizure and serious cerebral damage, even death, may ensue.

Vaso-vagal syncope (reflex syncope)

Most people have little difficulty in recognizing the uncomplicated faint when it occurs in appropriate circumstances and these patients are seldom sent to hospital. The adolescent boy who collapses in a crowded church with pallor and sweating after feeling hot and sick recovers rapidly in the vestry and is sent home. It is the most common form of syncope and is due to a combination of reflex vagal bradycardia and peripheral vasodilatation in the skeletal and visceral circulations (Sharpey–Schafer 1953, 1956). It can be precipitated in susceptible individuals by prolonged standing, a lordotic posture, hot stuffy surroundings, emotion, fatigue, pain or other unpleasant experiences. It is primarily a disorder of childhood and adolescence. Although there is a second peak of incidence in middle and late life adults who present with faints almost invariably give a history of similar episodes in

Table 17.2. Syncope: causes, potentiating and precipitating factors

'Vaso-vagal' syncope	Sudden postural change
	Prolonged standing
	Lordotic posture
	Pain (e.g. inju^y, injection)
	Unpleasant experience
	Acute emotion
	Excess heat
	Fatigue
	Anaemia
	Pregnancy
	Anoxia
Micturition syncope	Nocturnal micturition (males)
Cough syncope	Cßronic respiratory disease
Carotid sinus syndrome	Atherosclerosis of carotid sinus
Syncope associated with swallowing or defaecation	
Valsalva manoeuvre	Weight-lifting
	Wind instruments
	Prostatism
Disturbances of cardiac rhythm	Heart block
	Sino-atrial disease ('sick sinus syndrome')
	Tachyarrhythmias ($\pm$ postural change)
	Reflex asystole (pain-induced)
	Drug-induced
	Inadequate pacemaker
Structural cardiac disease	Aortic stenosis
	Hypertrophic obstructive cardiomyopathy
	Atrial myxoma
	Cardiac tamponade
Postural hypotension	Drugs
	Elderly
	Autonomic neuropathy (e.g. diabetes, Shy–Drager syndrome)
	Paraplegia
	Tabes dorsalis
	Convalescence from serious illness

their youth. Other factors that reduce cardiac filling may potentiate vaso-vagal syncope in the susceptible (Table 17.2).

Complications and variants

If syncope lasts more than ten seconds through failure to restore adequate cerebral blood flow, the deepening anoxia may be associated with one or two

clonic jerks and perhaps generalized rigidity ('tonic spasm') or even opisthotonous with clenched fists, dilated pupils and salivation ('convulsive syncope', Gastaut and Fischer–Williams 1957). There may be one or two
further jerks, but unlike a major convulsion, consciousness is rapidly
regained in a further five to ten seconds with little or no 'post-ictal'
confusion. Such 'tonic-anoxic' seizures may also occur secondary to short
periods of cardiac asystole or ventricular fibrillation.

The reflex anoxic seizure (Stephenson 1978) in which asystole is precipitated by pain, is a frequent source of alarm and erroneous diagnosis.

An 8-year-old girl has had several episodes of loss of consciousness with
rigidity and occasional incontinence usually occurring in the playground.
The patient, already on sodium valproate and with a diagnosis of
epilepsy, is referred to the clinic. Epilepsy is considered possible but
during tests a 'convulsion' is precipitated by venepuncture. There is
rapid recovery without confusion. A diagnosis of reflex anoxic seizures is
confirmed when an identical episode lasting 14 seconds is precipitated by
ocular compression and shown to coincide with cardiac asystole and
secondary slow waves on the EEG.

These attacks probably represent one end of the spectrum of vagally-
mediated reflex syncopes and have been estimated to occur in 8 per 1000
pre-school children (Lombroso and Lerman 1967). Up to 25 per cent have
been incorrectly diagnosed as epileptic. They are provoked by trivial injury
or a febrile illness. There is often no pallor and they are distinguished from
breathholding attacks by the cardiac asystole and the lack of cyanosis. They
can be prevented by long acting atropine preparations and may persist into
adult life.

Micturition syncope

The healthy adult male who collapses in the bathroom in the small hours
after passing urine is at considerable risk of being labelled epileptic. This
error is even more likely if he becomes wedged upright between wall and
bath where the resulting anoxic seizure is witnessed by an alarmed wife.

Although occasional 'cures' have been reported after surgical correction
of bladder neck obstruction (Eberhart and Morgan 1960), it is not a condition restricted to elderly men with prostatism. The peak incidence is
40–50 years (Gastaut and Gastaut 1956) but first attacks may occur in the
teens or may present for the first time in the sixth decade (Proudfoot and
Forteza 1959). The prevalence in healthy young men with a history of at least
one other simple faint has been reported to be about 4 per cent (Dermkisian
and Lamb 1958). Relevant physiological factors emphasized to varying
degrees by different authors include the sudden postural change, the relative
vasodilatation and low blood pressure resulting from increased vagal tone,

the Valsalva effect, the parasympathetic discharge associated with micturition and the loss of the pressor effect of the distended bladder.

Given the highly characteristic circumstances, investigations are seldom required and the usual management is to advise patients to get up slowly, and to pass urine sitting down. Such advice is presumably effective as few patients return to the clinic.

Cough syncope

The very high intrathoracic pressures which can be generated by violent coughing (200–300 mm Hg) impede venous return by an exaggerated Valsalva effect and may provoke a sudden peripheral vasodilatation via a baroreceptor reflex (Sharpey–Schafer 1953). Attacks may be precipitated by a single cough, nasal irritation or smoking and occur mainly in males with chronic respiratory disease. Some patients are amnesic for, or may deny the responsible coughing paroxysm and the accompanying twitching or secondary anoxic seizure may be confused with epilepsy. An eye witness is essential. Neurological examination should be carried out as *rare* cases with cerebral tumours or cerebrovascular disease may present in this way (Morgan–Hughes 1966). Providing anticonvulsants are avoided the condition is usually benign requiring only treatment of the chest condition and education of the patient on the dangers of severe coughing.

Carotid sinus syndrome

Hypersensitivity of the carotid sinus region to pressure is an occasional finding in patients presenting with dizzy attacks or syncope. In the affected middle aged or elderly patient head turning, carotid massage or sometimes the lightest touch may cause a severe bradycardia or prolonged asystole with profound hypotension. This has been considered to be due to atheroma of the carotid sinus but to what extent a hyperactive vagus or abnormally excitable sinus node may contribute is unknown. Some patients have evidence of cardiac conduction problems (Davies *et al.* 1979). Attacks may be prevented by anticholinergic drugs or pacemakers and in severe cases denervation of the carotid sinus (Hutchinson and Stock 1960).

Cardiac causes of 'funny turns'

Cardiac arrhythmias and their management are covered in detail in Chapter 5 and I shall limit my discussion to some aspects of symptomatology and the diagnostic problems posed by attacks with a cardiac basis.

While many cardiac conditions may precipitate episodes of altered awareness (Table 17.2) the common final mechanism is a reduction of cerebral blood flow due to a transient failure of cardiac output. Most episodes are due to disorders of rate or rhythm, but in some patients a structural abnormality may impair the ability of the heart to rapidly increase its output. Diagnostic difficulties are frequently due to the non-specificity of the syncopal symptoms and the transient nature of many arrhythmias. In some patients a combination of structural disorder and rhythm disturbance, or of pathological and physiological mechanisms, may be required to produce symptoms. For example, runs of paroxysmal tachycardia may be completely asymptomatic; resulting in a blackout only when they coincide with a postural change. Attacks associated with exertion or emotion in patients with restricted cardiac output may be due to reflex peripheral vasodilatation (Mark *et al.* 1973) superimposed on the outflow obstruction.

Structural cardiac lesions sufficiently severe to produce blackouts will usually be evident on examination or with echocardiography. Syncope may result from impaired atrial filling associated with a pericardial effusion, reduced ventricular filling due to an atrial myxoma or mitral stenosis, or obstruction to ventricular outflow in aortic stenosis or cardiomyopathy. However, the mere demonstration of such defects does not necessarily account for the funny turns. The risk of blackouts in hypertrophic cardiomyopathy may be related to ventricular arrhythmias that are commonly associated with this condition (McKenna *et al.* 1980), as it does not correlate with the degree of outflow tract obstruction (Doi *et al.* 1980). Funny turns in patients with mitral stenosis are more likely to be due to paroxysmal tachycardia than impaired ventricular filling and conduction defects are often present in cases of calcific aortic stenosis.

The most frequent symptoms produced by cardiac arrhythmias are dizziness, giddiness or blackouts. The complaint of palpitations does not significantly correlate with the finding of serious cardiac arrhythmias on long-term monitoring of· patients with funny turns at neurology clinics (Luxon *et al.* 1980). Their presence or absence are unreliable diagnostic features as they frequently go unnoticed or are not recalled after the event and may also occur with anxiety, epileptic or hypoglycaemic attacks. Other symptoms during episodic arrhythmias may closely resemble the aura of temporal lobe epilepsy (TLE). Some may be so bizarre that hysteria is considered. Strange feelings of disembodiment or distortions of body image have been reported in the dizzy attacks of chronic sino-atrial disease (Pearson 1945). Burning paraesthesiae and other odd visceral sensations may be described ascending from the stomach to chest, throat or head during attacks of atrioventricular (AV) block or paroxysmal ventricular fibrillation (Parkinson *et al.* 1941; Campbell 1944).

The classic example of the cardiac funny turn is the Stokes–Adams attack. In the typical triad, flushing follows the sudden loss of consciousness and pallor and the diagnosis is obvious when a slow pulse or typical ECG is found. However, flushing may be absent, minor attacks of dizziness are more common and heart block may occur on a background of sinus rhythm. Identical attacks may be caused by paroxysmal ventricular tachycardia or fibrillation and sinus arrest (Parkinson *et al.* 1941; Jensen *et al.* 1975). Minor attacks may go unnoticed by the patient unless items are dropped or injuries ensue (Pearson 1945). The arrhythmia may be triggered by noise, stooping, exertion, swallowing or defaecation, causing confusion with other forms of syncope.

Witnessed attacks during cardiac arrhythmias may be difficult to distinguish from temporal lobe epilepsy. There may be no more than a vacant expression with pallor and rapid recovery. One patient with periods of asystole due to sino-atrial disease would develop a look of fear followed by version of the head and eyes to the right with clenched teeth, repetitive swallowing and clutching of the hands (Pearson 1945). Such attacks may well be seizures secondary to previous ischaemic temporal lobe damage and triggered by the anoxia associated with reduced flow in the vertebrobasilar system, but simultaneous ECG and EEG data is not available in these reports. If loss of consciousness ensues, the patient is usually flaccid but a secondary anoxic seizure may occur as for any syncope. Tongue-biting was described in Stokes' original patient (Stokes 1846) and unequivocal tonic-clonic convulsions, even status epilepticus (Chaudron *et al.* 1976), may be a rare complication of cardiac arrhythmias (Singer *et al.* 1974).

Cardiac neurosis ('effort syndrome')

Syncope is a rare complication of this syndrome which may account for 10–15 per cent of all patients referred to cardiac departments (Kelly 1980). More typical features are the fear of death from a heart attack, palpitations, breathlessness, fatigue, dizziness and left submammary pain.

Iatrogenic

Drugs may cause dizzy attacks or blackouts by a variety of mechanisms including postural hypotension (e.g. L-dopa, hydrallazine, glyceryl trinitrate, nifedipine) cardiac arrhythmias (e.g. digoxin and tricyclic anti-depressants) lowered seizure threshold (e.g. phenothiazines, antidepressants) or increased conduction block (e.g. beta-blockers, verapamil, anticonvulsants). The ability of tricyclic antidepressants to precipitate both seizures and cardiac arrhythmias is a potential source of confusion. Moreover, the increased conduction block caused by tegretol and phenytoin (Rosen *et al.* 1967; Beerman *et al.* 1975) in patients with diseased conducting tissues may be a hazard for those who advocate 'therapeutic trials' for non-specific attacks.

Pacemakers may fail because the diagnosis is wrong, because of external electrical interference, because the loss of atrial systole may be important in the diseased heart or because of inhibition from skeletal muscle potentials during activity (Ohm *et al.* 1974).

Epilepsy

The management of epilepsy is covered in Chapter 18 and this section is limited to a brief consideration of some aspects of diagnosis.

Epilepsy is a symptom and not a disease so a complete diagnosis requires, in addition, the type and cause of the seizures in the individual patient. The main causes are listed in Table 17.3. Epileptic seizures are due to a sudden, excessive neuronal discharge in the central grey matter which tends both to recur and to have stereotyped effects. Occurrence may be random, but there is a tendency to cluster and onset in sleep or shortly after waking is common. In some patients, fits may be evoked by stress or fatigue, or a specific stimulus such as a flickering light or pattern, but most occur spontaneously without obvious triggers. Attention should be directed towards the aura or focal onset, the tonic phase (rigidity, forced cry), the clonic phase (rhythmic bilateral jerking of the limbs and tongue-biting) and the aftermath (drowsiness, confusion, headache, irritability, myalgia and incontinence).

Temporal lobe epilepsy

Diagnostic bewilderment often arises from the apparently endless variety of symptoms reported to occur in complex partial seizures and from the difficulties of the patients in describing them. The majority of such attacks present few diagnostic problems. Textbooks often lay much emphasis on the uncommon olfactory or gustatory aura but the most frequently encountered aura is the epigastric sensation which characteristically rises into the chest or throat. This is often accompanied by a dream-like sensation of familiarity (*déjà vu*) or one of unfamiliarity (*jamais vu*). There may be fear or panic, distortions of body image, vertigo and stereotyped and alarming hallucinations. In most attacks the patient will usually stop his activities, look blank and appear partially or wholly unresponsive. He may go pale or flush. Speech may arrest or become slurred or nonsensical. Automatic grimaces, lip-smacking, swallowing or chewing and repetitive movements of the limbs commonly occur without the patient's awareness. A brief period of confusion may follow and the patient may be amnesic for the whole episode. In some patients more complex, semi-purposeless behavioural patterns may occur. The patient may walk about, or abruptly and inappropriately leave the room or start folding newspapers. There may be prolonged spells of

Table 17.3. Main causes of epilepsy

Constitutional	Idiopathic
Local structural disease	Tumour Abscess Subdural haematoma Angioma
Infectious and demyelinating disease	Meningitis Acute infections ('febrile convulsions') Encephalitis Neurosyphilis Parasitic infestations Demyelination
Trauma	Perinatal injury or haemorrhage Head injury
Congenital	Tuberose-sclerosis, porencephaly
Degenerative and inborn errors of metabolism	Cerebral lipidoses Leukodystrophies Alzßeimer's disease
Vascular	Infarction Eclampsia Hypertensive encephalopathy
Exogenous poisons	Alcohol Barbiturates Tricyclic antidepressants Phenothiazines Local anaesthetics Amphetamine Monoamine-oxidase inhibitors
Anoxia	CO poisoning Nitrous oxide anaesthesia Severe anaemia
Metabolic and endocrine	Uraemia Hepatic failure Water intoxication Hypocalcaemia Hypokalaemia Porphyria Pyridoxine deficiency Alkalosis
Reflex epilepsy	Photosensitivity Gelastic Musicogenic Tactile epilepsy

confusion and unresponsiveness with odd behaviour (psychomotor fugue). The majority of attacks are over in several minutes or less and the aura, unlike the prolonged warning phase in presyncope or anxiety and 'hysterical attacks', lasts only a few seconds.

Other types of focal seizure include *Jacksonian motor epilepsy* in which rhythmic involuntary movements begin asymmetrically in one thumb or great toe or at the corner of the mouth. The attack may march up the limb and recede after seconds or minutes or end in a generalized convulsion. A transient weakness of the limb may follow the attack (Todd's paresis). *Sensory epilepsy* in which a similar anatomical march occurs is much less common. An epileptic discharge beginning in one frontal lobe may cause version of the head and eyes to the contralateral side (versive seizure).

Petit mal

This term should be strictly reserved for brief absences in which loss of awareness and arrest of activity lasts *no more than twenty seconds* (usually less) and is accompanied by a vacant stare and 3 cycle per sec spike and wave activity in the EEG. There may be slight pallor or flushing, blinking and one or two twitches in the limbs, but there are often no movements at all. The patient usually resumes activity immediately, often unaware of the gap and with no sequelae. It occurs for the first time only in childhood, but may persist into adult life.

Minor seizures

Some brief attacks do not fit neatly into the above categories. There may be a sudden fall with brief loss of consciousness but without convulsive movements (akinetic epilepsy). Other patients may have clonic jerks with incontinence but no fall. Some attacks which otherwise resemble *petit mal* may be followed by confusion or amnesia. Myoclonic jerks may occur without accompaniment, the outflung arm knocking over the milk at breakfast or the legs giving way without loss of consciousness.

Psychogenic or pseudoseizures ('hysterical attacks')

'. . . the moving womb when suddenly carried upwards violently compresses the intestines, the woman experiences a choking after the form of epilepsy but without convulsions'

Araeteus, Essay on hysteria. c.200 AD.

As many as 36 per cent of patients who present with 'episodes of uncertain mechanism' may be shown to have pseudoseizures by prolonged videographic recordings (King *et al.* 1982). In different studies of epileptic populations, between eight and twenty per cent have been reported to have *both* epileptic fits and pseudoseizures (Ramani *et al.* 1980; Desai *et al.* 1982). These patients are difficult to manage and tend to gravitate to specialized centres.

There are no specific diagnostic criteria for pseudoseizures and their differentiation from epilepsy on the basis of either history or observation is often difficult. King *et al.* (1982) found neurologists were correct in only 72 per cent of attacks observed on videotape without EEG or clinical information. Although the crudely imitated major convulsion will be obvious to the experienced observer, the resemblance to a major fit varies from case to case with the sophistication of the mimicry. Individual components may be very convincing but the overall pattern and sequence of events is often atypical and bizarre. When attacks occur without gross motor elements it is often more difficult to exclude epilepsy, particularly temporal lobe seizures.

The onset of a pseudoseizure is often vague and prolonged in contrast with the brief, sudden epileptic aura. Motor activity may be 'organized' or 'goal-directed', or composed of bizarre random asynchronous movements on either side of the body. Periods of unresponsiveness may alternate with episodes of motor or 'automatic' behaviour. In contrast to the forced expiration or grunts of a major seizure, opisthotonous may be accompanied by surprisingly well enunciated phrases, often vulgarities. Recovery may be rapid, even dramatic, perhaps with laughing or crying and a detailed recollection of events. Attacks may show a clear evolution with a continuously changing pattern, new features being added to old with a tendency to accumulate the more spectacular symptoms. In other patients, attacks may be quite stereotyped. The occurrence of tongue-biting, incontinence or a nocturnal onset seems controversial. Some authors maintain these features *never* occur in pseudoseizures (Riley and Massey 1980; Holmes *et al.* 1980), while a recent report suggests they are commonly encountered in this situation (Cohen and Suter 1982). In my own experience such features are rare and the contrary opinion may merely reflect the ease with which symptoms can be induced by suggestion in such patients when under intensive study.

Pseudoseizures frequently occur in front of an audience or in the clinic and may be precipitated by stress. Their onset is, in some cases, related to organic illness such as head injury or stroke (Liske and Forster 1964). They may occur in epidemics. In one outbreak at a comprehensive school which lasted twenty-one months, 447 blackouts occurred in sixty teenage girls and three boys (Mohr and Bond 1982). The affected girls showed a higher neurotic score and incidence of behavioural abnormalities than their non-affected classmates. When compared with control populations sufferers are statistically more likely to be single females with a family or personal history of depression or attempted suicide and high levels of 'morbid anxiety' (Roy 1979). Nevertheless, only a minority of patients with pseudoseizures display definite evidence of the 'hysterical personality' (Desai *et al.* 1982). Motives are unconscious in some patients but clearly intentional or wilful in others. This bimodality was thought to be reflected in the observation that during monitoring, attacks cease in some patients and continue unchanged in frequency in others (Holmes *et al.* 1980). Many patients have evidence of both conversion reaction and malingering (Skrabanek 1977). For these reasons, the terms psychogenic seizure (Desai *et al.* 1982) or pseudoseizure (Liske and Forster 1964; King *et al.* 1982) have been considered more appropriate than 'hysterical attacks'.

Attacks may be recorded after induction by hypnosis (Breuer and Freud 1955), mere suggestion (perhaps assisted by a tuning fork placed between the eyes) or saline injection (Cohen and Suter 1982). Videomonitoring with EEG will solve most difficult cases (King *et al.* 1982) and prolactin has been reported to be elevated in the serum 10–20 minutes after most major seizures, but not pseudoseizures (Trimble 1978). This test may prove to be less helpful where the attacks mimic complex partial seizures.

Firm pressure on one ovary was the treatment recommended by Charcot and found wanting by Gower (Lennox and Lennox 1960). Modern approaches seem similarly unsatisfactory and when pseudoseizures do remit other symptoms often take their place. Long term follow-up in hysterical patients suggests a 15 per cent reduction in life expectancy with a high incidence of suicide. Coexistent depression should be treated, although caution should be exercised if the patient is also epileptic. Serum drug levels should be checked. Toxic concentrations may produce both a deterioration in epileptic control and an increased frequency of pseudoseizures. If doubt persists, cautious weaning off anticonvulsants under close hospital observation is often helpful in coming to a decision.

Anxiety and hyperventilation attacks

Overbreathing in response to anxiety may produce tingling in the extremities and around the mouth, unpleasant sensations in the head or even tetany with muscle twitching and carpo-pedal spasm. Recognition of these real physical symptoms reinforces the victim's anxiety and increases the breathing further. As with a frightened squirrel in a cage each new symptom causes additional fear and more symptoms result. Most patients remain acutely alert throughout although it is claimed that loss of consciousness can occur. Symptoms may be reproduced by overbreathing and reversed by re-breathing into the traditional brown paper bag. The latter is still a surprisingly effective remedy in some patients but others may require tranquillizers or beta-blockers to break the vicious spiral.

Miscellaneous causes of episodic disturbed consciousness

Trauma

Brief loss of consciousness with amnesia for the event may result from head injury and cause diagnostic confusion. Head injury may also cause problems when it occurs secondary to seizures and syncopal attacks.

Migraine

Basilar migraine, which usually affects young women, may present with blackouts (Bickerstaff 1961). The prodromata of ataxia, dysarthria, paraesthesiae, confusion and visual symptoms which are due to brain stem ischaemia may be followed by gradual loss of consciousness for several minutes with a severe throbbing occipital headache and nausea on recovery. Migraine without loss of consciousness is usually present at other times. Treatment is usually ineffective and most symptoms eventually remit. Diagnostic problems may arise if the pain triggers off a vasovagal syncopal attack or very rarely an epileptic seizure, perhaps secondary to the ischaemia.

Transient global amnesia

Attacks take the form of a sudden loss of short-term memory, often lasting for several hours, during which the patient may be able to perform automatic tasks such as driving. More commonly he is disturbed by his loss of memory and asks repeated questions. There is no loss of identity or clouding of consciousness but the patient appears anxious and continues to ask about the time, his whereabouts and recent activities, despite repeated assurances. Abrupt recovery eventually occurs but the memory gap is permanent. Attacks may be precipitated in some by bathing or exercise. The pathological basis of these episodes is unknown, but is thought to be due to a transient ischaemic lesion of the temporal lobes. The patient can be reassured that recurrence is unlikely. These attacks may be confused with the amnesia of temporal lobe epilepsy.

Cerebrovascular disease

Basilar insufficiency is unlikely to be a cause of episodic loss of consciousness in the absence of other brain stem symptoms but it may account for occasional episodes in elderly patients with atherosclerosis. Compression of the vertebral artery in the neck with head movement must be a very rare cause of recurrent attacks of loss of consciousness.

Drop attacks

A sudden fall to the ground without loss of consciousness occurs in a rare form of *petit mal* and occasionally myoclonic epilepsy. A much more common condition of this type afflicts middle-aged women. The typical scenario is of a sudden inexplicable fall while out shopping which results in grazed knees and elbows. Fractures or head injuries may occur on occasion but most patients are aware of hitting the ground and put out their arms to break their fall. Therefore, any loss of consciousness is exceedingly brief. The patient is left shaken and embarrassed but without after effects. Despite intensive investigation no cause is found and the aetiology remains obscure (Stevens and Matthews 1973). Treatment is limited to reassurance of the benign nature of the condition and though attacks may recur over many years, the condition often remits.

Intermittent obstructive hydrocephalus

Acute obstruction of the CSF pathways, for example by the very rare colloid cyst of the third ventricle, may result in drop attacks with or without loss of consciousness and headaches. Mental changes and raised intracranial pressure may be present.

Vertigo

Consciousness may rarely be lost during severe attacks of aural vertigo. Coexistent deafness and tinnitus will usually make the diagnosis obvious. Vertigo is a more frequently encountered feature of the temporal lobe aura than is widely recognized (Kogeorgos *et al.* 1981).

Hypoglycaemia

A low blood sugar may be responsible for an almost infinite variety of neurological signs and symptoms and should always be kept in mind when presented with an acutely confused or comatose patient. Odd behaviour, ataxia, irritability and slurred speech due to hypoglycaemia has on occasion led to arrests on 'drunk and disorderly' charges. *Grand mal* seizures may be precipitated. The associated adrenalin secretion results in sweating, pallor, circumoral paraesthesiae, fear and palpitations. Most cases are due to insulin overdose but rarely these symptoms may be the presentation of an insulinoma. Patients with reactive hypoglycaemia, which may complicate gastric operations, may feel faint and giddy or even blackout after a heavy meal. The diagnosis may be established by a glucose tolerance test.

Narcolepsy

This disorder is characterized by an intermittent and overwhelming desire to sleep often in inappropriate circumstances. While the patient usually knows he is sleepy rather than 'having a blackout', it is often misdiagnosed as depression or hysteria. The sleep episodes are short and the patient can be readily aroused as from normal sleep. Associated diagnostic pointers include nocturnal insomnia, cataplexy, sleep paralysis and hypnagogic hallucinations. Treatment is with amphetamine derivatives and clomipramine.

Breathholding attacks

These alarming episodes occur in infants of less than three years of age and may be misdiagnosed as epileptic. They are characterized by arrest of respiration with limpness and cyanosis followed by clonic jerking. The EEG is normal and the clue to the diagnosis is the minor injury or painful episode which triggers the attack. They may be arrested at onset by a sharp slap.

Examination of the patient

Time spent on obtaining the history in minute detail is well spent as clues are often scarce when patients are examined between attacks. Nevertheless, full examination with close attention to the cardiovascular and nervous system is mandatory. Focal signs or signs of raised intracranial pressure will of course indicate the need for neurological investigation. Chronic respiratory disease and bouts of coughing may suggest cough syncope, and murmurs or irregularities of pulse, a cardiac cause. Postural hypotension should be excluded by taking the blood pressure lying and standing and if vasovagal syncope is suspected ocular pressure may precipitate a faint.

   While most funny turns will have resolved by the time the patient reaches hospital, valuable clues may be present in the aftermath. The patient's mental state should be assessed for residual confusion, disorientation, anxiety or drowsiness. The presence of injuries, particularly to tongue or head, should be sought and the temperature, pulse and respiratory rates noted. A transient pyrexia may occur after major seizures but does not complicate 'hysterical' or syncopal episodes. An extensor plantar response, or asymmetrical deep tendon jerks may be found in the post-ictal state, but rapidly resolve with recovery. Unilateral weakness may be a Todd's paresis or a chronic effect of neonatal brain damage.

   From time to time the casualty officer will have the opportunity to examine patients before they have recovered or even during their attacks. The usual examination of comatose patients should be carried out noting the depth of coma, pupillary responses, eye movements, corneal reflexes, response to pain, deep tendon jerks and the plantar responses. The blood should be taken for sugar examination and 50 grams of iv glucose given if there is doubt as to the cause of the attack. If a functional (pseudoseizure or hysterical) episode is suspected, various diagnostic pointers include the response to forced eye opening (resisted, positive Bell's sign), to restraining a jerking limb (force increases in proportion to degree of restraint), to obstruction of the airway by pinching off nose and mouth (terminates attack or provokes response(!)) (Riley and Massey 1980), and to turning the patient from one side to the other (eyes conjugately deviate towards ground despite 180° rotation) (Henry and Woodruff 1978).

Investigations

These can be tailored to the individual case to some extent, according to the reliability of the diagnosis, the age of onset and the severity of the complaint (Table 17.4). Three attacks in ten years can be investigated in the outpatient

Table 17.4. Investigations in patients with unexplained episodes of disturbed consciousness

	Mandatory	As indicated
X-rays	Chest, skull	CAT scan (e.g. focal symptoms or raised pressure)
Bloods:	Blood count ESR Sugar and calcium Urea and electrolytes Liver function tests WR	Blood sugar in attack Glucose tolerance test (reactive hypoglycaemia) Prolonged fast (insulinoma) Drug screen
Urine:	Routine analysis	VMA Porphyrins Amino acid/sugar screen (infants)
Cardiac:	Routine 12-lead ECG 24 hour ambulatory ECG monitoring	Repeated/prolonged ambulatory monitoring (continuing attacks) Carotid massage (carotid sinus syndrome) Treadmill test (exercise-induced attacks) Echocardiography (murmurs, left ventricular hypertrophy, etc.) Intracardiac electrophysiology
EEG	Routine 16-channel record including sleep, hyper- ventilation and photic stimulation	Long-term ambulatory EEG monitoring with simultaneous ECG Video (split-screen) telemetry techniques± activation procedures (suspected pseudoseizures or temporal lobe seizures)

clinic but the patient with two episodes of unexplained loss of consciousness in twenty-four hours should be admitted. In most funny turns diagnosis will be obvious from the history and investigations can be restricted to the essential. An EEG to confirm the diagnosis or demonstrate atypical features is all that can be justified in a straightforward case of *petit mal* epilepsy. As major seizures in children seldom have a structural cause, investigations other than simple screening of blood and urine and a skull X-ray and EEG are seldom warranted.

Less than half the adults presenting with epileptic seizures have structural lesions, but as the likelihood of acquired lesions increases with age, additional investigations including routine haematology, biochemistry, a chest X-ray, ECG and serology for syphilis should be performed. Of course focal seizures or signs would indicate the need for further tests, particularly a brain scan. In the absence of signs one's diagnostic enthusiasm should be tempered by the fact that many adult seizures remain unexplained even after extensive tests and a large proportion do not recur.

Patients with clearcut vasovagal or micturition syncope need advice rather than tests, although possible potentiating factors such as anaemia or ill health should be kept in mind. Patients suspected of carotid sinus syncope should have carotid massage carried out with ECG monitoring. Murmurs or unexplained ECG changes such as left ventricular hypertrophy should be pursued by echocardiography and an exercise tolerance test performed under careful supervision when attacks appear to be induced by exertion.

By far the majority of patients with unexplained attacks will have no abnormalities on examination, or on static laboratory tests. In these cases more intensive investigation may be required to exclude potentially treatable conditions (Table 17.4). Ambulatory monitoring of ECG or EEG (or both together) for long periods has been shown to be a useful technique for recording symptomatic events but it is time-consuming and presents considerable logistic problems. My present policy is to limit monitoring to a twenty-four hour baseline record if attacks are occurring somewhat less than once a week. If symptomatic events are occurring more frequently then monitoring should be continued (7–10 days is possible) until an attack is captured. Monitoring may need to be repeated on several occasions depending on attack frequency and severity.

The undiagnosable funny turn

After initial investigations have been carried out, a group of patients will remain whose attacks cannot be explained. Fortunately, these symptomatic episodes are often infrequent and in many cases soon remit without recurrence. If all baseline tests are negative a serious life-threatening condition is unlikely to have been missed. In some patients abnormalities may have been detected which may or may not require treatment in their own right, but to which the symptomatic episodes cannot be definitely related. Asymptomatic cardiac arrhythmias of doubtful significance are common in this population, increasing with age (de Bono *et al.* 1982). The prevalence of 'spikes' or paroxysmal discharges in the healthy population on long term EEG monitoring is as yet unknown. Artefacts which are difficult to distinguish from epileptic seizures are frequently encountered in such records (Blumhardt and Oozeer 1982a). Mistakes often occur with extrapolation from such asymptomatic findings and 'therapeutic trials' based on circumstantial evidence should be resisted. In my own experience patients with cardiac arrhythmias may find themselves on anticonvulsants while epileptics are considered for pacemakers. There is no substitute for relating captured symptomatic eventsœo simultaneous recordings and observations.

A female of 22 years (T.W.) gave a 5 year history of brief episodes in which she suddenly felt nauseated and weak with clammy hands. Although aware of surroundings throughout, she was unable to speak for 3 to 4 minutes, during which she would grip tightly on to any nearby support with eyes closed and was seen to be pale and trembling. After a further 10 minutes of mild malaise recovery was rapid.

An identical twin sister (T.T.) had very similar, though less frequent attacks. After two 'blackouts', a bundle of His abnormality was detected. A pacemaker was inserted. Attacks continued infrequently and irregularly despite the pacemaker.

Investigations in T.W., including ECG, EEG, bundle of His studies and CT scan, were all normal. Ambulatory ECG monitoring captured several attacks but showed only a sinus tachycardia of approximately 140/minute.

Simultaneous ECG and EEG ambulatory monitoring was then carried out for 120 hours and several typical attacks were captured. At the onset of each episode seizure activity occurred over the right hemisphere spreading to the left and accompanied by a sinus tachycardia (Fig. 17.1). A diagnosis of temporal lobe epilepsy was made and attacks ceased after commencement of carbamazepine.

Attacks continue in T.T. but are too infrequent to record at present.

However, in 64 per cent of patients with undiagnosed attacks the ECG and EEG appear normal during typical symptomatic events (Blumhardt and Oozeer 1982b). Such results are reassuring, ruling out cardiac arrhythmia as a cause of the symptoms and providing strong evidence, at least in dramatic attacks, against an epileptic convulsion. Nevertheless, long term follow-up studies are required to establish the significance of the findings. It should always be kept in mind that a negative result in one attack does not exclude a diagnosis of epilepsy, as seizures and pseudoseizures frequently co-exist.

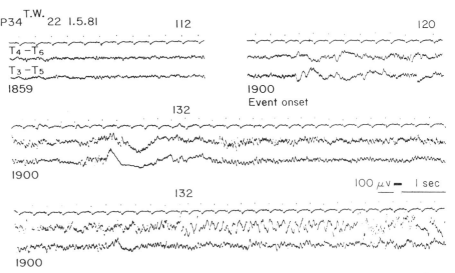

Fig. 17.1a. Simultaneous ECG and EEG recordings during onset of 'undiagnosed' attack. Top traces show events immediately prior to, and coinciding with, the onset of symptoms. Sequential traces below show the progressive build-up of epileptic seizure, with semi-rhythmic 5–6 cps slow activity over the right hemisphere accompanied by an increase in heart rate.

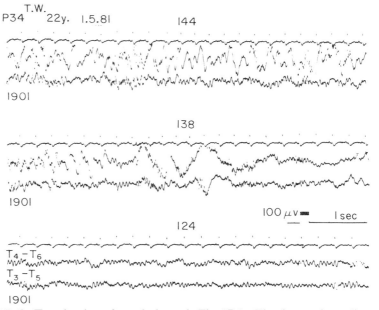

Fig. 17.1b. Termination of attack shown in Fig. 17.1a. The sinus tachycardia gradually subsides while slow EEG activity is now seen bilaterally but with greater amplitudes on the right side. The EEG rapidly returns to normal.

It is more difficult to exclude epilepsy as a cause of minor symptomatic episodes as ictal activity obtained from depth recordings may not be seen in surface traces (Crandall *et al.* 1963; Lieb *et al.* 1976). Ninety-five per cent of temporal lobe auras produce no detectable abnormality in surface EEG recordings (Ives and Woods 1980).

If unexplained attacks are continuing, the indication for more intensive investigations must be guided by the severity of the symptoms and their effect on the patient's day to day activity. Further assessment of the history from patient and witness is often helpful. Repeated monitoring or special tests may be indicated by new developments. When funny turns are frequent, admission for close observation and intensive monitoring, perhaps during supervised drug reduction, is often diagnostic.

Further reading

Beerman B., Edhag O. and Vallin H. (1975) Advanced heart block aggravated by carbamazepine. *British Heart Journal* **36**, 668–671.

Bickerstaff E.R. (1961) Basilar artery migraine. *Lancet* **1**, 15–17.

Blumhardt L.D. and Oozeer R. (1982a) Problems encountered in the interpretation of ambulatory EEG recordings in: *Proceedings of Symposium on Mobile Long Term EEG Monitoring* Bonn May 14–15, 1982. Stefan, H. and Burr, W. (eds) pp. 37–54. Springer Verlag.

Blumhardt L.D. and Oozeer R. (1982b) Simultaneous ambulatory monitoring of the EEG and ECG in patients with unexplained transient disturbances of consciousness in: *International Symposium of Ambulatory Monitoring 1981* Stott F.D. *et al.* (eds), pp. 171–182. Academic Press, London.

Breuer J. and Freud S. (1955) On the psychical mechanism of hysterical phenomena in Strachey J. (transl.) Studies on Hysteria vol. 2 in: *The Complete Works of Sigmund Freud.* Hogarth Press, London.

Campbell M. (1944) Complete heart block. *British Heart Journal* **6**, 69–89.

Charcot J.M. (1876) *Leçons sur les localisations dans les maladies de Cerveaux,* **1**, 1, Paris aux Bureaux du Progrès Médical.

Chaudron J.M., Heller F., Van den Berghe H.B. and Le Bacq E.G. (1976) Attacks of ventricular fibrillation and unconsciousness in a patient with prolonged QT interval. *American Heart Journal* **91**, 783–791.

Cohen R.J. and Suter C. (1982) Hysterical seizures: suggestion as a provocative EEG test. *Annals of Neurology* **11**, 391–395.

Crandall P., Walter R. and Rand R. (1963) Clinical applications of studies on stereotactically implanted electrodes in temporal lobe epilepsy. *Journal of Neurosurgery* **21**, 827–840.

Davies A.B., Stephens M.R. and Davies A.G. (1979) Carotid sinus hypersensitivity in patients presenting with syncope. *British Heart Journal* **42**, 583–586.

de Boer S. (1952) On the origin and essence of the Morgagni–Adams–Stokes syndrome. *Annals of Internal Medicine* **37**, 48–64.

de Bono D.P., Hyman N.M. and Warlow C.P. (1982) Cardiac rhythm abnormalities in patients presenting with transient non-focal neurological symptoms: a diagnostic gray area? *British Medical Journal* **284**, 1437–1439.

Dermkisian G. and Lamb L. (1958) Syncope in a population of healthy young adults. *Journal of American Medical Association* **168**, 1200–1207.

Desai B.T., Porter R.J. and Penry J.K. (1982) Psychogenic seizures. *Archives of Neurology* **39**, 202–209.

Doi Y.L., McKenna W.J., Chetty S., Oakley C.M. and Goodwin J.F. (1980) Prediction of mortality and serious ventricular arrhythmia in hypertrophic cardiomyopathy. *British Heart Journal* **44**, 150–157.

Eberhart C. and Morgan J.W. (1960) Micturition syncope. *Journal of American Medical Association* **174**, 2076–2077.

Gastaut H. and Fischer–Williams M. (1957) Electro-encephalographic study of syncope, its differentiation from epilepsy. *Lancet* **2**, 1018–1025.

Gastaut H. and Gastaut Y. (1956) Etude electro-encephalographique des syncopes. *Revue Neurologique* **95**, 420–421.

Henry J.A. and Woodruff G.H.A. (1978) A diagnostic sign in states of apparent unconsciousness. *Lancet* **2**, 920–921.

Holmes G.L., Sackellares J.C., McKiernan J., Ragland M. and Dreifuss F.E. (1980) Evaluation of childhood pseudoseizures using EEG telectomy and videotape monitoring. *Journal of Paediatrics* **97**, 554–558.

Hutchinson E.C. and Stock J.P. (1960) The carotid sinus syndrome. *Lancet* **11**, 445–449.

Ives J.R. and Woods J.F. (1980) A study of 100 patients with focal epilepsy using a 4 channel ambulatory cassette recorder in Stott F.D. *et al.* (eds) *International Symposium on Ambulatory Monitoring* pp. 383–392. Academic Press, London.

Jensen G., Sigurd B. and Sandoe E. (1975) Adams–Stokes seizures due to ventricular tachydysrhythmias in patients with heart block. *Chest* **67**, 43–48.

Kelly D. (1980) Cardiac neurosis. *Medicine*, 3rd Series, **36**, 1846–1849.

King D.W., Gallagher B.B., Murvin A.J., Smith D.M., Marcus D.J., Hartlage L.C. and Ward C. (1982) Pseudoseizures: diagnostic evaluation. *Neurology* **32**, 18–23.

Kogeorgos J., Scott D.F. and Swash M. (1981) Epileptic dizziness. *British Medical Journal* **282**, 687–689.

Lennox W.G. and Lennox W.A. (1960) *Epilepsy and Related Disorders*, Vol. 1. Little Brown & Co, Boston.

Lieb J., Walsh G., Babs T., Walter R.D. and Crandall P.H. (1976) A comparison of EEG seizure patterns recorded with surface and depth electrodes in patients with temporal lobe epilepsy. *Epilepsy* **17**, 137–160.

Liske E. and Forster F.M. (1964) Pseudoseizures: a problem in the diagnosis and management of epileptic patients. *Neurology* **14**, 41–49.

Lombroso C.T. and Lerman P. (1967) Breath-holding spells (cyanotic and pallid infantile syncope) *Pediatrics* **39**, 563–581.

Luxon L.M., Crowther A., Harrison M.J.G. and Coltart D.J. (1980) Controlled study of 24-hour ambulatory electrocardiagraphic monitoring in patients with transient neurological symptoms. *Journal of Neurology, Neurosurgery and Psychiatry* **43**, 37–41.

McKenna W.J., Chetty S., Oakley C.M. and Goodwin J.F. (1980) Arrhythmia in hypertrophic cardiomyopathy: exercise and 48 hour ambulatory assessment with and without beta adrenergic blocking therapy. *American Journal of Cardiology* **45**, 1–5.

Mark A.L., Kiosclios M., Aboud F.M., Heistad D.D., Schmid P.G. and Burr J.W. (1973) Abnormal vascular responses to exercise in patients with aortic stenosis. *Journal of Clinical Investigation* **52**, 1138–1146.

Mohr P.D. and Bond M.J. (1982) A chronic epidemic of hysterical blackouts in a comprehensive school. *British Medical Journal* **284**, 961–962.

Morgan–Hughes J.A. (1966) Cough seizures in patients with cerebral lesions. *British Medical Journal* **2**, 494–496.

Ohm O.-J., Bruland H., Pedersen O.M. and Waerness E. (1974) Interference effect of myopotentials on function of demand pacemakers. *British Heart Journal* **36**, 77–84.

Parkinson J., Papp C. and Evans W. (1941) The electrocardiogram of the Stokes–Adams attack. *British Heart Journal* **3**, 171–199.

Pearson R.S.B. (1945) Sinus bradycardia with cardiac asystole. *British Heart Journal* **7**, 85–90.

Proudfit W.L. and Forteza M.E. (1959) Micturition syncope. *New England Journal of Medicine* **260**, 228–231.

Ramani S., Quesney L., Olson D. and Gumnit R. (1980) Diagnosis of hysterical seizures in epileptic patients. *American Journal of Psychiatry* **137**, 705–709.

Riley T.L. and Massey C.W. (1980) Pseudoseizures in the military. *Military Medicine* **145**, 614–619.

Rosen M., Lisak R. and Rubin I.K. (1967) Diphenylhydantoin in cardiac arrhythmias. *American Journal of Cardiology* **20**, 674–678.

Roy A. (1979) Hysterical seizures. *Archives of Neurology* **36**, 447.

Sharpey–Schafer E.P. (1953) The mechanism of syncope after coughing. *British Medical Journal* **2**, 860–863.

Sharpey–Schafer E.P. (1956) Emergencies in general practice: syncope. *British Medical Journal* **1**, 506–509.

Singer P.A., Crampton R.S. and Bass N.H. (1974) Familial QT prolongation syndrome: convulsive seizures and paroxysmal ventricular fibrillation. *Archives of Neurology* **31**, 64–66.

Skrabanek P. (1977) Briquet's syndrome or hysteria? *Lancet* **1**, 1261–1262.

Stephenson J.B.P. (1978) Reflex anoxic seizures ('white breath-holding'): non-epileptic vagal attacks. *Archives of Diseases in Childhood* **43**, 193–200.

Stevens D.D. and Matthews W.B. (1973) Cryptogenic drop attacks: an affliction of women. *British Medical Journal* **1**, 439–442.

Stokes W. (1846) Observation in some cases of permanently slow pulse. *Dublin Quarterly Journal of Medical Science* **2**, 73–85.

Trimble M.R. (1978) Serum prolactin in epilepsy and hysteria. *British Medical Journal* **2**, 1682.

18 · Epilepsy

C. P. WARLOW

There are three fairly distinct situations in which epilepsy presents an urgent problem:

(1) A patient, who may or may not be known to have epilepsy, who has a single seizure.
(2) A patient who has a series of seizures in rapid succession, or who has a very prolonged single seizure.
(3) An unconscious patient who has had seizures in the past.

The diagnosis and differential diagnosis of epilepsy has already been covered in Chapter 17 and this chapter will focus on emergency and early management. It cannot be over emphasized that epilepsy of any type is a symptom and not a disease and, while treatment is being initiated, all the various causes of epilepsy must be kept in mind (Table 18.1). More than half the patients will have no identifiable cause for their seizures, in which case the epilepsy is deemed to be idiopathic.

A single seizure

It is usually the generalized tonic–clonic seizure (*grand mal* convulsion) which presents urgently to the general practitioner (GP) or casualty department whilst other less visibly dramatic forms of epilepsy (focal motor, focal sensory, temporal lobe, *petit mal* absences etc.) tend to be dealt with in the surgery or out-patients. However, a single *grand mal* convulsion does not necessarily demand urgent referral to hospital if the patient has recovered and there is no sign of head injury or acute neurological or other disease. Many such patients are best referred for a specialist opinion as an out-patient, provided of course that any waiting time is reasonably short.

First aid

The patient should be placed on the floor, or on a bed from which he or she cannot fall. Furniture and other objects which might result in injury should be moved away, any constricting clothing around the neck loosened and the patient placed in the semi-prone position as soon as it is feasible to achieve this. It is usually quite impossible to insert anything between the teeth during the tonic phase and if anything is going to be used later (which is seldom

Table 18.1. Causes of epilepsy

Infection	Encephalitis
	Meningitis
	Cerebral abscess
	Neurosyphilis
	Septicaemia
	Rubella
	Infectious mononucleosis
	Cytomegalovirus
	Toxoplasmosis
	Malaria
	Toxocara
	Cysticercosis
	Hydatid
	Post-immunization
	Febrile convulsions
Trauma	Head injury
	Subdural haematoma
	Neurosurgical procedure in the head
	Burns in childhood
Neoplasms	Primary, e.g. meningioma
	astrocytoma
	oligodendroglioma
	microglioma
	neurofibromatosis
	Secondary tumour
	Hamartoma
Metabolic disorders	Anoxia
	Electrolyte and water imbalance, e.g. hyponatraemia
	Hypoglycaemia
	Hyperosmolar non-ketotic hyperglycaemia
	Hypocalcaemia
	Hypomagnesaemia
	Hepatic failure
	Kernicterus
	Reye's syndrome
	Uraemia
	Hyperthyroidism
	Porphyria
	Amino-acidurias
	Galactosaemia
	Pyridoxine deficiency
	Eclampsia

Table 18.1. Causes of epilepsy *continued*

Cerebrovascular disorders	Intracranial haemorrhage
	Cerebral infarction
	Hypertensive encephalopathy
	Arteriovenous malformation
	Cortical venous thrombosis
	Vasculitis, e.g. systemic lupus erythematosus
	Migraine
Drugs and toxins	Alcohol
	Aminophylline
	Amphetamine
	Analeptics
	Anticholinergics
	Antihistamines
	Cephalosporins
	Cocaine
	Cycloserine
	Disopyramide
	Hypoglycaemic drugs
	Indomethacin
	Iodinated contrast media
	Isoniazid
	Lead
	Lignocaine
	Lithium
	Mianserin
	Naladixic acid
	Penicillins
	Phenothiazines
	Tricyclic antidepressants
	TRH
Drug withdrawal	Alcohol
	Barbiturates
	Benzodiazepines
	Other anticonvulsants
Miscellaneous	Multiple sclerosis
	Tuberous sclerosis
	Sturge–Weber syndrome
	Neurolipidoses
	Cortical dysplasias

necessary) it must be soft—a bitten tongue is more acceptable than bitten fingers and broken teeth which so often result from misguided attempts to insert metal spoons and such like. Dentures should be removed as soon as possible. When the clonic phase subsides the tongue should be brought forward and any mucous, blood, or vomitus cleared away so that an adequate airway can be maintained. No emergency anticonvulsant medication is necessary unless another seizure occurs within a matter of minutes or hours. The patient should be allowed to sleep and relatives or friends reassured. Analgesics may be useful if there is headache or muscle pains.

Reasons for a single seizure

If a patient has never had epilepsy before then the cause of the first seizure will need to be considered (Table 18.1) and the appropriate investigations instituted. Normally this does not have to be done as an emergency, unless the patient is obviously ill with some kind of neurological or other disease, and early referral to neurological out-patients is all that is necessary. Immediate anticonvulsant therapy is seldom required, an exception being the presence of definite intracranial disease. My own treatment preferences for the various types of epilepsy are shown in Table 18.2.

Table 18.2. Anticonvulsant treatment for various types of seizure

Type of seizure	First choice	Daily dose*	Daily dose in children	Second choice
Generalized tonic–clonic (*grand mal*) Focal motor, or focal sensory	Phenytoin	200 mg → 250 mg	5–10 mg/kg	Carbamazepine Phenobarbitone Valproate
Temporal lobe (complex partial)	Carbamazepine	200 mg → 400 mg	10–20 mg/kg	Phenytoin Phenobarbitone Valproate
Petit mal (absence attacks)	Ethosuxamide	500 mg → 750 mg	20 mg/kg	Valproate
Myoclonic seizures	Clonazepam	1.0 mg → 2.0 mg	0.1 mg/kg	Nitrazepam

*The daily dose should usually be divided and taken morning and evening. To minimize adverse effects the dose in the first column should be used for the first week and then increased to the dose in the second column. Thereafter the dose should be adjusted on the basis of seizure frequency, adverse effects and—with circumspection—blood levels.

If a patient has had seizures before, it is important to determine why another seizure has occurred and then to act accordingly. There are various possibilities:

1. Difficult control

In some patients epilepsy is, for various reasons, exceedingly difficult to control and such patients will often be brought to casualty departments following seizures. Usually the patient will be under the care of a specialist to whom he should be referred back with a letter explaining what has happened. If there are any difficulties (for example, not knowing the patient's exact medication) a telephone call will normally sort them out. Most neurologists subscribe to the 'one patient, one doctor, one drug' doctrine for the treatment of epilepsy and would far rather be consulted by telephone than have the patient appear in the next clinic on another, or worse still an additional, anticonvulsant. It is often helpful to the specialist if the casualty officer arranges for a blood level of the appropriate anticonvulsant just after the seizure.

2. Erratic drug-taking

A seizure may occur if a patient suddenly stops anticonvulsant medication, or is erratic with tablet taking. Of course a deliberate and recent change in medication may also be the explanation. A blood level just after the seizure will be particularly helpful in this situation.

3. Drug interactions

There are many drugs which increase the blood level and/or pharmacological effect of anticonvulsants (particularly of phenytoin, which is the most frequently prescribed and best studied) and which, when started, will precipitate anticonvulsant toxicity. If the anticonvulsant dose is reduced to counter this situation and then subsequently the other drug stopped, the anticonvulsant effectiveness will obviously be less. There are rather few interactions which reduce the effectiveness of anticonvulsants—possibly the use of antacids in patients taking phenytoin is an example.

4. Precipitating events

Patients with epilepsy may be sensitive to one or more events which increase the likelihood of seizures. For example:

    Photic stimulation (particularly television)
    Psychological stress
    Alcohol
    Withdrawal of drugs, particularly alcohol (Table 18.1)
    Physical stress (late nights, lack of food, infections, fever)
    Menstruation

Diarrhoea
Malabsorption
Epileptogenic drugs (Table 18.1)

5. Head injury

Patients with epilepsy are at risk of head injury; acute brain damage or a
subdural haematoma may increase seizure frequency.

6. Underlying cause

The underlying cause of epilepsy may be getting worse, so increasing seizure
frequency.

Early management

The first essential is a good history (usually from a witness but also, if
necessary, from a relative or friend, as well as from the patient) of exactly
what happened. It may be necessary to telephone the patient's general
practitioner or specialist to find out about medication, compliance and any
underlying disease. Examination of the nervous system is no more or less
important than examination of the rest of the patient and, in cases of
diagnostic doubt, evidence of a *grand mal* convulsion should be sought: for
example, a bitten tongue or inside cheek, petechial haemorrhages over the
upper trunk and neck, and urinary incontinence. A careful check for any
sign of head injury is most important, particularly if the patient is not
showing signs of regaining consciousness within an hour. Investigations can
be initiated, particularly if the patient has never previously had a seizure,
and include a full blood count, erythrocyte sedimentation rate, biochemical
screen, blood glucose, syphilis serology, chest and skull X-rays and an
electrocardiogram. If there is no sign of intracranial disease the need for an
electro-encephalogram (EEG) and computerized X-ray tomography of the
head (CT-scan) can be assessed later, usually by a specialist in out-patients.

Hospital admission is seldom necessary for patients who are known to
have epilepsy, indeed they often resent any such action. An exception is if
there is a significant head injury. Even a patient with a first seizure does not
need admission, provided there is complete recovery of consciousness, no
evidence of neurological or other disease and someone to look after the
patient at home. However, it is essential that the GP is informed that the
patient is going home, and an early appointment with a specialist must be
made so that the diagnosis and management can be reviewed—the patient
should take along a witness to the attack if one is available. Some night
sedation may be helpful for a few days if the patient is particularly anxious.

Status epilepticus

Repetitive generalized tonic–clonic seizures without return of consciousness between seizures, or a very prolonged tonic–clonic seizure (more than thirty minutes) is referred to as status epilepticus. The mortality is about 10 per cent although most, but not all, of the deaths are due to the underlying disease. The patient is at risk of injury, anoxia and pulmonary inhalation. In addition, continuing epileptic discharges almost certainly cause damage to the brain itself with subsequent neurological or mental deterioration. The management of a patient with several seizures in a few hours, albeit with return of consciousness between seizures, is hardly any less urgent and in both situations admission to hospital is necessary, preferably into an intensive care unit where neurological facilities and expertise are available. All anticonvulsants will, when used in the large doses necessary to supress severe epilepsy (e.g. 20 mg or more of diazepam given over a few minutes), have a tendency to depress respiration and one should be very alert to the potential need for ventilatory support.

The causes of status epilepticus

Status epilepticus is almost always a sign of significant intracranial disease if there has been no past history of epilepsy. The usual causes are infection, tumour, head trauma and cerebrovascular disease. If the patient is known to have had epilepsy before, the most likely explanation is irregularity or alteration in anticonvulsant medication, but the other reasons already mentioned in the discussion of a single seizure should not be forgotten. Of course it may not be very easy to discover if a patient has had previous seizures but there should be some clues: anticonvulsant, other drugs, or a prescription in the patient's clothes, drugs brought in by the ambulancemen if a patient was admitted from home, a bracelet or necklace indicating the diagnosis, an out-patient appointment card, or perhaps the characteristic facies and gums of a patient taking phenytoin. Also it is always worth considering a telephone call to relatives, friends, or the patient's GP.

Early management (Table 18.3)

First aid

The patient should be stripped, put in a loose gown, and placed on a bed with secure cot sides with enough padding to avoid injury. The semi-prone position is best and can usually be achieved between seizures at which time a plastic (*not* metal) pharyngeal airway should be inserted and secured. Care of the airway is crucial and suction will be necessary to clear mucous, blood,

Table 18.3. The management of status epilepticus (adults)

First aid   Airway and suction
                   Protect from self-injury
                   Semi-prone
                   Establish secure i.v. line

First line i.v. anticonvulsant treatment

	1. Diazepam	10 mg over 1–2 minutes. Repeat as necessary and/or diazepam infusion
or	2. Clonazepam	1 mg over 1–2 minutes. Repeat as necessary
or	3. Lorazepam	4 mg over 2 minutes. Repeat as necessary

Start, or continue long-term anticonvulsant treatment
      Take blood for drug levels
      Loading dose of phenytoin: 10 mg/kg oral (nasogastric tube)
      Tail off i.v. anticonvulsants

Treat any underlying cause

Second line anticonvulsant treatment

1. i.m. Paraldehyde	10 ml. Repeat as necessary, or i.v. infusion
2. i.v. Chlormethiazole	0.8 per cent solution 50–100 ml in 10 minutes, then up to 100 ml/hour
3. i.v. Phenytoin	50 mg/minute up to 1000 mg. ECG monitor

Last ditch anticonvulsant treatment
      i.v. Thiopentone, plus muscle relaxants and ventilation if necessary. Monitor EEG

General measures
      1. Nursing care
      2. Fluid and electrolyte balance
      3. Feeding via nasogastric tube if prolonged unconsciousness
      4. Monitor respiration, heart rate and BP, conscious state
      5. Control hyperpyrexia
      6. Watch for complications:
          Anoxia
          Acidosis
          Hypoglycaemia
          Head injury
          Renal failure

---

or vomitus. An intravenous line needs to be set up and secured particularly well. Although intravenous infusions are often necessary it is important not to add anticonvulsants to 500 ml of dextrose and allow it to run in slowly since someone may inadvertently increase the rate of delivery. It is better to use a system which can only deliver a small quantity at a time so that such an accident cannot occur.

Immediate treatment

The seizures must be stopped as soon as possible and three mistakes are commonly made:

(1) to give anticonvulsant drugs in an inadequate dosage,
(2) to give the drugs intramuscularly,
(3) to delay starting oral anticonvulsants.

Not surprisingly there are few clinical trials in this area and the treatment recommendations are always influenced by personal experience. If treatment is started out of hospital it is essential to send a note of the drug, route of administration, and dose. Apart from paraldehyde, *intramuscular drugs should never be used* since their absorption can be erratic and delayed: *intramuscular benzodiazepines are particularly useless.*

Intravenous diazepam

Diazepam is made up in 10 mg or 20 mg ampoules. Ten mg should be given i.v. over one or two minutes. If the seizures do not stop within about five minutes a further dose should be given. If, after about 40 mg have been given over twenty minutes, there is no response, then this drug should be abandoned and clonazepam tried (see below), remembering that the side effects are likely to be additive with the preceding diazepam. In children, the i.v. dose is 0.2 to 0.3 mg per kg. If the bolus does stop the seizures but they then recur after fifteen to thirty minutes (the effective half life of diazepam being quite short when given intravenously) a diazepam drip should be used. However, there is no point in using a drip if the boluses have been ineffective. 100 mg of diazepam can be made up in 500 ml of dextrose or dextrose–saline and infused at a rate high enough to control the seizures. However, anything more than 40 mg per hour is likely to cause unacceptable adverse effects, particularly suppression of respiration and hypotension. As mentioned previously, a properly controlled infusion system must be used to avoid the possibility of the fluid being run in too quickly. The diluted solution should be used within six hours. Sedation is almost inevitable but of no particular importance at first.

Intravenous clonazepam

The dose of clonazepam is one-tenth that of diazepam and its effect may be even better and possibly longer lasting. There seems to be little experience with i.v. infusions but 6 mg can be made up in 500 ml of dextrose or dextrose–saline and is usable for up to twelve hours. However, there is some uncertainty as to the stability of clonazepam in dilute solution. The regime for i.v. boluses and the side effects are the same as for diazepam.

Intravenous lorazepam

There is little experience with this benzodiazepine but in some recent studies it has proved very effective. A 4 mg bolus should be given over two minutes and it can be repeated after fifteen minutes if necessary.

Second line anticonvulsants

If i.v. benzodiazepines are ineffective then one of the 'second line' anticonvulsants should be used. My own preference is paraldehyde and, if this fails, chlormethiazole. In the United States intravenous phenytoin is particularly popular. If all else fails thiopentone has to be used.

Paraldehyde

Paraldehyde is an unfashionable but remarkably effective anticonvulsant. In an adult, 5 ml should be given by intramuscular injection into each buttock. A glass syringe should be used if possible since paraldehyde dissolves certain types of plastic. However, in an emergency a plastic syringe is usually safe if the drug is drawn up and injected immediately. The dose may be repeated every few hours as necessary but frequent i.m. injections can cause muscle necrosis and an alternative is to use an i.v. infusion. A 6 per cent solution in dextrose–saline (30 ml in 500 ml) can be used in a dosage of up to 100 ml of the diluted solution per hour. As usual, the rate is governed by the therapeutic response and any adverse effects, usually depressed respiration.

Chlormethiazole

This drug has a short half life and has to be given as an intravenous infusion. It is available in 0.8 per cent (8 mg per ml) solution in dextrose and should be used in a dose high enough to stop the seizures but not so high that respiration is depressed. The initial dose is 50 to 100 ml over ten minutes, and then up to 100 mg per kg per hour which is about 100 ml per hour in an adult. It can cause rather prolonged sedation which may lead to diagnostic confusion.

Intravenous phenytoin

Phenytoin may be given as i.v. boluses directly into a vein or into an i.v. line provided this is flushed through. It tends to crystallize out in dilute solution and should never be used in intravenous infusion fluids. Nor should i.m. phenytoin be used since its absorption is unpredictable. It should not be given at a rate of more than 50 mg per minute since the propylene glycol solvent can cause hypotension. It is probably wise to monitor the electrocardiogram since phenytoin is a cardiac depressant and may cause various types of conduction abnormalities. Up to 1000 mg in twenty minutes can be given to an adult in this fashion. However, if the patient is already taking phenytoin the suitable dose is extremely difficult to calculate even when rapid blood level estimations are available. If the seizures recur, a further bolus of up to 500 mg can be given but blood levels must be used as a guide.

Intravenous thiopentone

If all else fails intravenous thiopentone can be used. To suppress very severe seizures an anaesthetic dose is usually required which will almost inevitably mean the need for assisted ventilation. If curare is used under these circumstances, and some would say even if it is not, continuous monitoring of the electro-encephalogram is mandatory since there is no longer any visible indication of continuing seizure activity within the brain. An initial i.v. bolus of 100 to 250 mg of thiopentone is given and then 50 mg every two to five minutes until seizure activity disappears from the EEG. At this stage the maintenance dose, to keep the EEG seizure free, is usually about 0.5 to 1.5 ml per minute of a 0.5 per cent solution (5 mg per ml). Despite the problem of circulatory overload, this is probably better made up in normal saline than dextrose since thiopentone is strongly alkaline and dextrose, which is acid, may reduce therapeutic effectiveness. Naturally this treatment requires close monitoring of arterial oxygen tension and blood pressure.

Starting, or continuing, long-term anticonvulsants

Sooner or later, it will be necessary to establish adequate long-term oral anticonvulsant prophylaxis so that i.v. therapy can be tailed off and stopped. Oral anticonvulsants can and must be started, usually by nasogastric tube, while the status epilepticus is being brought under control, usually within half an hour or so of hospital admission. An early start is important since it takes some hours to attain therapeutic blood levels. If a patient is already having anticonvulsants blood needs to be taken for drug levels and the normal regime continued by nasogastric tube, assuming it to be reasonable. If there are any problems with gastro-intestinal absorption the best plan is to use phenytoin in slow i.v. boluses.

Any inadequacies in the normal regime can be sorted out in the first few days, probably in consultation with the specialist looking after the patient. If the patient is not receiving anticonvulsants, a loading dose of oral phenytoin should be given (10 mg per kg, and then 5 mg per kg per day in two divided doses) and later doses adjusted in the light of therapeutic response, side effects, and blood levels. Oral carbamazepine or phenobarbitone are alternatives to phenytoin. Whichever drug is used, it should be given orally, started soon, and the blood levels built up quickly so that the intravenous drugs can be tailed off and stopped.

General measures

The complications of status epilepticus are listed in Table 18.4. To avoid them it is not only important to control the seizures as quickly as possible but also to have available good nursing, attention to the airway, adequate oxygenation, and satisfactory fluid balance. It is very easy to forget about fluid balance and the fact that large quantities of infusion fluid are often being used as a vehicle for anticonvulsants. Hyperpyrexia can develop during prolonged seizures and should be treated with tepid sponging and aspirin. In difficult cases monitoring of blood gases will be needed and

Table 18.4. The complications of status epilepticus

Head, or other injury
Respiratory obstruction
Respiratory depression (usually drug induced)
Inhalation pneumonia
Anoxia
Circulatory failure (usually drug induced)
Hyperpyrexia
Water and electrolyte imbalance
Acidosis
Hypoglycaemia
Hyperuricaemic acute renal failure
Pneumoperitoneum

Table 18.5. Monitoring of the following may be required in status epilepticus

Conscious level
Seizure frequency
Pulse and blood pressure
Temperature
Respiratory rate and depth
Fluid balance
Blood urea, uric acid and electrolytes
Blood glucose
Blood gases and pH
Blood levels of anticonvulsants
Electrocardiogram
Electro-encephalogram

occasionally intubation is required even if assisted ventilation is not. Some, many, or all of the variables in Table 18.5 may need to be monitored and none should be forgotten.

Treatment of the underlying cause

As soon as the immediate first aid has been given and intravenous anticonvulsants started, thought should be directed to the possible causes of status epilepticus, particularly if the patient has not previously had seizures. A history from a witness, friend, or relative is crucial and also as full an examination as possible under the circumstances. An increase in body temperature, because of the intense and prolonged muscle activity, and a neutrophil-leucocytosis are quite common. In fact there may even be a modest rise in the cell count in the cerebro-spinal fluid (very rarely more than 50 polymorphs or mononuclear cells per cubic millimetre) and cerebro-spinal fluid protein (never more than 1.0 g per litre). Naturally these findings must not be attributed to the status epilepticus until a search for infection has been negative. As soon as possible, blood will be needed for a full blood count, erythrocyte sedimentation rate, urea and electrolytes, anticonvulsant levels if the patient is already taking them, and at least a skull X-ray if not a chest X-ray should be done. If there is any hint of an underlying neurological disease a CT-scan of the head is required and this MUST be done before lumbar puncture if there is a possibility of raised intracranial pressure or a cerebral abscess. If the CT-scan does not show a mass lesion and the ventricles are of normal size, then lumbar puncture is safe and should be done if there is a possibility of encephalitis or meningitis. An electro-encephalogram will probably be needed quite early, and urgently if encephalitis is a possibility.

Within an hour or two it should be possible to have some idea of the underlying disorder, if any, to have instituted treatment, and—if necessary—to transfer the patient to a neurological or neurosurgical centre. Meanwhile, the specific and general measures for status epilepticus must be continued.

Focal and *petit mal* status epilepticus

Forms of epilepsy other than generalized tonic–clonic seizures may occur continuously and, although not as dramatic, require urgent treatment. For example, focal motor epilepsy may be so unremitting that the patient becomes exhausted, even though consciousness is retained. Both temporal lobe epilepsy and *petit mal* absences can be prolonged and the 'dreaminess' and confusion look very similar—an electro-encephalogram is necessary to differentiate between the two although in an adult *petit mal* status is exceedingly rare. The immediate treatment is, like major status epilepticus, intravenous benzodiazepines accompanied by the appropriate oral anticonvulsant, depending on the seizure type (Table 18.2).

The unconscious patient who has epilepsy

It is not unusual for an unconscious patient who is known to have epilepsy to be brought to the casualty department and the cause assumed to be 'post-ictal'. Post-ictal coma rarely if ever lasts more than an hour or two and within that period of time the patient should be showing signs of recovery. If this does not happen, the following possibilities need to be considered:

(1) Over-sedation.
(2) Overdose of anticonvulsants.
(3) Head injury.
(4) Progression of the underlying cause of the epilepsy.
(5) Temporal lobe or *petit mal* status.
(6) Other causes of coma.

A common problem is inadvertent over-sedation with anticonvulsants by either the GP or casualty officer. In this situation there should be no focal neurological signs and the coma should lighten within a few hours provided no further sedation, apart from the patient's usual anticonvulsants, is given. Anticonvulsant blood levels, if they can be obtained quickly, are obviously helpful here. The deliberate self-administered overdose of either anticonvulsants or some other drug is a possibility, particularly in a patient with epilepsy who, as is often the case, has behaviour problems, or who may even be schizophrenic. Head injury is common in patients with epilepsy and the skull should be carefully examined and X-rayed. If there is any hint of head injury, or focal neurological signs, a CT-scan may reveal intracerebral haemorrhage or subdural haematoma. It may also reveal a structural underlying cause for epilepsy (e.g. a tumour) which may have advanced and lead to coma. Finally, the usual causes of coma should not be forgotten (Chapter 2); epilepsy is no protection against, for example, diabetic keto-acidosis.

Further reading

Edie M.J. and Tyrer J.H. (eds) (1980) Pharmacological basis and practice: in *Anticonvulsant Therapy*. Churchill Livingngstone, Edinburgh.

Laidlaw J. and Richens A. (eds) (1982) *A Textbook of Epilepsy*, 2nd edition. Churchill Livingstone, Edinburgh.

Tryer J.H. (ed.) (1980) *The Treatment of Epilepsy*. MTP Press, Lancaster.

19 · Subarachnoid Haemorrhage

P. J. TEDDY

The exact incidence of spontaneous subarachnoid haemorrhage (SAH) in the United Kingdom is uncertain but is probably in the order of 15/100,000 per year. The principal underlying causes for all subarachnoid bleeds are:

1. Rupture of a cerebral arterial ('berry') aneurysm.
2. Bleeding from a cerebral or spinal arteriovenous malformation.
3. Trauma.
4. Bleeding into the subarachnoid space in patients who are anticoagulated or who suffer from blood dyscrasias.
5. Subarachnoid extension of a primary intracerebral haematoma and spontaneous 'hypertensive' SAH.

In about 15 per cent of patients investigated angiographically no cause can be found.

Bleeds from ruptured cerebral arterial aneurysms and arteriovenous malformations occur most frequently and certainly pose the most important problems in management. They occur with roughly equal probability up to the age of twenty but thereafter a ruptured aneurysm becomes increasingly the single most likely cause for the bleed. In general, unless there is strong evidence to the contary (e.g. a clear relation of SAH to trauma, uncontrolled anticoagulant therapy, a child or young adult presenting with an obvious intracranial bruit) all patients presenting with SAH should be suspected as having a ruptured aneurysm until proved otherwise. This is extremely important as improvements in the early diagnosis and management of these cases are critical factors which could lead to a reduction of the appallingly high mortality and morbidity rates associated with bleeds from aneurysms (Drake 1981).

The immediate mortality from a ruptured cerebral arterial aneurysm is about 40–45 per cent. Un-operated, 35 per cent of the survivors would be expected to die from recurrent haemorrhage within the first year. The great majority of these would die within the first three weeks, there being a mortality rate of roughly 8 per cent per week. Fifty-one per cent of the survivors would be dead within five years (Pakarinen 1967) and thereafter there is an annual rebleed rate of about 3 per cent.

Twenty years ago there was considerable doubt as to the efficacy of surgery in the treatment of ruptured aneurysms (McKissock *et al.* 1960). However, modern microsurgical techniques and improved neuro-anaesthesis have combined to reduce the operative mortality and morbidity to levels which should make occlusion of the aneurysmal sac the treatment of choice, whenever possible, to prevent fatal rebleeds.

Yet despite these advances, surgical treatment has not led to any dramatic fall in overall mortality and morbidity from this disease over the past two decades (Drake 1981; Adams *et al.* 1981).

There are two important reasons for this. The first is that as yet, we have made little progress in the prevention of either early recurrent haemorrhage or the treatment of cerebral arterial spasm occurring before or after operation.

One of the chief risks of operating on ruptured aneurysms is that of the development of postoperative cerebral arterial spasm. This occurs irregularly and unpredictably but once established is very resistant to treatment and may lead to severe ischaemic brain deficit and death.

The mechanism of production of vasospasm is unknown but may be in part due to the release of unidentified vaso-active substances into the CSF at the time of the bleed with their subsequent reactivation or further release combined with increased vascular sensitivity induced by surgery.

Neurosurgeons are still unable to agree upon the optimum time for operation following the haemorrhage. For several years a widely held view has been that the greatest risk of provoking postoperative vasospasm is brought about by operating within the first week to ten days following the haemorrhage (Adams *et al.* 1976). Thus many surgeons, and this includes probably the great majority in the United Kingdom, prefer to delay operation for at least a week in most cases and for even longer in patients with hypertension or other 'high risk' factors. Similarly, some neuroradiologists believe that cerebral angiography carried out within the first week may be detrimental. They prefer to delay such investigation, particularly in older hypertensive patients and those with a profound neurological deficit. However, several recent reports have suggested that operating strictly within the first forty-eight hours after the bleed does not carry this high risk of inducing postoperative vasospasm and, of course, means that many of those patients who would otherwise have died from a rebleed whilst awaiting surgery can be saved (Kassell *et al.* 1981; Ljunggren *et al.* 1981; Hugenholtz and Elgie 1982). Furthermore, those patients who do develop postoperative spasm after early operation can be treated more energetically knowing that the aneurysm has been occluded.

However, early operation following SAH can be technically much more difficult and hazardous and until such operations can convincingly be shown to be associated with a lower morbidity and mortality, the general attitude will probably be that of continuing to defer surgery, accepting that in the interim some patients may die or deteriorate to a level at which surgery cannot be contemplated.

The second reason for the continuing high mortality rate is that surgeons are seeing only a small fraction of all the patients suffering from SAH each year (estimated in various series as between thirteen and thirty per cent). Even allowing for the high immediate mortality this means that at the very best only half of the early survivors of a ruptured aneurysm come to surgery. Whilst some patients would never reach a stage where they might be considered for operation many others succumb for want of an early diagnosis and a prompt neurosurgical referral. If the morbidity rates are to be improved, the key must lie in the immediate recognition of the first bleed and in the provision of optimum early conservative treatment. Management must be aimed at minimizing the risk of recurrent haemorrhage particularly if neurosurgical investigations and operation are to be delayed, and at improving the condition of 'poor risk' patients such that they may later be considered for surgery. The remainder of this chapter is concerned with the diagnosis and medical management of SAH from suspected rupture of a berry aneurysm.

Diagnosis

History

Classically, SAH is characterized by sudden severe headache (frequently described as the worst headache the patient has ever had)—often occipital, frontal or behind the eyes—followed by nausea and vomiting. There is a variable effect on the level of consciousness, some patients carrying on with their work, others being rendered immediately deeply unconscious. Some patients complain of neck stiffness and of photophobia. Occasionally the onset is accompanied by a fit. Rarely the patient may present with sudden back pain and bilateral sciatica. The clinician should ask specifically about:

Previous history of similar headaches.
Previous epileptic fits (cerebral arteriovenous malformations (AVMs) commonly present with epilepsy).
Hypertension, eclampsia.
Trauma.
Anticoagulant therapy.

Signs

These will to some extent depend on the severity and site of the haemorrhage and on the time interval between the haemorrhage and presentation.
The critical sign is that of meningeal irritation (neck stiffness and positive Kernig's sign). The conscious level may be unimpaired or depressed to a variable degree. There may be photophobia, a niggling pyrexia, hypertension (in a previously normotensive patient) and retinal or subhyaloid

haemorrhages. If subhyaloid haemorrhages are present they are virtually pathognomonic of SAH. Papilloedema may develop over the few days subsequent to the bleed. Focal neurological signs may or may not be present. Listen for an intracranial bruit.

Suspect SAH in any case of sudden (not necessarily severe) headache which is unusual for the patient. Look for the signs described above. This cannot be over-emphasized as patients suffering a second SAH have a 64 per cent mortality rate and for a third haemorrhage the mortality rate is 86 per cent (Pakarinen 1967).

Differential diagnosis

The chief differential diagnoses to consider are:

Migraine

This may generally be excluded in cases of SAH by the absence of previous similar headaches, aura, teichopsia and family history and by the presence of neck stiffness.

Intracerebral haemorrhage/infarction

This is not usually accompanied by neck stiffness unless there is greatly elevated intracranial pressure or the clot has ruptured through the cortex. Focal/lateralizing neurological signs are generally prominent.

Cerebellar haematoma

This may be spontaneous in the elderly hypertensive, or associated with cerebellar AVMs in younger patients. It is usually accompanied by or preceded by cerebellar symptoms/signs (dizziness, ataxia, nystagmus) and if the clot is of large size, by 'coning' with profound impairment of consciousness and evidence of brainstem compression.

Bacterial meningitis

The main concern is to exclude this. Although the headache is usually of gradual onset, bacterial meningitis can develop extraordinarily rapidly. The signs may be identical with SAH and in a confused patient the history may not be sufficiently accurate to differentiate.

Confirming the diagnosis

Normally done by lumbar puncture which is mandatory to exclude bacterial meningitis. CT scanning may show blood in the subarachnoid space within the first few days but this should not be used (unless immediately available) to establish the diagnosis, except in those cases where there is a real doubt about the history or findings, e.g. papilloedema or evidence suggesting a posterior fossa mass lesion. There is still a substantial mortality from pneumococcal meningitis and time lost in its early treatment by transferring patients to distant scan facilities may be fatal. The principal uses of the CT scan in the management of SAH are in the demonstration of intracerebral and intraventricular clots, cerebellar haematomas and hydrocephalus and in indicating which aneurysm may have bled when several are later identified. If there is any doubt regarding the advisability of lumbar puncture then neurosurgical advice should be sought first.

The CSF obtained should be sent for microbiological examination and examined on the ward for uniformity of blood staining *and* xanthochromia of the supernatant which is normally present after about eight hours. Allow the red cells to sediment out and hold the supernatant up against a white card in natural light. *Always* look for xanthochromia yourself as it may be the only definite confirmatory evidence that an SAH has occurred. If it is absent in a doubtful case the patient may be spared unnecessary angiography, an investigation not without its own risks.

However, most cases of SAH present no diagnostic difficulty and after confirmation by lumbar puncture a neurosurgical opinion should be promptly sought.

Management

The period of medical management required will depend on the practice adopted by the regional neurosurgical unit and on the condition of the patient. The following suggested programme of treatment outlines the chief priorities.

Resuscitation

In the unconscious patient attention must immediately be directed toward:

Protection of the airway—if necessary intubate and, if the respiratory effort is inadequate, consider ventilation.
Preventing aspiration of vomit—keep the patient on his side and horizontal.
Fits—these should be aborted *promptly* with intravenous diazepam (10 mg) and if a single injection fails follow this with paraldehyde (5 ml i.m. in each buttock). Prophylactic anticonvulsants (diphenylhydantoin 300 mg daily, preferably given orally or by nasogastric tube) should then be started.

Assessment

The history and full neurological and general examination should include the points already listed in considering and confirming the diagnosis. Some idea of prognosis and candidacy for surgery may be gained by recording the patient's condition by means of a grading system such as that of Hunt and Hess (1968), e.g.:

Grade 1 asymptomatic or minimal headache and slight neck stiffness.
Grade 2 moderate to severe headache and neck stiffness with no neuro-
         logical deficit other than cranial nerve palsy.
Grade 3 drowsiness, confusion or mild focal deficit.
Grade 4 stupor, profound hemiparesis, decerebrate rigidity.
Grade 5 moribund.

Normally, only patients in Grades I and II are considered good operative risks.

General measures

These are aimed at treating symptoms of headache and of vomiting and photophobia and at preventing hypoxia, sudden changes in intracranial pressure and blood pressure and monitoring the neurological state.

The patient should be nursed horizontally on his side, preferably in a single but easily observed room in which direct bright light can be avoided. Neurological observations (pupil size and reaction, blood pressure, pulse, respiration rate, level of consciousness and limb movement) should be carried out by the nursing staff at four-hourly intervals, or more frequently if the clinical condition is poor. The patient should be kept quietly in bed and excessive visiting should be discouraged.

Headache should be treated with codeine phosphate (60 mg 4–6 hourly prn), DF118 or paracetamol. *Do not* give morphine, diamorphine, pethidine or any other drug which might impair respiration, alter the level of consciousness or mask neurological signs. Pentazocine can be a potent emetic and should not be given.

For nausea and vomiting we generally give metoclopramide 10 mg i.m. or prochlorperazine 12.5 mg i.m.

Although strict bed rest should be maintained most patients find using a bedpan is awkward. Straining at stool should be avoided and a suitable compromise is to allow the patient up only to use the commode. If there is evidence of constipation—and there frequently is in view of the use of large amounts of codeine—then suitable laxatives should be given. Patients should be commenced on oral fluids (1500 ml daily) and feeds (1000–1500 calories/day) as soon as they are able to take these, otherwise fluids, food and drugs are best given by nasogastric tube. Clearly, in some patients fluid and electrolyte deficits may have to be replaced by intravenous infusion. Blood urea and electrolytes should be checked regularly as electrolyte disturbances—particularly hyponatraemia—are common following SAH. These can profoundly affect the neurological state.

It is important to prevent patients becoming hypoxic as this may lead to cerebral vasodilatation and brain swelling thereby increasing the intracranial pressure and impairing the level of consciousness. Patients should be examined regularly for evidence of chest infection and treated promptly should this occur. Those patients at particular risk for developing deep venous thromboses should be supplied with anti-embolism stockings.

Preventing the recurrent haemorrhage

There are at present two specific lines of treatment (neither of which has achieved universal adoption) which are used in an attempt to prevent rebleeding. The first is that of treatment of hypertension and general control of the blood pressure and the second is the use of antifibrinolytic agents to prevent clot lysis in and around the aneurysm sac.

Many previously normotensive patients who suffer an SAH have moderate elevation of blood pressure on admission. This may well settle spontaneously but some surgeons maintain that pre-operative hypertension (taken as being systemic blood pressure higher than 140/90) carries a poor prognosis and advise that any patient who is found to be hypertensive on admission should be treated with antihypertensive agents and surgery should be delayed (Artiola I. *et al.* 1980). Others suggest that all patients with suspected ruptured aneurysms be put on a beta-blocking agent (Propranolol 20 mg tds) unless there is a specific contra-indication such as asthma. They feel that this helps to prevent swings in blood pressure in the pre-operative phase and particularly at periods of potential danger such as the induction of anaesthesia. The beta-blocking agent should be discontinued if the patient develops a significant bradycardia or a fall in the diastolic blood pressure below 80 mm of mercury in a previously normotensive patient. The treatment is stopped after operation. However, it is equally important not to produce rapid and profound falls in blood pressure in the pre-operative phase as this can lead to impaired cerebral circulation and the risk of cerebral ischaemic deficit. For this reason drugs such as hydrallazine, diazoxide and sodium nitroprusside are to be avoided.

In view of the continuing uncertainty regarding the role of antihypertensive agents in the early management of SAH perhaps the best course to suggest is that patients who are normotensive or who exhibit only a moderate elevation of blood pressure on admission (and who have no previous history of hypertension) may be treated initially with bed rest and analgesics as outlined above. If the blood pressure fails to return to normal levels over twenty-four hours then gradual control should be introduced, using a beta-blocking agent and/or a diuretic and aiming at a diastolic pressure of no less than 80 mm of mercury in the previously normotensive subject. It would be wise to check at an early stage on the views held by the surgeons on the regional neurosurgical unit so that this regime could be altered accordingly. Most conscious patients have a lot of headache and are only too willing to lie quietly in bed. Sedatives are best avoided altogether but if really necessary a small dose of phenobarbitone (30–60 mg orally or i.m.) may be used. Chlorpromazine should be avoided as this can cause a profound drop in blood pessure.

There has been a recent vogue for the use of antifibrinolytic agents in patients with subarachnoid haemorrhage. The validity of this treatment is still contentious as almost all the numerous trials carried out to evaluate their use have been poorly controlled or have involved very small numbers of patients. The most recent data suggest that antifibrinolytic therapy may reduce the incidence of recurrent haemorrhage over the first two weeks but becomes less effective thereafter. The risk of cerebral ischaemic deficit does seem to be increased by their use (Fodstad et al. 1981; Kassell et al. 1984). These most recent papers showed that although patients with antifibrinolytic therapy had a significantly lower rebleeding rate, they had higher rates of ischaemic deficits and hydrocephalus. The net result was no difference in mortality in the first month following the initial SAH. Although further trials are necessary to determine the overall effects of antifibrinolytic therapy, the best course at present is to advise against antifibrinolytic agents, except in good grade patients presenting with their second or subsequent bleed. Again, there will be different neurosurgical opinion regarding this. If it is decided to treat with antifibrinolytic agents then tranexamic acid (1.5 g 6-hourly initially i.v. then orally as recommended by the manufacturer) should be given until operation, or for the first three weeks after the bleed if no operation is planned. Antifibrinolytic therapy should not be given to patients at high risk of DVT/pulmonary emboli and is discontinued in those patients who develop side effects, the most common being profuse diarrhoea.

Antifibrinolytic agents are not used in the treatment of a bleed from a known cerebral AVM as the risk of early recurrent haemorrhage is not as high as that following rupture of a cerebral arterial aneurysm.

Dealing with neurological deterioration/other complications

Sudden recurrent severe headache or a rapid deterioration in the conscious level usually heralds a recurrent haemorrhage. Unfortunately, aside from general supportive measures and maintaining an airway, breathing and circulation there is little that can be done specifically to help. The rebleed may be confirmed by a repeat lumbar puncture but if the CSF is already heavily bloodstained this might not be of value. Recurrent haemorrhage will normally mean that surgery has to be postponed such that it would then be undertaken a week to ten days from the second bleed. Attempts at immediate 'salvage' operations are all too frequently disastrous.

A less acute but sometimes rapidly accelerating deterioration particularly associated with progressive focal neurological deficit may be caused by cerebral arterial spasm. No specific agent has yet been found which will reverse this condition but there is some evidence that aggressive control of the circulating blood volume and the blood pressure by means of transfusion with plasma expanders and infusions of aminophylline and isoprenaline may be of value in reducing the cerebral ischaemic sequelae of the vasospasm (Fleischer and Tindall 1980; Sundt 1975). This should be carried out with monitoring of the central venous pressure in an intensive care or neuro-surgical unit.

There is no good evidence to show that the administration of dexa-methazone has any significant effect in reducing the brain swelling associated with cerebral arterial spasm. With the attendant risks of inducing gastro-intestinal haemorrhage and of elevating the blood pressure and prompting fluid retention there is no real place for the use of steroids in the management of these cases.

Many patients suffering SAH subsequently develop some degree of communicating hydrocephalus. Normally this will settle down spontaneously and requires no specific treatment. However, it can occasionally show rapid progression and since it may be relatively easily treated it is important not to miss the diagnosis. Suspect hydrocephalus in any patient developing progressively more severe headache with gradual or variable lowering of the level of consciousness, incontinence and increasing papilloedema. The optic fundi should be checked daily. The diagnosis may be confirmed by CT scanning and as the patient might require some form of shunt procedure he should be transferred to neurosurgical care.

Most patients treated in the manner outlined above who are clinically in Grade 1 or Grade 2 stabilize and are subsequently able to undergo investigation by CT scan and by two or four vessel angiography. Surgery can then be planned accordingly. Until neurosurgical techniques can be further refined to make early operation on ruptured aneurysms safer, the real advances in the treatment of SAH must be made in emergency medical care and treatment during the first critical week after the haemorrhage.

Summary

SAH is a common condition the most important cause of which is the rupture of an aneurysm on the circle of Willis. Probably the best treatment in the long-term is surgical occlusion of the aneurysm sac. The essential problems in management are making an early diagnosis and preventing a fatal rebleed which is most likely to occur in the first three weeks, often before surgery can be undertaken. Therefore:

1. Suspect SAH in any case of sudden headache or collapse.

2. Look for signs of meningeal irritation.
3. Confirm the diagnosis by lumbar puncture unless there is evidence of raised intracranial pressure or posterior fossa pathology when a CT scan is valuable. Look for blood *and* xanthochromia in the CSF.
4. Maintain strict bed rest, treat headache and vomiting but do not give drugs which will lower conscious level or mask neurological signs.
5. Control blood pressure without inducing hypotension.
6. Consider the use of antifibrinolytic agents.
7. Watch closely for the development of hydrocephalus.
8. Obtain an early neurosurgical opinion.

Further reading

Adams C.B.T., Loach A.B. and O'Laoire S.A. (1976) Intracranial aneurysms: analysis of results of microneurosurgery. *British Medical Journal* 2, 607–609.
Adams H.P., Kassell N.F., Torner J.C., Nibbelink D.W. and Sahs A.L. (1981) Early management of aneurysmal subarachnoid haemorrhage. A report of the cooperative aneurysm study. *Journal of Neurosurgery* 54, 141–145.
Artiola I., Fortuny L., Adams C.B.T. and Briggs M. (1980) Surgical mortality in an aneurysm population: effects of age, blood pressure and pre-operative neurological state. *Journal of Neurology, Neurosurgery and Psychiatry* 43, 879–882.
Drake C.G. (1981) Management of cerebral aneurysm. *Stroke* 12, 273–283.
Fleischer A.S. and Tindall G.T. (1980) Cerebral vasospasm following aneurysm rupture. A protocol for therapy and prophylaxis. *Journal of Neurosurgery* 52, 149–152.
Fodstad H., Forssell A., Liliequist B. and Schannong M. (1981) Antifibrinolysis with tranexamic acid in aneurysmal subarachnoid haemorrhage: A consecutive controlled clinical trial. *Neurosurgery* 8, 158–165.
Hugenholtz H. and Elgie R.G. (1982) Considerations in early surgery on good risk patients with ruptured intracranial aneurysms. *Journal of Neurosurgery* 56, 180–185.
Hunt W.E. and Hess R.M. (1968) Surgical risk as related to time of intervention in the repair of intracranial aneurysms. *Journal of Neurosurgery* 28, 14–20.
Kassell N.F., Boarini D.J., Adams H.P., Sahs A.L., Graf C.J., Torner J.C. and Gerk M.K. (1981) Overall management of ruptured aneurysm. Comparison of early and late operation. *Neurosurgery* 9, 120–128.
Kassell N.F., Torner J.C. and Adams H.P. (1984) Antifibrinolytic therapy in the acute period following aneurysmal subarachnoid hemorrhage. *Journal of Neurosurgery* 61, 225–230.
Ljunggren B., Brandt L., Kagström E. and Sundbärg G. (1981) Results of early operations for ruptured aneurysms. *Journal of Neurosurgery* 54, 473–479.
McKissock W., Paine K. and Walsh L. (1960) An analysis of the results of ruptured intracranial aneurysms. *Journal of Neurosurgery* 17, 762–767.
Pakarinen S. (1967) Incidence, aetiology and prognosis of primary subarachnoid haemorrhage. *Acta Neurologica Scandinavica* 43, Suppl. 29.
Sundt T.M. Jr. (1975) Management of ischaemic complications after subarachnoid haemorrhage. *Journal of Neurosurgery* 43, 418–425.

20 · Meningitis and Encephalitis

PRIDA PHUAPRADIT

Meningitis is a medical emergency which requires prompt recognition, rapid identification of the causative organism and the earliest possible appropriate treatment. Headache with photophobia, fever and stiff neck are the hallmarks of the meningitic syndrome. In adults the clinical features are common to all forms of meningitis, but are modified by the acuteness and severity of the disease. Bacterial and viral meningitides usually present acutely while tuberculous and fungal meningitides usually have a subacute onset.

Bacterial meningitis

The relative frequencies with which different bacteria cause meningitis are related to the patient's age and the presence of predisposing conditions. The three most common causes of bacterial meningitis are *Streptococcus pneumoniae, Neisseria meningitides* and *Haemophilus influenzae* type B. Bacterial meningitis in the neonate is often caused by Gram-negative bacilli, in particular *E. coli* strains containing K_1 capsular antigen and group B streptococci. In infants four to twelve weeks of age, group B streptococci and *Streptococcus pneumoniae* are the leading causes. From three months to five years of age *Haemophilus influenzae* type B, *Neisseria meningitides* and *Streptococcus pneumoniae* are the common organisms. *Neisseria meningitides* and *Streptococcus pneumoniae* are the most common causes of primary bacterial meningitis in children over five years of age and in adults. The former is uncommon in patients over fifty years of age.

Meningococcal meningitis occurs sporadically or in outbreaks particularly in military recruits. *Haemophilus influenzae* meningitis is encountered almost exclusively in children between three months and five years of age. Pneumococcal meningitis is associated with pneumonia, acute otitis media and acute sinusitis. Conditions predisposing to pneumococcal infections and meningitis are sickle cell anaemia, multiple myeloma, alcoholism, splenectomy, CSF rhinorrhoea following head injury, pregnancy and hypogammaglobulinaemia. Shunt infection in patients with hydrocephalus is often caused by *Staphylococcus epidermidis* and *Staphylococcus aureus* (Schoenbaum *et al.* 1975). Gram-negative bacillary meningitis in adults is usually hospital-acquired and occurs in patients following neurosurgical procedure, head injury with open skull fractures and those with debilitating diseases. *Listeria monocytogenes* causes acute meningitis in the newborn and in the immunosuppressed or alcoholic adult (Cherubin *et al.* 1981).

Manifestations

In adults there is usually an abrupt onset of fever, severe headache with photophobia and vomiting, stiff neck, confusion and impairment of consciousness. Signs of meningeal irritation, of which stiff neck is the most reliable, are present in most patients, but they may be absent in infants, and in very old or unconscious patients. Petechiae are seen in more than half of patients with meningococcal meningitis (Whittle and Greenwood 1976). They are rare in meningitis caused by other bacteria and its presence almost always indicates meningococcal infections. Papilloedema and signs of focal cerebral damage are uncommon in bacterial meningitis. Their presence raises the possibility of brain abscess, tuberculous meningitis, occlusion of major venous sinuses or space occupying lesions.

In infants, meningitis develops with none of the signs familiar in an adult. Fever, feeding difficulty, irritability, drowsiness, convulsions and distension of the fontanelle are the manifestations.

Diagnosis

Cerebrospinal fluid (CSF) examination is the most essential investigation to establish the diagnosis, the causative organism and the choice of antibiotics. The CSF is often under elevated pressure. The fluid is turbid or frankly purulent. The cell counts usually range between 1000 to 10,000 per cubic millimetre. Neutrophils constitute most of the white cells. Rarely, the cell counts may be less than 100 per cubic millimetre and the fluid contains a suspension of bacteria with very few cells (Moore and Ross 1973). CSF glucose, which must be analysed promptly with the simultaneously taken blood glucose, is usually reduced below 2.2 mmol/l or less than 40 per cent of the blood glucose. The protein content is usually raised between 1–5 g/l. Gram stains of the CSF sediments are positive in the majority of the patients. Pretreatment with antibiotics in the usual out-patient dosages, may reduce the yield of the Gram smears and cultures of the CSF, but seldom significantly alter other abnormalities of the fluid (Harter 1963; Dalton and Allison 1968; Jarvis and Saxena 1972; Davis *et al.* 1975). If no organism is found in the Gram smear, detection of bacterial antigen by counter current immuno-electrophoresis may rapidly identify the pathogen. The available sera include those against *Haemophilus influenzae* type B, *Neisseria meningitides, Streptococcus pneumoniae,* group B β-haemolytic streptococci and *E. coli* K_1. Failure to detect these antigens does not exclude bacterial meningitis because the antisera may not be sensitive enough to detect small concentration of bacterial antigens in some patients. The limulus lysate test of the CSF can be used as a rapid diagnostic adjunct to detect endotoxin produced by Gram-negative bacteria, notably *Haemophilus influenzae* type B, *Neisseria meningitides* and *E. coli* K_1 (Nachum *et al.* 1973).

Blood cultures should always be performed because they are positive in about half of the patients. X-rays of the chest and skull may reveal evidence of pneumonia or septic foci. Hyponatremia suggests the possibility of inappropriate secretion of antidiuretic hormone, which not uncommonly occurs in bacterial meningitis.

Treatment

Antibiotics are the mainstay of therapy and should be given as early as possible. Specific treatment can be given from the beginning, if the Gram stain of the CSF sediment reveals the causative organism.

The treatment of choice of meningococcal and pneumococcal meningitis is large doses of intravenous benzyl penicillin 20–24 million units, in six divided doses (400,000 units/kg/day) for a period of ten days. Although benzyl penicillin does not penetrate the meninges exceptionally well, this dose provides CSF levels that far exceed the minimal bactericidal concentration for these organisms throughout the course of treatment (Hieber and Nelson 1977). In view of the recent emergence of penicillin-resistant pneumococcal strains, antibiotic sensitivity testing should be routinely performed. Fortunately these strains are rare and have not become widespread. In patients allergic to penicillin, chloramphenicol 100 mg/kg/day (not more than six grams per day) should be given intravenously in four divided doses for ten days. It has been shown that chloramphenicol is bactericidal against *Haemophilus influenzae* type B, *Neisseria meningitides* and, to a lesser extent, *Streptococcus pneumoniae* (Rahal and Simberkoff 1979).

Since the emergence of plasmid-mediated ampicillin-resistant strains of *Haemophilus influenzae* type B, the treatment of this type of meningitis has changed to intravenous chloramphenicol 100 mg/kg/day either alone or in combination with intravenous ampicillin 300–400 mg/kg/day until the result of a sensitivity test is available. Theoretical antagonism between ampicillin and chloramphenicol is not observed in clinical and experimental *Haemophilus influenzae* meningitis (Feldman 1978; Rahal 1978). Recently cefuroxime 200–250 mg/kg/day has been found to be effective in the treatment of meningitis, caused by rare strains of *Haemophilus influenzae*, which are resistant to both ampicillin and chloramphenicol (Sirinavin *et al.* 1984).

If the microscopy of the Gram smear is negative, the initial therapy must be broad enough to cover the most likely organism. In a previously healthy adult with acute bacterial meningitis, benzyl penicillin alone is the treatment of choice. In patients with conditions that might predispose them to infection with unusual organisms, chloramphenicol should be added. Children over three months of age with meningitis, in whom the cause is not yet determined, should be treated with intravenous ampicillin 300–400 mg/kg/day and chloramphenicol 100 mg/kg/day, pending the result of the culture of the CSF.

The treatment of Gram-negative bacillary meningitis has been difficult and rather disappointing. The antibiotics commonly used in the treatment of this type of meningitis are chloramphenicol, ampicillin and aminoglycosides. The use of chloramphenicol has been limited by its potential toxicity in the neonates, and the failure to effectively treat Gram-negative bacillary meningitis in adults because it does not produce a bactericidal effect in spite of an adequate CSF concentration against many of the Gram-negative bacilli (Cherubin et al. 1981). In addition, the organisms can develop resistance to chloramphenicol during the course of treatment. The use of ampicillin is also limited, because about one-third of the strains of the Gram-negative bacilli causing neonatal meningitis and the majority of the strains in adults with meningitis are ampicillin resistant (McCracken and Mize 1976; Berk and McCabe 1980).

The role of intraventricular aminoglycosides in the treatment of Gram-negative bacillary meningitis remains unclear at present in view of conflicting evidence. Gentamicin penetrates into the CSF poorly and even lumbar intrathecal treatment does not result in adequate ventricular concentration of the antibiotic (Kaiser and McGee 1975; McCracken and Mize 1976). Careful study of intraventricular gentamicin in neonatal meningitis was found to be associated with an increased mortality rate when compared to systemic treatment alone (McCracken et al. 1980). Its use, both in the neonatal period and in adults, must be restricted to selected instances, such as persistence of the organisms in the CSF for 24–48 hours after the treatment or in gravely ill patients. Administration of an aminoglycoside into the ventricle via a reservoir with careful monitoring of the CSF levels and adjustment of the intraventricular dose may result in a favourable outcome (Wright et al. 1981).

The next development in the treatment of the Gram-negative bacillary meningitis will probably be the systemic use of new bactericidal drugs that can produce effective levels in the CSF. Recently it has been demonstrated that the new generation of cephalosporins or cephalosporin-type antibiotics, notably cefotaxime and moxalactam are effective in the treatment of Gram-negative bacillary meningitis in patients of various age groups with excellent bactericidal activity in the CSF (Belohradsky et al. 1980; Landesman et al. 1980; Olson et al. 1981; Landesman et al. 1981; Mullaney and John 1983).

Viral meningitis

Viral meningitis usually occurs in children and young adults. The onset is sudden with intense headache, fever and stiffness of the neck. Prodromal symptoms of flu-like illness may be present in some patients. The patient does not look as ill as one with bacterial meningitis. Cranial nerve palsy and focal neurological signs are rare. A maculopapular rash suggests infection with Echo or Coxsackie virus. The CSF pressure is usually normal. The CSF contains mainly lymphocytes which may vary from 10 to 500 per cubic millimetre. Cell counts above 1000 per cubic millimetre are seen in lymphocytic choriomeningitis. In the early stages of viral meningitis some patients have a polymorphonuclear cell response in the CSF. In such cases repeat lumbar puncture after six to twelve hours of close observation will show a change from a predominance of neutrophils to mononuclear cells (Feigin and Shackelford 1973). In contrast to other types of meningitis, the CSF glucose concentration is usually normal. However, low CSF glucose level may occasionally be found, particularly in mumps and zoster meningitis (Wilfert 1969; Reimer and Reller 1981). The CSF protein is mildly elevated and usually less than 1.5 g/l. In addition to viruses, similar abnormalities of the CSF are found in meningovascular syphilis, lepto-spirosis, brain abscess, mycoplasma infection, cerebral cysticercosis and parameningeal suppuration. Although non-specific, quantitative measurement of C-reactive protein in the serum and CSF may be a sensitive and practical test to differentiate bacterial from non-bacterial meningitis (Corrall et al. 1981; Peltola 1981). The levels of C-reactive protein, both in the serum and CSF, are far above the normal limits in bacterial meningitis, but normal or only slightly raised in viral meningitis.

The management of viral meningitis is symptomatic. Bed rest, analgesics, repletion of fluid and electrolytes usually suffice. Most patients recover within a period of one to two weeks without sequelae.

Tuberculous meningitis (TBM)

Although tuberculous meningitis is now relatively rare in the United Kingdom, it still occurs, particularly in children and Asian immigrants (Naughten et al. 1981; Swart et al. 1981). Clinicians should have high index of suspicion of tuberculous meningitis in any patient with lymphocytic meningitis and low glucose levels in the CSF. Failure to recognize this condition and delay in treatment result in tragic consequences. The history is usually more prolonged than in purulent meningitis. Headache, pyrexia and systemic symptoms, such as night sweats and anorexia are the usual presentation. In advanced cases there is impairment of consciousness, increasing to coma. Papilloedema and paralysis of the sixth cranial nerve are common.

In miliary tuberculosis, choroidal tubercles are occasionally seen. Arteritis affecting large intracranial vessels may produce focal neurological signs such as hemiparesis. Paraparesis from spinal arachnoiditis is a rare complication. Evidence of active tuberculosis may be found in the chest, bones and kidneys. As in miliary tuberculosis, the tuberculin test may give negative results in some patients with TBM.

The CSF is usually under increased pressure and contains 20–500 white cells per cubic millimetre. Cell counts in the CSF of more than 1000 per cubic millimetre are exceptionally rare. Both lymphocytes and neutrophils are present and the latter can be as high as 70 per cent of the total cell count. The protein of the CSF is raised and ranges from 1 to 5 g/l. Levels of more than 10 g/l indicates a spinal block. The glucose level of the initial CSF examination is low (below 2.2 mmol/l) in about 90 per cent of the patients. A large amount of CSF (10 ml) should be collected for Ziehl–Neelson stain and culture. When the CSF is left standing, a fine cobweb may be seen. The acid fast bacilli must be carefully sought in the stain of the CSF sediment.

The Bromide partition test is useful as an adjunct in differentiating tuberculous from viral meningitis (Taylor and Smith 1954; Crook *et al.* 1960; Mandal *et al.* 1972). However, it is a non-specific test with five to ten per cent false positivity and false negativity (Taylor and Smith 1954). The test is also abnormal in meningeal carcinomatosis, spinal block, cryptococcal meningitis, mumps meningo-encephalitis and cerebral malaria.

Treatment

Owing to the lack of appropriate clinical trials, treatment of tuberculous meningitis has been based mainly on known pharmacokinetic and anti-bacterial properties of the drugs. Isoniazid, rifampicin, streptomycin and pyrazinamide are effective drugs against tuberculosis. Isoniazid and pyra-zinamide are useful drugs in view of their bactericidal effect on the myco-bacteria, and excellent penetration through the inflamed and normal meninges (Fletcher 1953; Forgan-Smith *et al.* 1973). Ethambutol, rifampicin and streptomycin cross the blood–brain barrier and produce appreciable concentrations in the CSF only when the meninges is inflamed (Pilheu *et al.* 1971; Bobrowitz 1972; D'Oliveira 1972; Sippel *et al.* 1974; Forgan-Smith *et al.* 1973). Para-aminosalisylic acid should not be used in the treatment of tuberculous meningitis, because the drug does not enter the CSF.

The prognosis of patients who are alert and have no signs of focal cerebral damage is very good. Treatment in these patients should consist of isoniazid 300–400 mg/day orally (20 mg/kg/day in children), rifampicin 600 mg/day orally (15 mg/kg day in children), pyrazinamide 1.5–2.0 g/day (40 mg/kg/day in children) and streptomycin 1.0 g/day intramuscularly (30 mg/kg/day in children). Streptomycin and pyrazinamide are given for two to three months and the first two drugs for eighteen months.

Patients who are seriously ill with stupor or focal neurological signs have a grave prognosis. Intensive treatment of these patients with isoniazid, rifampicin, ethambutol, pyrazinamide and streptomycin are justified in the acute stage. The role of intrathecal streptomycin in TBM is controversial. It is not necessary in patients who are alert and should be reserved only for patients who are very ill. Intrathecal streptomycin, 25–50 mg/day, can be given via the lumbar route or 25 mg/day intraventricularly via an Ommaya reservoir. Appropriate clinical trials of corticosteroid in the treatment of TBM are lacking (Editorial, *Lancet* 1982). Its use is indicated in patients with raised intracranial pressure, communicating hydrocephalus and spinal arachnoiditis.

Communicating hydrocephalus is common and should be suspected in all patients with TBM who develop an impaired level of consciousness, or who fail to respond to the treatment (Newman *et al.* 1980). Repeated lumbar punctures, corticosteroids and the use of acetazolamide may be successful in the treatment of the hydrocephalus (Visudhiphan and Chiemchanya 1979). In patients who abruptly deteriorate, ventricular drainage or early insertion of a shunt may be necessary. Cerebral tuberculoma may rarely complicate tuberculous meningitis and should be suspected in patients who develop focal neurological signs or seizures (Lees *et al.* 1980).

The result of the treatment of TBM depends largely on the early diagnosis and treatment before permanent damage in the central nervous system takes place.

Cryptococcal meningitis

This is the most common form of fungal meningitis. Although the majority of the patients have underlying conditions, in which immunity is impaired, it can occur in previously healthy subjects. Clinical manifestations and CSF abnormalities are similar to those of tuberculous meningitis. It should be suspected in all patients, who present with subacute lymphocytic meningitis and low CSF glucose level.

The encapsulated yeast form can be seen in more than half of the patients by examination of a fresh India Ink smear of CSF sediment. The organism may be mistaken for lymphocytes or red blood cells if India Ink is not used. Detection of the capsular antigen in the CSF by latex agglutination gives a positive result in about 90 per cent of the patients. Chest X-ray may reveal pulmonary lesions mimicking tuberculosis. Communicating hydrocephalus and cerebral granulomata may complicate the meningitis.

Cryptococcal meningitis should be treated with amphotericin B, 0.3 mg/kg/day, by intravenous infusion in combination with oral flucytosine 150 mg/kg/day in four divided doses (Bennett *et al.* 1979). Side effects of amphotericin B are common. These include chills, fever, nausea and vomiting during the infusion, nephrotoxicity, renal tubular acidosis and anaemia. Flucytosine may cause bone marrow depression, particularly in patients with impaired renal function. In such patients the dose of flucytosine should be reduced (Dawborn *et al.* 1973). The treatment is continued for at least six weeks. In patients who fail to respond to amphotericin B and flucytosine, treatment with miconazole, a new antifungal agent may be successful (Graybill and Levine 1978; Weinstein and Jacoby 1980).

Viral encephalitis

The clinical feature of viral encephalitis is that of an acute onset of pyrexia, headache, confusion, impairment of conscious level and signs of focal or diffuse cerebral damage. In a recent British series the identified viruses causing encephalitis are herpes simplex, mumps, influenza and Epstein–Barr virus (Kennard and Swash 1981). Arthropod-borne viral encephalitis is endemic in Japan, Southeast Asia, America and central Europe. Syndromes similar to viral encephalitis may be caused by acute demyelination of the central nervous system following exanthemata or smallpox vaccination.

Herpes simplex encephalitis is the most common form of sporadic severe encephalitis in the United Kingdom (Illis 1977). The virus has a predilection to cause haemorrhagic necrosis of the temporal lobes, producing focal neurological signs. Clinically, the disease presents as a rapidly progressing neurological disorder with personality change and memory disturbances as early features. This may be quickly followed by headache, seizures, focal neurological signs, such as hemiparesis and aphasia and increasing impairment of conscious level. Electro-encephalogram often shows slow or sharp waves localized in one or both temporal lobes. The EEG abnormalities may dramatically change from day to day. A computerized tomographic scan of the brain frequently shows low density abnormalities in one or both temporal lobes, often with a shift of the mid-line structures and slight degree of contrast enhancement (Kaufman *et al.* 1979).

The CSF is normal in about 10 per cent of the patients on first examination (Illis 1977). It is usually under increased pressure and contains lymphocytes or mixed pleocytosis with a moderate rise of protein and normal glucose level. Red cells and xanthochromia may be found. Early diagnosis and treatment before the development of stupor or serious neurological deficit are essential. Rapid diagnosis can be made by brain biopsy and demonstration of the viral antigen by immunofluorescent staining. A sensitive and specific radio-immunosorbent assay for serum and CSF IgG antibody against herpes simplex has recently been described and evaluated as a rapid and non-invasive diagnostic test for herpes simplex encephalitis (Klapper *et al.* 1981).

The treatment of herpes simplex encephalitis has been far from satis-factory. The mortality rate in untreated patients approaches 70 per cent and those who survive are left with serious disability (Whitley *et al.* 1977). The use of antiviral agents, idoxuridine and cytarabine has been disappointing. A recent controlled study in the United States showed that adenine arabinoside, given early in the course of the disease before the onset of coma, reduced the mortality from 70 per cent to 28 per cent, but many of those who survived, were left with serious disability (Whitley *et al.* 1977). Although the results have been inconclusive, dexamethasone and mannitol should be given in patients who develop cerebral oedema. The use of acyclovir has been advocated in the treatment of herpes simplex encephalitis (Chin and Edis 1982). Due to its low toxicity and the poor results of other therapy, this agent is now being used in many centres to treat this condition. Moreover, a recent controlled trial has found a significant reduction in mortality and in morbidity at six months in patients treated with acyclovir compared to those treted with vidarabine (Skoldenberg *et al.* 1984).

Further reading

Belohradsky B., Bruch K., Geiss D., Kafetzis D., Marget W. and Peters G. (1980) Intravenous cefotaxime in children with bacterial meningitis. *Lancet* 1, 61–63.

Bennett J.E., Dismukes W.E., Duma R.J., Medoff G., Sande M.A., Gallis H., Leonard J., Fields B.T., Bradshaw M., Haywood H., McGee Z.A., Cate T.R., Cobbs C.G., Warner J.F. and Alling D.W. (1979) A comparison of amphotericin B alone and combined with flucytosine in the treatment of cryptococcal meningitis. *New England Journal of Medicine* 301, 126–131.

Berk S.L. and McCabe W.R. (1980) Meningitis caused by gram-negative bacilli. *Annals of Internal Medicine* 93, 253–260.

Bobrowitz I.D. (1972) Ethambutol in tuberculous meningitis. *Chest* 61, 629–632.

Cherubin C.E., Marr J.S., Sierra M.F. and Becker S. (1981) Listeria and gram-negative bacillary meningitis in New York city, 1972–1979. *American Journal of Medicine* 71, 199–209.

Chin D. and Edis R. (1982) Acyclovir for herpes simplex encephalitis: the price of survival? *Lancet* 2, 870.

Corrall C.J., Pepple J.M., Moxon E.R. and Hughes W.T. (1981) C-reactive protein in spinal fluid of children with meningitis. *Journal of Pediatrics* 99, 365–369.

Crook A., Duncan H., Gutteridge B. and Pallis C. (1960) Use of Br^{82} in differential diagnosis of lymphocytic meningitis. *British Medical Journal* 1, 705–706.

Dalton H.P. and Allison M.J. (1968) Modification of laboratory results by partial treatment of bacterial meningitis. *American Journal of Clinical Pathology* 49, 410–413.

Davis S.D., Hill H.R., Feigl P. and Arnstein E.J. (1975) Partial antibiotic therapy in Haemophilus influenzae meningitis. *American Journal of Diseases of Children* 129, 802–807.

Dawborn J.K., Page M.D. and Schiavone D.J. (1973) Use of 5-fluorocytosine in patients with impaired renal function. *British Medical Journal* 4, 382–384.

D'Oliveira J.J.G. (1972) Cerebrospinal fluid concentration of rifampicin in meningeal tuberculosis. *American Review of Respiratory Disease* **106**, 432–437.

Editorial. (1982) Steroid in bacterial meningitis, helpful or harmful? *Lancet* **1**, 1164.

Feigin R.D. and Shackelford P.G. (1973) Value of repeat lumbar puncture in the differential diagnosis of meningitis. *New England Journal of Medicine* **289**, 571–574.

Feldman W.E. (1978) Effect of ampicillin and chloramphenicol against *Haemophilus influenzae* meningitis. *Pediatrics* **61**, 406–409.

Fletcher A.P. (1953) CSF isoniazid level in tuberculous meningitis. *Lancet* **2**, 694–696.

Forgan-Smith R., Ellard G.A., Newton D. and Mitchison D.A. (1973) Pyrazinamide and other drugs in tuberculous meningitis. *Lancet* **2**, 374.

Graybill J.R. and Levine H.B. (1978) Successful treatment of cryptococcal meningitis with intraventricular miconazole. *Archives of Internal Medicine* **138**, 814–816.

Harter D.H. (1963) Preliminary antibiotic therapy in bacterial meningitis. *Archives of Neurology* **9**, 31–35.

Hieber J.P. and Nelson J.D. (1977) A pharmacologic evaluation of penicillin in children with purulent meningitis. *New England Journal of Medicine* **297**, 410–413.

Illis L.S. (1977) Encephalitis. *British Journal of Hospital Medicine* **18**, 412–422.

Jarvis C.W. and Saxena K.M. (1972) Does prior antibiotic treatment hamper the diagnosis of acute bacterial meningitis? Analysis of a series of 135 childhood cases. *Clinical Pediatrics* **11**, 201–204.

Kaiser A.B. and McGee Z.A. (1975) Aminoglycoside therapy of gram-negative bacillary meningitis. *New England Journal of Medicine* **293**, 1215–1220.

Kaufman D.M., Zimmerman R.D. and Leeds N.E. (1979) Computed tomography in herpes simplex encephalitis. *Neurology* **29**, 1392–1396.

Kennard C. and Swash M. (1981) Acute viral encephalitis. Its diagnosis and outcome. *Brain* **104**, 129–148.

Klapper P.E., Laing I. and Longson M. (1981) Rapid non-invasive diagnosis of herpes simplex encephalitis. *Lancet* **2**, 607–609.

Landesman S.H., Corrado M.L., Cleri D. and Cherubin C.E. (1980) Diffusion of a new beta-lactam (LY 127935) into the cerebrospinal fluid. Implications for therapy of gram-negative bacillary meningitis. *American Journal of Medicine* **69**, 92–98.

Landesman S.H., Corrado M.L., Shah P.M., Armengaud M., Barza M. and Cherubin C.E. (1981) Past and current roles for cephalosporin antibiotics in treatment of meningitis—emphasis on use in gram-negative bacillary meningitis. *American Journal of Medicine* **71**, 693–703.

Lees A.J., MacLeod A.F. and Marshall J. (1980) Cerebral tuberculomas developing during treatment of tuberculous meningitis. *Lancet* **1**, 1208–1211.

Mandal B.K., Evans D.I.K., Ironside A.G. and Pullan B.R. (1972) Radio-active bromide partition test in differential diagnosis of tuberculous meningitis. *British Medical Journal* **4**, 413–415.

McCracken G.H. and Mize S.G. (1976) A controlled study of intrathecal antibiotic therapy in gram-negative enteric meningitis of infancy. *Journal of Pediatrics* **89**, 66–72.

McCracken G.H., Mize S.G. and Threlkeld N. (1980) Intraventricular gentamicin therapy in gram-negative bacillary meningitis of infancy. *Lancet* 1, 787–791.

Moore C.M. and Ross M. (1973) Acute bacterial meningitis with absent or minimal cerebrospinal fluid abnormalities. *Clinical Pediatrics* 12, 117–118.

Mullaney D.T., John J.F. (1983) Cefotaxime therapy, evaluation of its effect on bacterial meningitis, CSF drug levels, and bactericidal activity. *Archives of Internal Medicine* 143, 1705–1708.

Nachum R., Lipsey A. and Siegel S.E. (1973) Rapid detection of gram-negative bacterial meningitis by the limulus lysate test. *New England Journal of Medicine* 289, 931–934.

Naughton E., Weindling A.M., Newton R. and Bower B.D. (1981) Tuberculous meningitis in children. Recent experiences in two English Centres. *Lancet* 2, 973–975.

Newman P.K., Cumming W.J.K. and Foster J.B. (1980) Hydrocephalus and tuberculous meningitis in adults. *Journal of Neurology, Neurosurgery and Psychiatry* 43, 188–190.

Olson D.A., Hoeprich P.D., Nolan S.M. and Goldstein E. (1981) Successful treatment of gram-negative bacillary meningitis with moxalactam. *Annals of Internal Medicine* 95, 302–305.

Peltola H.O. (1981) C-reactive protein for rapid monitoring of infections of the central nervous system. *Lancet* 1, 980–982.

Pilheu J.A., Maglio F., Cetrangolo R. and Pleus A.D. (1971) Concentrations of ethambutol in the cerebrospinal fluid after oral administration. *Tubercle* 52, 117–122.

Rahal J.J. (1978) Antibiotic combinations: the clinical relevance of synergy and antagonism. *Medicine (Baltimore)* 57, 179–195.

Rahal J.J. and Simberkoff M.S. (1979) Bactericidal and bacteriostatic action of chloramphenicol against meningeal pathogens. *Antimicrobial Agents and Chemotherapy* 16, 13–18.

Reimer L.G. and Reller B.L. (1981) CSF in herpes zoster meningo-encephalitis. *Archives of Neurology* 38, 668.

Schoenbaum S.C., Gardner P., Shillito J. (1975) Infections of cerebrospinal fluid shunts: Epidemiology, clinical manifestations and therapy. *Journal of Infectious Diseases* 131, 543–552.

Sippel J.E., Mikhall I.A., Girgis N.I. and Youssef H.H. (1974) Rifampicin concentrations in cerebrospinal fluid of patients with tuberculous meningitis. *American Review of Respiratory Disease* 109, 579–580.

Sirinavin S., Chiemchanya S., Visudhipan P. and Lolekha S. (1984). Cefuroxime treatment of bacterial meningitis in infants and children. *Antimicrobial Agents and Chemotherapy* 25, 273–275.

Sköldenberg B. and Swedish Study Group (1984) Acyclovir versus vidarabine in herpes simplex encephalitis. *Lancet* ii, 707–711.

Swart S., Briggs R.S. and Millac P.A. (1981) Tuberculous meningitis in Asian patients. *Lancet* 2, 15–16.

Taylor L.M. and Smith H.V. (1954) The blood-CSF barrier to bromide in diagnosis of tuberculous meningitis. *Lancet* 1, 700–702.

Visudhiphan P. and Chiemchanya S. (1979) Hydrocephalus in tuberculous meningitis in children: Treatment with acetazolamide and repeated lumbar puncture. *Journal of Pediatrics* 95, 657–660.

Weinstein L. and Jacoby I. (1980) Successful treatment of cerebral cryptococcoma and meningitis with miconazole. *Annals of Internal Medicine* **93**, 569–571.

Whitley R.J., Soong S.J., Dolin R., Galasso G.J., Ch'ien L.T., Alford C.A. and the Collaborative Study Group. (1977) Adenine arabinoside therapy of biopsy-proved herpes simplex encephalitis. *New England Journal of Medicine* **297**, 289–294.

Whittle R.C. and Greenwood B.M. (1976) Meningococcal meningitis in the northern savana of Africa. *Tropical Doctor* **6**, 99–104.

Wilfert C.M. (1969) Mumps meningo-encephalitis with low cerebrospinal fluid glucose, prolonged pleocytosis and elevated protein. *New England Journal of Medicine* **280**, 855–859.

Wright P.F., Kaiser A.B., Bowman C.M., McKee K.T., Trujillo H. and McGee Z.A. (1981) The pharmacokinetics and efficacy of an aminoglycoside administered into the cerebral ventricles in neonates: implications for further evaluation of this route of therapy in meningitis. *Journal of Infectious Diseases* **143**, 141–147.

21 · Acute Inflammatory Polyneuropathy and Myasthenia Gravis

R. C. ROBERTS

Acute inflammatory polyneuropathy (Guillain–Barré syndrome)

Guillain defined a syndrome involving ascending paralysis with a high cerebrospinal fluid (CSF) protein from which recovery might occur (Guillain *et al.* 1916; Guillain 1936). He excluded similar fatal cases such as those of Landry (1859). The subsequent controversy surrounding the definition of the 'Guillain–Barré syndrome' in the first half of this century (Haymaker and Kernohan 1949) persists to the present day (Asbury *et al.* 1978; Posner 1981). However, there is no difficulty in recognizing the typical case and diagnosis depends on clinical, CSF and electrophysiological criteria.

Diagnosis

Clinical presentation

Most cases of acute inflammatory polyneuropathy present with weakness beginning in the legs and spreading to the arms and trunk. The weakness may be more marked proximally or distally and may be asymmetrical. It progresses over a few days or weeks but not usually for more than four weeks. Tendon reflexes are almost invariably absent and their preservation should cast doubt on the diagnosis. Straight leg raising may be limited due to lumbosacral root irritation. Sensory symptoms are commonly present from the outset with tingling in the fingers and toes. Nevertheless, sensory signs may be absent and when they are present there is usually a mild distal impairment of joint position sense and vibration sense. In occasional patients there is severe sensory involvement. Pain in the limbs may be distressing. Lower motor neurone facial weakness occurs in about 50 per cent of patients. Bulbar weakness and extra-ocular muscle involvement may occur and 10–23 per cent of patients will require assisted ventilation. Autonomic involvement may occur (Tuck and McLeod 1981). A few, otherwise typical, cases have signs of involvement of the central nervous system, the commonest being extensor plantar responses. Papilloedema occurs rarely and has been ascribed to raised CSF protein (Denny–Brown 1952) and to cerebral oedema (Davidson and Jellinek 1977). Ataxia of apparent cerebellar origin (rather than due to weakness and sensory impairment) may occur. In addition, the Miller Fisher syndrome in which ataxia is combined with external ophthalmoplegia and areflexia, is probably rightly considered a variant of acute inflammatory polyneuropathy (Fisher 1956).

Cerebrospinal fluid

The CSF protein is typically elevated by the end of the first week of the illness without any increase in cells (Guillain's 'dissociation albumino-cytologique'). The absence of an increase in CSF protein does not exclude the diagnosis and in occasional cases up to 50 lymphocytes/mm^3 may be present. Electrophoresis may reveal 'oligoclonal bands' in the gamma globulin region (Link 1978).

Electrophysiology (McLeod 1981)

Early in the illness it is sometimes not possible to find any electro-physiological abnormalities, and if present they may be confined to pro-longation of F-wave and H-reflex latencies due to proximal demyelination in the nerve roots. Later, marked slowing of conduction peripherally and prolongation of terminal motor latencies may be found due to segmental demyelination. If electromyography reveals evidence of axonal degener-ation, recovery is liable to be slow and possibly incomplete.

Differential diagnosis

Acute diptheritic neuropathy and poliomyelitis, although now rare, should still be considered. An acute neuropathy may rarely occur in systemic lupus erythematosus (SLE). Polymyositis is differentiated by the absence of sen-sory involvement and preservation of tendon reflexes. Neuropathies due to volatile solvents, drugs, chemicals, lead and porphyria should also be con-sidered. When the symptoms and signs are confined to the legs, cauda equina compression by an acute lumbar disc is an important differential diagnosis. Some patients initially thought to have the Guillain–Barré syn-drome will turn out to have a chronic relapsing polyneuropathy or a chronic progressive inflammatory polyneuropathy.

Aetiology

It seems likely that the Guillain–Barré syndrome is caused by an auto-immune reaction against the patient's peripheral nerve and root myelin. This is probably triggered by a preceding 'immunological insult' (usually a viral infection). However, there remains considerable debate and uncertainty about the nature of the auto-immune reaction and the antigen against which it is directed remains unidentified. There is evidence to support involvement of both cell mediated and humoral immune mechanisms (Iqbal *et al.* 1981; Cook and Dowling 1981). Pathological examination of peripheral nerve has revealed the macrophage to be the major effector of the demyelination (Prineas 1981).

Symptoms suggestive of a viral illness precede the onset of weakness in 50–70 per cent of cases. This illness is usually respiratory and occasionally gastro-intestinal. The causative infective agent commonly remains obscure. Dowling and Cook (1981) have recently reported evidence of acute cytomegalovirus infection in 15 per cent of patients and of acute Epstein–Barr virus infection in 8 per cent. Other identified preceding viral infections occur at much lower frequencies and include measles, chicken pox, rubella, mumps, influenza, hepatitis and enterovirus infections. The aetiological significance of these infections is less certain. Of non-viral infections only mycoplasma pneumoniae has so far been strongly linked with the Guillain–Barré syndrome, occurring in about 5 per cent of cases. Other triggering factors have been surgical operations and vaccinations. Vaccination with the A/New Jersey influenza vaccine in the United States in 1976–77 was associated with just under one excess case of Guillain–Barré syndrome per 100,000 vaccinations. This may be compared with the overall incidence of the disease, which is about 1/100,000/year. The incidence is slightly increased in patients with Hodgkin's disease and lymphomas.

Treatment and prognosis

Most patients (about 60 per cent) with the Guillain–Barré syndrome make a complete recovery. Only about 5 per cent remain significantly handicapped and between 2 per cent and 6 per cent die (Wiederholt *et al.* 1964; Dowling *et al.* 1977; Löffel *et al.* 1977). Recovery usually begins between two and four weeks after progression has ceased but may be more delayed. In most patients it takes about six months but in some it takes much longer. Management is aimed at preventing complications that might arise from the paralysis while spontaneous recovery is awaited. The role of 'immunological treatments' (steroids, immunosuppressive agents, plasma exchange) is controversial.

The major causes of death are complications arising from respiratory and bulbar muscle weakness, sudden cardiovascular collapse presumed to be associated with autonomic involvement and pulmonary embolism. All of these are potentially preventable or treatable. Patients suspected of having the Guillain–Barré syndrome should be admitted to a hospital where facilities are available for assisted ventilation. The vital capacity should be regularly recorded, as often as hourly if the rate of deterioration is rapid.

Between 10 and 23 per cent of patients will require assisted ventilation. The point at which endotracheal intubation is indicated depends partly on the rate of fall of the vital capacity. If the rate of fall is rapid, preparation for assisted ventilation as the vital capacity falls towards 1 litre will be wise. If it is slower, occurring over many days, and progression seems to be levelling out, then vital capacities as low as 700 ml may be acceptable. Associated severe bulbar weakness may require endotracheal intubation to protect the airway, and the passing of a nasogastric tube to administer nourishment and drugs. If assisted ventilation is likely to be necessary for more than a few days, a tracheostomy should be performed. Regular chest physiotherapy is essential. The electrocardiogram and blood pressure are monitored to detect arrhythmias and/or hypotension. Deep vein thrombosis may be discouraged by prophylactic anticoagulation with subcutaneous low dose heparin. Hyponatraemia may occur and usually responds to fluid restriction. Intensive and expert nursing is clearly essential during a prolonged period of paralysis if complications such as bed sores and pressure palsies are to be avoided. The severely affected patient will be unable to communicate and the nature of his disease should be fully discussed with him before it has progressed too far. He will need constant reminding of the good prognosis. Limb pain may be distressing and may respond to quinine if ordinary analgesics fail. As muscular power returns, active physiotherapy will hasten recovery.

There is no specific therapy of proven benefit. Since most cases recover spontaneously, many agents have appeared to be effective. Guillain's remedies included sodium salicylate, quinine, methenamine, colloidal silver, strychnine and extracts of adrenal cortex (perhaps the first use of steroids!) and he obtained good results. Optimistic reports on the effect of steroids appeared in the 1950s. Subsequently it became widely accepted that although steroids did not affect the eventual outcome of the disease, they arrested the progress and hastened the onset of improvement. However, more recent retrospective studies showed little effect of steroids (Hughes *et al.* 1981) and a randomized controlled trial showed, if anything, a detrimental rather than a beneficial effect (Hughes *et al.* 1978). The dose of prednisolone used in this trial was 60 mg daily for one week, 40 mg daily for four days, 30 mg daily for three days and the drug was then continued or reduced at discretion. Whether or not much higher doses of steroids given for longer might be effective remains uncertain, but the potential side effects of such aggressive therapy might be greater than the hazards of the disease itself. Furthermore, there is a suspicion that the use of steroids may increase the chances of subsequent relapse. There is little data on the use of other immunosuppressants; again the potential side effects have discouraged their use in a disease with a favourable prognosis. Anecdotal reports have recently been appearing on the use of plasma exchange and good results have been claimed in some patients. Clearly, the significance of these observations must await the outcome of randomized controlled trials. It may finally be noted that, whereas steroids and immunosuppressants appear to have no role in the treatment of acute inflammatory polyneuropathy, they may be beneficial in chronic relapsing and chronic progressive inflammatory polyneuropathies (Dalakas and Engel 1981).

Myasthenia gravis

Myasthenia gravis is now established as an auto-immune disease. In about 90 per cent of patients, antibody can be detected to the nicotinic acetylcholine receptors of the post-synaptic membrane of neuromuscular junctions of skeletal muscle (Lindstrom *et al.* 1976). It is a heterogeneous IgG antibody which reduces the number of functional acetylcholine receptors and thus interferes with neuromuscular transmission. The prevalence of the disease lies between 1 in 10,000 and 1 in 50,000 of the population. The age of onset is usually between ten and seventy with the peak incidence in the third decade. Under the age of forty, females are affected two or three times more commonly than males. There is evidence for disease heterogeneity (Compston *et al.* 1979; Sagar *et al.* 1980a,b).

Clinical presentation

Myasthenia is characterized by weakness, which appears or is exacerbated by repeated or prolonged contraction. The extra-ocular, facial, bulbar and neck muscles are particularly vulnerable and one or more of these groups is usually involved first. Patients may present with drooping eyelids and double vision, with difficulty chewing and swallowing towards the end of a meal, with weak nasal speech, or with inability to hold the head up. The symptoms are intermittent and their significance is often not initially recognized, leading to delay in diagnosis. As the disease progresses the limb muscles (proximal greater than distal) and respiratory muscles may become involved. The onset of symptoms is usually insidious and they may have been present many months on initial presentation. A more rapid onset or exacerbation may be associated with infection, pregnancy, the puerperium, anaesthesia, or drugs (quinidine, propranolol, lithium).

Examination may reveal a 'fatiguable ptosis' with continuous upgaze for two to three minutes. The extra-ocular movements may be impaired, usually asymmetrically, and the weakness of the extra-ocular muscles may be exaggerated by prolonged gaze in one direction. There is usually weakness of the facial muscles with a 'myasthenic snarl' on attempted smiling. Characteristically, weakness of jaw closure leads the patient to prop the jaw up with his hand. Palatal movement may be impaired and the speech nasal. Fatigue of shoulder muscles may be demonstrated and monitored by recording the time for which the patient is able to hold his arms extended in front of him. The degree of respiratory muscle involvement is assessed by measurement of the vital capacity.

Diagnosis

The diagnosis of myasthenia gravis depends initially on clinical suspicion. Patients with mild intermittent symptoms and no definite signs are all too often labelled at first as 'functional' or 'hysterical'. It is important that the diagnosis is also considered in patients with a fixed deficit (ptosis, ophthalmoplegia), as fatigue is not always demonstrable. Laboratory confirmation of a clinical suspicion can usually be obtained by an electrophysiological examination, Tensilon test and assay of serum acetylcholine receptor antibodies.

Electrophysiological tests

In myasthenia gravis a rapid reduction (decrement) may be found in the amplitude of compound muscle action potentials evoked by repetitive stimulation of nerves at low frequencies (usually 3/second). A brief period of isometric exercise or tetanic stimulation may result in post activation facilitation (increase in amplitude of the compound action potential with decreased decrement) and then exhaustion (decrease in amplitude of the compound action potential with increased decrement). If examination of distal muscles is negative, that of facial muscle may be positive. However, repetitive stimulation studies are negative in 30–40 per cent of unselected myasthenic patients, mostly those with mild or purely ocular disease. In recent years single-fibre electromyography has been shown to be a very sensitive method of detecting abnormalities of neuromuscular transmission and abnormalities may be found when repetitive stimulation studies are normal (Stålberg et al. 1974; Stålberg 1980). The potentials from pairs of muscle fibres belonging to the same motor unit are studied. There may be an increase in 'jitter' (variability of the inter-potential intervals) and there may be an increase in the proportion of fibre pairs displaying 'blocking' (intermittent failure of conduction to one of the fibres). These abnormalities are not specific for myasthenia and routine needle electromyography is necessary to exclude other causes (e.g. polymyositis, motor neurone disease).

Tensilon test

This is performed by injecting intravenously 10 mg of edrophonium (Tensilon), a short acting anticholinesterase. Careful observation is made for any improvement in the patient's ptosis, ophthalmoplegia or other signs. A test dose of 2 mg is given initially, and the remaining 8 mg about thirty seconds later. There is a very small risk of cardiac arrest, and it is wise to have atropine (0.6 mg) drawn up ready for i.v. administration if necessary. Slight degrees of improvement may be difficult to assess and the test is thus best performed 'blind'. The observer is given two identical syringes, one containing edrophonium and the other normal saline, and both are injected in the same manner. Improvement following edrophonium occurs within one minute and lasts four to five minutes.

Acetylcholine receptor antibody assay

This is positive in about 90 per cent of patients with myasthenia of all degrees of severity (Lindstrom *et al.* 1976; Compston *et al.* 1980) and in about 70 per cent of patients with mild generalized or ocular myasthenia gravis (Kelly *et al.* 1982). A positive titre is virtually diagnostic, although a few false positives have been reported in patients treated with snake venom (Mittag and Caroscio 1980). The assay is performed by only a few specialized laboratories and considerable delays may occur in obtaining the results.

None of these tests are positive in all cases of myasthenia gravis, but they are complementary, and most patients will have the diagnosis confirmed if all of them are employed (Kelly *et al.* 1982). They will also help to differentiate other diseases such as the Eaton Lambert syndrome and chronic progressive external ophthalmoplegia.

About 10 per cent of patients with myasthenia gravis, especially older males, will have thymomas. Most of these are revealed by routine posteroanterior (PA) and lateral chest X-rays. Recently, the role of other methods of detecting thymomas, including CT scanning, has been discussed (Keesey *et al.* 1980). About 5 per cent of patients have coincident thyrotoxicosis and there is also an association with rheumatoid arthritis and SLE. Myasthenia, indistinguishable from the spontaneous syndrome, may be induced by penicillamine but it usually resolves when the drug is withdrawn.

Acute management

Patients presenting acutely with myasthenia gravis will either be new cases or previously established cases who have deteriorated. The new cases will usually have mild symptoms and the diagnosis can be established before commencing treatment with oral anticholinesterase medication. Patients presenting with severe bulbar and respiratory muscle weakness are usually established cases who have deteriorated and they are the medical emergencies.

Anticholinesterases

Therapy with anticholinesterases was introduced in the early 1930s. The two preparations now commonly used are neostigmine (Prostigmin) and pyridostigmine (Mestinon). Pyridostigmine has a more prolonged action and weaker muscarinic effects than neostigmine but it is a little slower to take effect. The initial dose is one tablet (pyridostigmine 60 mg, neostigmine 15 mg) three or four times a day, which may be increased as necessary up to twenty or more tablets distributed throughout the day. Muscarinic side effects (abdominal cramps, diarrhoea, nausea, vomiting and increased salivation) may necessitate the addition of oral atropine. Overdosage will lead to progressive pupillary constriction and 'cholinergic crisis', with muscular cramps, fasciculation and generalized weakness due to depolarization of the nicotinic receptors. Measurement of serum anticholinesterase levels has not proved clinically helpful.

Severe respiratory and bulbar weakness

When a patient presents with breathlessness, severe dysphagia, a weak voice and dangling chin, they must be admitted immediately to a unit (intensive care or respiratory) where facilities for assisted ventilation and intensive nursing are available. Since the patient is usually already on treatment with anticholinesterases, it may be unclear as to whether the deterioration is due to a relapse of the myasthenia or to a 'cholinergic crisis'. If he is tiring and has a vital capacity below one litre and falling, this is immaterial to the immediate management. Endotracheal intubation (unless the patient already has a tracheostomy) and elective positive pressure ventilation will usually be necessary. A tracheostomy may subsequently be required. A nasogastric tube should be passed to allow the administration of drugs and nourishment. A chest X-ray should be done to detect infection or pulmonary collapse, and appropriate therapy should be given. If muscarinic side effects are not obvious, a Tensilon test can be performed to elucidate whether the patient is over- or under-dosed with anticholinesterase. This should only be done after full preparations for ventilation as the patient's respiratory weakness will be exacerbated if he is in 'cholinergic crisis'. Sometimes there will be improvement in function of one group of muscles but deterioration in another. If anticholinesterase overdose seems likely, the medication should be stopped for at least twenty-four hours and then reintroduced at a lower level. In severe myasthenia consideration should be given to the use of plasma exchange. This may produce rapid and dramatic clinical improvement in association with a fall in circulating acetylcholine receptor antibodies (Pinching et al. 1976; Newsom-Davis et al. 1978). However, the effects are temporary and one of the other 'immunological' therapies discussed below should be instituted at the same time.

Long-term management

In patients with persistent significant symptoms, treatment aimed at reducing the levels of circulating acetylcholine receptor antibodies is indicated. This involves either thymectomy or treatment with steroids (with or without other immunosuppressant drugs).

Thymectomy is most effective in patients under the age of forty without a thymoma, although those with a thymoma will obviously also have to undergo surgery (Simpson 1958; Buckingham et al. 1976). There have been no prospective controlled trials of its effects but the data available suggest that 25 per cent of this group will obtain a remission and up to a further 50 per cent will improve. The improvement usually occurs during the first postoperative year. The effectiveness of thymectomy may be related to the removal of thymic cells which enhance acetylcholine receptor antibody production by lymphocytes (Newsom-Davis et al. 1981). The thymus itself is not the major site of antibody production (Scadding et al. 1981).

Prednisolone now has an established place in treatment with remission or improvement occurring in at least 80 per cent of patients (Mann et al. 1976). When treatment is initiated with high doses, deterioration may take place during the first two weeks before improvement begins. This effect may be minimized by using an alternate day regime and gradually incrementing doses (Seybold and Drachman 1974). Nevertheless, it is wise to start treatment in hospital in patients with generalized weakness or bulbar symptoms. A suitable regime is to start with 25 mg prednisolone on alternate days and to increase the dose by 25 mg increments every four days up to 100 mg on alternate days. The alternate day regime may reduce long-term side effects. However, the addition of a small dose of prednisolone on the non-steroid day may be necessary in a few patients to iron out fluctuations in weakness. Improvement occurs over several months and the dose is gradually reduced to the minimally effective maintenance level. It is not usually possible to completely withdraw treatment, except in patients who subsequently have a good response to thymectomy.

In recent years, azathioprine has been used increasingly in association with prednisolone. It seems effective (Mertens et al. 1981), but no randomized controlled trials have been reported. It may allow the maintenance dose of prednisolone to be decreased and it certainly seems indicated when this is unacceptably high. The usual dose is 3 mg/kg. Improvement occurs slowly over the course of three to twelve months. Its long-term use has, of course, serious potential side effects. Cyclophosphamide has also been used (Perez et al. 1981). Plasma exchange though useful in the short-term in the seriously ill patient, probably has no role in the long-term management (Hawkey et al. 1981). In patients who obtain a remission with 'immunological' therapy, it is often possible to withdraw anticholinesterase medication.

Further reading

Asbury A., Arnason B., Karp H. and McFarlin D. (1978) Criteria for diagnosis of Guillain–Barré syndrome. *Annals of Neurology* **3**, 565–566.

Buckingham J.M., Howard F.M., Bernatz P.E., Spencer-Payne W., Harrison E.G., O'Brien P.C. and Weiland L.H. (1976) The value of thymectomy in myasthenia gravis. *Annals of Surgery* **184**, 453–458.

Compston D.A.S., Vincent A., Newsom-Davis J. and Batchelor J.R. (1980) Clinical, pathological, HLA antigen and immunological evidence for disease heterogeneity in myasthenia gravis. *Brain* **103**, 579–601.

Cook S.D. and Dowling P.C. (1981) The role of auto-antibody and immune complexes in the pathogenesis of Guillain–Barré syndrome. *Annals of Neurology* **9** (Suppl.), 70–79.

Dalakas M.C. and Engel W.K. (1981) Chronic relapsing (dysimmune) polyneuropathy: pathogenesis and treatment. *Annals of Neurology* **9** (Suppl.), 134–145.

Davidson D.L.W. and Jellinek E.H. (1977) Hypertension and papilloedema in the Guillain–Barré syndrome. *Journal of Neurology, Neurosurgery and Psychiatry* **40**, 144–148.

Denny-Brown D.E. (1952) The changing pattern of neurological medicine. *New England Journal of Medicine* **246**, 839–846.

Dowling P.C. and Cook S.D. (1981) Role of infection in Guillain–Barré syndrome: Laboratory confirmation of Herpes viruses in 41 cases. *Annals of Neurology* **9** (Suppl.), 44–55.

Dowling P.C., Menonna J.P. and Cook S.D. (1977) Guillain–Barré syndrome in Greater New York, New Jersey. *Journal of the American Medical Association* **238**, 317–318.

Fisher M. (1956) An unusual variant of acute idiopathic polyneuritis (syndrome of ophthalmoplegia, ataxia and areflexia). *New England Journal of Medicine* **255**, 57–65.

Guillain G. (1936) Radiculoneuritis with acellular hyperalbuminosis of the cerebrospinal fluid. *Archives of Neurology and Psychiatry* (Chicago) **36**, 975–990.

Guillain G., Barré J.A. and Strohl A. (1916) Sur un syndrome de radiculo-névrite avec hyperalbuminose du liquide céphalo-rachidien sans réaction cellulaire: Remarque sur les caractéres cliniques et graphiques des réflexes tendineux. *Bulletin Société Médicale des Hôpitaux de Paris* **40**, 1462–1470.

Hawkey C.J., Newsom-Davis J. and Vincent A. (1981) Plasma exchange and immunosuppressive drug treatment in myasthenia gravis: no evidence for synergy. *Journal of Neurology, Neurosurgery and Psychiatry* **44**, 469–475.

Haymaker W. and Kernohan J.W. (1949) The Landry–Guillain Barré syndrome: A clinico-pathologic report of fifty fatal cases and a critique of the literature. *Medicine (Baltimore)* **28**, 59–141.

Hughes R.A.C., Kadlubowski M. and Hufschmidt A. (1981) Treatment of acute inflammatory polyneuropathy. *Annals of Neurology* **9** (Suppl.), 125–133.

Hughes R.A.C., Newsom-Davis J., Perkin G.D. and Pierce J.M. (1978) Controlled trial of prednisolone in acute polyneuropathy. *Lancet* **ii**, 750–753.

Iqbal A., Oger J.J. and Arnason B.G.W. (1981) Cell-mediated immunity in idiopathic polyneuritis. *Annals of Neurology* **9** (Suppl.), 65–69.

Keesey J., Bein M., Mink J., Sample F., Sarti D., Mulder D., Herrmann C. and Peter J.B. (1980) Detection of thymoma in myasthenia gravis. *Neurology* **30**, 233–239.

Kelly J.J., Daube J.R., Lennon V.A., Howard F.M. and Younge B.R. (1982) The laboratory diagnosis of mild myasthenia gravis. *Annals of Neurology* **12**, 238–242.

Landry O. (1859) Note sur la paralysie ascendante aigue. *Gazette Hebdomadaire Medicale de Paris* **6**, 472–474.

Lindstrom J.M., Seybold M.E., Lennon V.A., Whittingham S. and Duane D.D. (1976) Antibody to acetyl choline receptor in myasthenia gravis—Prevalence, clinical correlates and diagnostic value. *Neurology* **26**, 1054–59.

Link H. (1978) Demonstration of oligoclonal immunoglobulin G in Guillain–Barré syndrome. *Acta Neurologica Scandinavica* **52**, 111–120.

Löffel N.B., Rossi L.N., Mumenthaler M., Lütschg J. and Ludin H.P. (1977) The Landry–Guillain–Barré syndrome—complications, prognosis and natural history in 123 cases. *Journal of the Neurological Sciences* **33**, 71–79.

McLeod J.G. (1981) Electrophysiological studies in the Guillain–Barré syndrome. *Annals of Neurology* **9** (Suppl.), 20–27.

Mann J.D., Johns T.R. and Campa J.F. (1976) Long-term administration of corticosteroids in myasthenia gravis. *Neurology* **26**, 729–740.

Mertens H.G., Hertel G., Reuther P. and Ricker K. (1981) Effect of immuno-suppressive drugs (azathioprine). *Annals of New York Academy of Sciences* **377**, 691–698.

Mittag T.W. and Caroscio J. (1980) False positive immuno-assay for acetylcholine receptor antibody in amyotrophic lateral sclerosis. *New England Journal of Medicine* **302**, 868.

Newsom-Davis J., Pinching A.J., Vincent A. and Wilson S.G. (1978) Function of circulating antibody to acetylcholine receptor in myasthenia gravis: investigation by plasma exchange. *Neurology* **28**, 266–272.

Newsom-Davis J., Willcox N. and Calder L. (1981) Thymus cells in myasthenia gravis selectively enhance production of acetylcholine receptor antibody by autologous blood lymphocytes. *New England Journal of Medicine* **305**, 1313–18.

Perez M.C., Buot W.L., Mercado-Danguillan C., Bagabaldo A.G. and Renales L.D. (1981) Stable remissions in myasthenia gravis. *Neurology* **31**, 32–37.

Pinching A.J., Peters D.K. and Newsom-Davis J. (1976) Remission of myasthenia gravis following plasma exchange. *Lancet* **ii**, 1373–76.

Posner C.M. (1981) Criteria for the diagnosis of the Guillain–Barré syndrome. A critique of the NINCDS guidelines. *Journal of the Neurological Sciences* **52**, 191–199.

Prineas J.W. (1981) Pathology of the Guillain–Barré syndrome. *Annals of Neurology* **9** (Suppl.), 6–19.

Sagar H.J., Gelsthorpe K., Milford-Ward A. and Davies-Jones G.A.B. (1980a) Clinical and immunological associations in myasthenia gravis 1: autoantibodies. *Journal of Neurology, Neurosurgery and Psychiatry* **43**, 967–970.

Sagar H.J., Davies-Jones G.A.B. and Allonby I.D. (1980b) Clinical and immunological associations in myasthenia gravis 2: cell mediated immunity. *Journal of Neurology, Neurosurgery and Psychiatry* **43**, 971–977.

Scadding G.K., Vincent A., Newsom-Davis J. and Henry K. (1981) Acetylcholine receptor antibody synthesis by thymic lymphocytes: correlation with thymic histology. *Neurology* **31**, 935–943.

Seybold M.E. and Drachman D.B. (1974) Gradually increasing doses of prednisolone in myasthenia gravis. *New England Journal of Medicine* **290**, 81–84.

Simpson J.A. (1958) An evaluation of thymectomy in myasthenia gravis. *Brain* **81**, 112–144.

Stålberg E. (1980) Clinical electrophysiology in myasthenia gravis. *Journal of Neurology, Neurosurgery and Psychiatry* **43**, 622–633.

Stålberg E., Ekstedt J. and Broman A. (1974) Neuromuscular transmission in myasthenia gravis studied with single fibre electromyography. *Journal of Neurology, Neurosurgery and Psychiatry* **37**, 540–547.

Tuck R.R. and McLeod J.G. (1981) Autonomic dysfunction in Guillain–Barré syndrome. *Journal of Neurology, Neurosurgery and Psychiatry* **44**, 983–990.

Wiederholt W.C., Mulder D.W. and Lambert E.H. (1964) The Landry–Guillain–Barré–Strohl syndrome or polyradiculoneuropathy-Historical review, report on 97 patients and present concepts. *Mayo Clinic Proceedings* **39**, 427–451.

22 · Spinal Cord and Cauda Equina Compression

P. J. TEDDY

This subject is mentioned briefly here not because it normally presents any great difficulty in diagnosis or management but because so often there is a failure to deal with the problem with the necessary urgency. Delay in diagnosis and definitive treatment may result in otherwise avoidable paraplegia and loss of sphincter control.

For a full and useful account of the diagnosis and management of this problem the reader is referred to the article by Uttley in the *British Journal of Hospital Medicine,* December 1981.

Probably the commonest causes of subacute spinal cord compression encountered by the physician are those of extradural metastases from primary lesions in lung, breast and prostate and, less commonly, infection within the spinal canal in patients with septicaemia or those prone to serious generalized infections. The metastatic deposits in the spinal canal occur almost invariably in the thoracic or lumbar regions.

Any patient who presents with evidence of a progressive weakness and sensory level in the limbs or trunk should be considered to have spinal cord or cauda equina compression until proved otherwise. These clinical features may quickly be followed or sometimes preceded by sphincter disturbance (usually painless urinary retention with overflow, and constipation). Often there is a previous history of back pain.

Once this working diagnosis has been made, prompt investigation is required and immediate steps must be taken to provide some form of spinal decompression. These patients often develop very rapid acceleration of their symptoms and a paraparesis may progress to an irreversible paraplegia within twenty-four hours. Loss of sphincter control may become permanent after only eight to twelve hours.

The following is an outline of the essentials of management necessary to prevent such disasters.

Ask for

History of trauma.
Back pain—if sudden may represent vertebral collapse. May be associated with rapid worsening of symptoms.
Root pains.
Symptoms suggesting pre-existing malignant disease or infection.

Look for

Spinal tenderness—much more severe with abscesses.

Spinal angulation.

Tone/power in limbs—spastic or flaccid weakness will depend on level of compression.

Sensation—sensory level or root distribution of sensory impairment.

    —sacral sparing; this may imply a better prognosis regarding sphincter control.

    —saddle anaesthesia, implying lower sacral root compression.

Sphincter dysfunction—usually painless retention with overflow and constipation.

Investigations

Having made a clinical diagnosis of cord compression do *not* carry out a lumbar puncture. This is generally not helpful and can make subsequent myelography difficult. CSF may be obtained for analysis and microbiology at the time of myelography.

Blood, urine, sputum cultures where appropriate.

Chest X-ray.

Plain spinal X-rays—look for bony metastatic deposits or infection.

    —paravertebral masses.

    —collapse of vertebral bodies.

    —erosion of pedicles.

    —calcification and narrowing of disc spaces.

Myelography—this should be carried out after consultation with a neurosurgeon and performed by a radiologist experienced in such work in a unit with easy access to a neurosurgical theatre.

    —look for partial or complete obstruction to flow of contrast material and for multiple lesions.

    —this investigation should be carried out at the earliest available opportunity once the diagnosis of cord compression has been made.

CT scan—now of increasing value *when* rapidly available

Interim treatment

Pain—give adequate analgesia.

Urinary retention—catheterize as necessary.

Steroids—dexamethazone may be of some value in treating cord compression due to metastatic lesions particularly when radiotherapy is to be given as an adjunct or as an alternative to surgery. Be sure to exlude an infective aetiology before such treatment is given.

Anxiety—many patients are naturally extremely distressed by their condition and a calm, careful explanation of the anticipated course of management goes a long way to allaying fear and anxiety.
Obtain an urgent neurosurgical opinion.

Further reading

Uttley D. (1981) Diagnosis not to be missed. Spinal cord compression. *British Journal of Hospital Medicine* **26**, 6:607–610.

23 · Upper Gastro-intestinal Haemorrhage

H. J. KENNEDY

Upper gastro-intestinal haemorrhage is a common emergency. It was found to be the seventh most common of all the medical emergencies in the survey presented in the introduction to this book. There were 202 admissions for upper gastro-intestinal haemorrhage during the year surveyed. There was a survey of haematemesis and melaena in Oxford spanning the years 1953 to 1967 (Schiller *et al.* 1970) and a further survey is in preparation. These studies demonstrate that the mortality rate remains at about nine per cent despite the advances that have been made in diagnosis and medical care. Several other centres have reported similar mortality rates (Allen and Dykes 1976; Mayberry *et al.* 1981). It should be possible to reduce this mortality. It is the aim of this chapter to summarize the current state of knowledge and suggest ways in which this improvement might be achieved.

Source of the haemorrhage

This section is included to show the approximate frequency of bleeding from different sites. The figures in Table 23.1 represent the findings in Oxford between 1968 and 1977. There are several important observations to make about these results. First, there are many patients in whom the cause was not known, most of these patients had minimal bleeding and therefore they were not investigated. In this study, separate categories for bleeding from Mallory–Weiss tears and oesophagitis were not included but they are often a cause of minor bleeding and sometimes of severe blood loss. Secondly, there

Table 23.1. Final diagnosis in 1604 patients with upper gastro-intestinal haemorrhage

Diagnosis	No of patients	Per cent
Duodenal ulcer	526	32.8
Gastric ulcer	303	18.9
Acute erosions	178	11.1
Oesophageal varices	41	2.6
Stomal ulcer	31	1.9
Carcinoma of stomach	29	1.8
Cause unknown	317	19.8
Miscellaneous	179	11.2

is a relatively large percentage of patients bleeding from gastric erosions. This is a very important diagnosis to make as surgery is usually contra-indicated in such patients. Endoscopy is the best method of diagnosis, as erosions are difficult to diagnose radiologically even with double contrast studies. Thirdly, bleeding from oesophageal varices is not a common source of upper gastro-intestinal haemorrhage in Britain, although it is more common in parts of Europe and the United States of America. Nevertheless, even in the United Kingdom, this is a substantial problem. Bleeding from this source is frequently torrential and the prognosis remains poor. The final but most important point to stress is that in ten to twenty-five per cent of patients there is more than one lesion present (Thomas *et al.* 1978). This must always be remembered during the diagnosis and management of all patients presenting with gastro-intestinal haemorrhage.

Clinical features and patient assessment

Presenting features

A precise assessment of every patient must be made on admission. A detailed history and examination are necessary with particular attention being paid to the past medical history, drug ingestion, smoking and alcohol consumption. On examination, a careful search should be made for signs of heart failure, chronic lung disease, renal failure and chronic liver disease.

Identification of the high risk patient

The factors shown in Table 23.2 have all been shown to increase the risk of mortality. Avery Jones (1956) demonstrated a twelvefold increase in mortality in patients having a recurrent haemorrhage following admission to hospital. The factors reported to increase the risk of rebleeding are shown in

Table 23.2. Factors shown to increase the risk of mortality in patients with an upper gastro-intestinal haemorrhage

Recurrent haemorrhage
Age > 60 years
Chronic rather than acute ulcers
Bleeding oesophageal or gastric varices
Concurrent cardiac, respiratory, renal or liver disease
Initially severe bleed as judged by hypotension, low
    haemoglobin or large transfusion required

Table 23.3. Factors reported to increase the risk of rebleeding after an upper gastrointestinal haemorrhage

Oesophageal or gastric varices
Initial severe haemorrhage
Haematemesis versus melaena alone
Endoscopic finding of: fresh bleeding
adherent clot in an ulcer
visible vessel in base of ulcer
central spot in an ulcer

Table 23.3. It may be possible to reduce the mortality rate if all the patients demonstrating factors known to increase mortality receive special attention from a skilled team (Hunt *et al.* 1979). However, it is far from certain which is the best form of treatment in any patient and particularly in those who are elderly with diseases of other systems. This problem is discussed later in the chapter.

Drugs as a cause of upper gastro-intestinal bleeding

Despite many reports and many firmly held views, the role of drugs in causing *significant* upper gastro-intestinal bleeding remains unclear. It has now been well documented that aspirin causes occult microbleeding in a high proportion of people (Salter 1968). Similar findings have been reported with indomethacin. However, the data relating to other nonsteroidal anti-inflammatory drugs and the corticosteroids is less certain.

Aspirin has also been fairly strongly implicated as causing significant bleeding when consumed in substantial amounts (Levy 1974). Similar data does not exist for any other drug (Conn and Blitzer 1976; Dronfield and Langman 1978). Indeed, even with aspirin it has been suggested that the drug was being taken because of symptoms due to gastro-intestinal lesions rather than causing them.

Therefore, with the present state of knowledge, any patient presenting with an upper gastro-intestinal haemorrhage should have a careful drug history taken. If possible, any suspected drugs should be stopped during the acute period. Subsequently, the balance of benefit and risk for any particular drug has to be judged in each individual.

Investigation and management

A schematic representation of investigation and management is given in Fig. 23.1.

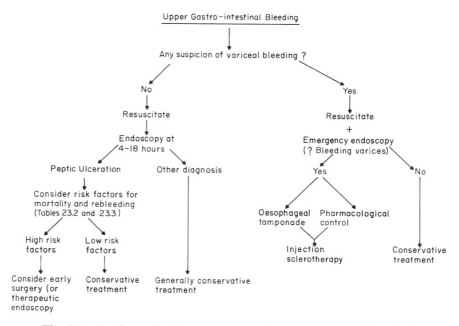

Fig. 23.1. A scheme for the management of acute upper gastro-intestinal haemorrhage.

Immediate management

The initial aims are to replace the lost circulating volume and to stop the bleeding if massive haemorrhage continues. As soon as it is recognized that the patient is bleeding, the following measures should be undertaken:

1. Blood taken for grouping and cross-matching, full blood count, pro-thrombin time (coagulation screen), urea, electrolytes, biochemical profile and blood glucose.

2. Insertion of an intravenous cannula and in cases of severe haemor-rhage, a central venous pressure line.

3. Replace lost circulating volume. The two questions that arise are: what fluid should be used and how much should be given (see below).

4. Monitor pulse, blood pressure, exact fluid balance and if possible the initial body weight of the patient.

5. Measure blood gases and then supply added oxygen in suitable quantity in elderly, ill and shocked patients.

6. A chest X-ray and electrocardiogram are required in patients with significant bleeding.

Restoration of blood volume

The type of fluid

There is no doubt that blood is the fluid replacement of choice in every patient requiring transfusion. An urgent cross-match can be completed in about thirty minutes. However, this time may be longer if the staff undertaking the cross-match are not immediately available or if the cross-match is not straight forward. Most patients require only a small volume of alternative fluid before cross-matched blood becomes available. Nevertheless, there is a group of patients with massive haemorrhage who require a considerable volume of fluid replacement before any blood can be cross-matched urgently. The choice of fluid in these circumstances can be very important.

In general, initial replacement with electrolyte solutions is recommended as they are readily available, cheap and they restore effective circulating volume. Sodium chloride (0.9 per cent) should be used rather than Ringer's lactate, as this fluid results in the production of lactic acid which may accumulate in the circulation. The sodium and water load may be harmful in the elderly and in patients with salt retaining conditions such as chronic liver disease or cardiac failure. Replacement of these fluids by cross-matched blood is particularly urgent in these patients. In desperate situations, it is occasionally justified to give group O Rhesus negative blood to a patient. If the blood group of the patient is definitely known, it is preferable to use blood of his own group.

In addition to the electrolyte solutions, colloids such as plasma, plasma fractions, albumin or plasma substitutes may be used. These fluids are efficient at restoring the circulating volume but they are less readily available and more expensive than the electrolyte solutions. Moreover, in sustained shock the capillary wall may become permeable to particles with a molecular weight up to 240,000 (Holcroft and Trunkey 1975). In this situation, both the electrolyte solutions and the colloids pass rapidly into the extra-vascular space in a few hours but the colloids may take as long as seven to ten days to be removed. This may result in intractable tissue oedema causing particular difficulty in the brain and lungs (Virgillio *et al.* 1979). The plasma fractions carry the added danger of transmitting hepatitis viruses and most of the colloid solutions contain as much sodium per unit volume as 0.9 per cent sodium chloride.

The most commonly used plasma substitutes are the Dextrans with average molecular weight of 70,000 and 40,000. These Dextrans can interfere with the cross-matching of blood and some patients are allergic to them. We favour the use of Haemaccel which is degraded gelatin (molecular weight 35,000) in 0.9 per cent sodium chloride. This does not interfere with the cross-matching of blood. The problems related to fluid replacement in shock are considered in more detail in Chapter 9.

Assessment of blood loss and volume of fluid replacement

The volume of blood lost is frequently difficult to determine. Haematemesis together with melaena usually indicates more severe bleeding than melaena alone. Most patients who have had a significant upper gastro-intestinal haemorrhage have lost more than half of their circulating volume (Tudhope 1958). A patient who has collapsed with poor peripheral perfusion, a pulse rate of greater than 100 beats per minute and a systolic blood pressure of less than 90 mm of mercury has always bled significantly. However, these parameters measured individually are not reliable. In particular, the pulse rate may be rapid due to anxiety and conversely, the blood pressure may be maintained, especially in young people, despite a considerable haemorrhage. A postural drop in blood pressure is sometimes found in these patients, which may be helpful. A urine output of below 0.5 ml/kg/hour and the measurement of plasma and urinary osmolarity may be useful guides to the degree of hypovolaemia. The initial blood haemoglobin concentration and haematocrit are poor guides to the extent of the blood loss because it takes several hours for haemo-dilution to occur. Nevertheless, a haemoglobin of less than 10 g/dl in a previously healthy individual suggests that transfusion is required.

A central venous pressure line should be inserted in those patients suspected of having a severe haemorrhage. It must be stressed that the line must be correctly positioned and read. Sequential measurements of pressure are of more value than a single reading. However, a pressure of less than 2 cm of water, measuring from the mid-axillary line with the patient supine, indicates a reduced venous return to the heart. The aims of fluid replacement should be to achieve a stable situation with good peripheral perfusion, the systolic blood pressure being greater than 100 mm Hg, a urine output of greater than 0.5 ml/kg/hr and a central venous pressure of about 5–10 cm of water. A fall in the central venous pressure has been found to be an early sign of recurrent bleeding (Northfield and Smith 1970).

Patient monitoring and general management

Frequent clinical examination should be carried out in all patients requiring fluid replacement. Over-enthusiastic transfusions can cause cardiac failure particularly in elderly patients.

Mobilization

Patients who have had an upper gastro-intestinal haemorrhage should be mobilized as soon as possible as this minimizes the risk of deep vein thrombosis and pulmonary embolism. Even those patients who have required transfusion may be sent home after six days provided they have had no complications as, by this time, their risk of rebleeding is very low (Cotton and Russel 1977).

Nasogastric intubation

This is best avoided because the tube itself or aspiration through the tube can cause damage to oesophageal varices, result in gastric erosions and displace a clot on an ulcer. In addition, it is uncomfortable for the patient, it increases the risk of respiratory complications and can easily become blocked. The use of gastric lavage is considered later.

Adequate ventilation

This is another aspect of management which can easily cause difficulty, particularly in the elderly and in those with chronic obstructive airways disease. An initial arterial sample of blood should be taken for analysis of the blood gases and acid : base status in any patient with a significant haemorrhage. Added oxygen should not be given without knowledge of the blood gas analysis. A suitable concentration of oxygen may then be given and further arterial samples taken to monitor the response.

Aspiration of gastric contents may easily occur in critically ill patients. Therefore, early endotracheal intubation is recommended in these patients to avoid the complication and ensure adequate ventilation.

Sedation

Upper gastro-intestinal haemorrhage is frightening and sedation may be required. Small doses of benzodiazepines are recommended. These should only be given when necessary and care needs to be taken not to oversedate the patient. Inadequate ventilation and aspiration of stomach contents into the lungs are more likely if too much sedation is given. Patients with chronic liver disease are more sensitive to any form of sedation and hepatic encephalopathy may be precipitated.

Oral intake

Oral fluid intake is encouraged in patients who are well enough and who are not requiring endoscopy or surgery. Antacids, as required, may help to relieve gastric pain.

Identification of the source of the bleeding

There is now general agreement that a skilled endoscopist can more accurately determine the source of bleeding (80–95 per cent) than can be achieved by a double contrast barium meal (up to 80 per cent) (Stevenson *et al.* 1976). Nevertheless, the skill of the available staff is paramount. Both investigations are difficult in patients who have had a significant haemorrhage. A double contrast barium meal carried out by an expert can provide more information than a gastroscopy undertaken by an unskilled endoscopist.

Endoscopy

Endoscopy must be carried out under optimal conditions in any patient who has had a significant upper gastro-intestinal haemorrhage. Not only must the endoscopist be skilled but he needs support from skilled nursing and endoscopy staff. If possible, the procedure should be performed in a fully equipped endoscopy room. In any case, adequate suction facilities and resuscitation equipment must be immediately available to manage cardiac arrest, respiratory arrest and inhalation of gastric contents. It is our practice to always consult the surgical team prior to endoscopy.

Normally, endoscopy should be undertaken within four to eighteen hours after the haemorrhage. Prior to this the patient needs to be resuscitated and by waiting four hours, sufficient time elapses for the blood to be at least partly cleared from the stomach. It also means that the procedure can normally be carried out during the working day when full support facilities are readily available. The main exception to this role is in patients suspected of having portal hypertension. Where there is a risk of haemorrhage from oesophageal or gastric varices *emergency* endoscopy is required so that blood loss can be controlled. If endoscopy is delayed much more than eighteen hours, the diagnostic yield begins to fall.

Frequently, the stomach still contains a considerable amount of clot. This lies on the greater curve when the patient is in the left lateral position. The endoscope can usually be passed down the lesser curve of the stomach over the clot in these circumstances. This allows inspection of the duodenum, antrum, lesser curve and oesophagus. Bleeding from the greater curve is unusual and so even if this area is not seen most lesions are visualized. Nevertheless, the greater curve can sometimes be seen by moving the patient into the right lateral position. Gastric lavage through a wide bore (32–38 French gauge) tube can be useful in removing clot from the stomach.

When lesions are found at endoscopy, inspection should be made for signs of recent haemorrhage. These are a visible vessel, adherent clot and dark slough in the base of an ulcer. It must be remembered that in 10–25 per cent of patients there is more than one lesion and so detailed examination of the remainder of the upper gastro-intestinal tract must be made, even when one lesion has been found.

Radiology

The double contrast barium meal can be used as an alternative investigation to an endoscopy and in skilled hands can give a high diagnostic yield. The patient must be resuscitated and prepared for the examination in the same way as for endoscopy. The less blood present in the stomach by the time of the examination the better. For examination of the small bowel beyond the second part of the duodenum, a small bowel enema is the investigation of choice (Nolan 1979). Selective angiography is of value in patients with continuing severe bleeding from an obscure source. The patient must be actively bleeding at the rate of at least 0.5 ml/min. Good results can only be obtained if the appropriate vessel can be selectively catheterized. This should include catheterization of the left gastric, gastroduodenal, splenic and superior mesenteric arteries. Angiography may also occasionally demonstrate an arteriovenous malformation in a patient who has stopped bleeding.

Specific treatment in non-variceal bleeding

Medical measures in patients bleeding from peptic ulceration

H_2 receptor antagonists and other agents known to heal ulcers

Controlled trials of both cimetidine (Pickard et al. 1979) and ranitidine (Dawson and Cokel 1982) have shown no overall benefit for the use of H_2 receptor antagonists in the treatment of upper gastro-intestinal bleeding from peptic ulceration.

However, they are probably the agents of choice to aid ulcer healing and should be started as soon as possible after the haemorrhage. Some centres initially give intravenous cimetidine but this is not usually justified. There are now several other agents that have been shown to aid ulcer healing, including pirenzepine, carbenoxolone, colloidal bismuth, sucralfate and intensive antacid therapy. There is no reason why one of these agents should not be used in place of an H_2 receptor antagonist providing their various side effects are considered.

Other agents

There is some evidence that vasopressin may control bleeding from peptic ulcers but its effect is temporary and it is not widely used for this purpose.

Tranexamic acid has antifibrinolytic activity and has been shown to reduce the transfusion requirement and the incidence of emergency surgery (Briggs et al. 1976). This agent requires further evaluation.

Somatostatin has also been used in the treatment of bleeding ulcers with some benefit (Kayassen et al. 1980).

Medical measures in the treatment of erosions and stress-induced ulcers

The aetiology of gastric erosions is unknown. They may be associated with aspirin ingestion. Bleeding from erosions usually stops spontaneously with general medical management. Where the erosions are thought to be associated with aspirin ingestion they usually heal spontaneously after the drug is cleared from the stomach. There is a small percentage of patients who continue to bleed from erosive gastritis. This is a serious condition which has a poor prognosis. Surgery should only be attempted as a last resort. There are no controlled clinical trials of therapy in this condition due to its rarity. The aim of treatment is to provide full supportive general medical care and to keep the gastric pH above five by the intravenous administration of an H_2 receptor antagonist. In addition, tranexamic acid is also thought to be of benefit. Vasopressin infusion has been found to arrest haemorrhage at least temporarily (Athanasoulis et al. 1974). When vasopressin either fails to control, or only temporarily controls haemorrhage, selective arterial embolization has been employed.

The aetiology of stress ulcers is unknown. They can occur in patients who are severely ill from any cause. They carry a high mortality. No therapy has been shown to be effective once an ulcer has formed. However, intravenous H_2 receptor antagonists, given to keep the gastric pH above five, may be helpful. Surgery has to be used as a last resort but carries a high mortality in these severely ill patients. There is no doubt that the prophylactic use of H_2 receptor antagonists is currently the most effective management in these patients. Several controlled studies have shown that cimetidine substantially reduces the risk of upper gastro-intestinal haemorrhage when it is given prophylactically to severely ill patients (Basso et al. 1979; MacDougall et al. 1977).

Therapeutic endoscopy in non-variceal haemorrhage

The value of various endoscopic therapeutic manoeuvres is under study and none of the techniques are being widely used. Laser photocoagulation, mono and bipolar electrocoagulation, electrohydrothermoprobes, clips and endoscopic spray techniques are all being assessed. The use of lasers has received the most publicity; it is expensive and with the information currently available its benefit is uncertain (Laurence *et al.* 1980). Bipolar electrocoagulation and the electrohydrothermoprobe are the most promising of the other techniques.

Surgery in non variceal haemorrhage

Operation is seldom required for Mallory–Weiss tears and is only used as a last resort in severe bleeding from gastric erosions and stress ulceration. However, surgery remains the only definitive method of stopping recurrent or persistent haemorrhage from peptic ulceration. Early surgery has often been recommended in patients over sixty exhibiting increased risk factors, as shown in Tables 23.2 and 23.3. These patients do badly if rebleeding occurs. However, they also have a high operative morbidity and mortality. As yet, there are no controlled clinical trials to determine whether early operation is the best form of management in elderly patients with increased risk factors. Some trials are now underway and some preliminary results from Birmingham suggest that early surgery is beneficial in this group but not in young patients. An open mind must be kept on this subject but it is our current policy to recommend early surgery in elderly patients at risk. However, it is important to consider each individual case and for full liasion between physicians and surgeons to take place. It is also very important that these emergency operations are carried out by experienced surgeons.

Specific treatment of upper gastro-intestinal haemorrhage in patients with portal hypertension

The first priority in the management of these patients is to restore the circulating volume as soon as possible as was discussed in detail earlier in this chapter. The next requirement is to undertake an emergency endoscopy to determine the site of bleeding. There is considerable controversy concerning the frequency of bleeding from sites other than the varices in patients with portal hypertension (Mitchell *et al.* 1982). In our experience acute bleeding in these patients arises from varices in about 50 per cent of patients and from other sources in the remaining 50 per cent. In patients bleeding from varices, emergency control of haemorrhage is imperative. Currently, the two methods advocated are the intravenous administration of vasopressin or its analogue, Glypressin and oesophageal tamponade by a modified Sengstaken tube or a Minnesota tube.

Vasopressin and glypressin

Lysine-vasopressin is widely available and the usual method of administration has been to give 20 units in 100 ml of 5 per cent dextrose over 10 minutes. More recently, a continuous infusion of 0.4 units/minute of vasopressin into a peripheral vein has been recommended (Johnson *et al.* 1977). This study found that intravenous administration of vasopressin was as effective as intra-arterial administration (controlling bleeding in 56 per cent of patients). Recently, the use of triglycyl lysine vasopressin (glypressin), 2 mg 6 hourly as an intravenous bolus, has been advocated (Freeman *et al.* 1982). This substance acts as a depot from which vasopressin is slowly released. At the moment, this agent is expensive and not widely available.

Oesophageal tamponade

Balloon tamponade is an effective way of achieving early control of bleeding varices and can be successful in up to 85–90 per cent of cases (Teres *et al.* 1978). However, serious complications can occur including respiratory obstruction, aspiration pneumonia and laceration, ulceration or rupture of the oesophagus. This procedure should only be undertaken by doctors and nurses familiar with the technique. The complications can be reduced to a minimum by scrupulous care and attention to detail. These tubes should only be inserted either in a fully equipped endoscopy room with a tipping bed and suction apparatus or in an operating theatre.

The tube should have a gastric and an oesophageal balloon. The four channel Minnesota or Sengstaken–Blakemore tubes are suitable. That is, one channel to fill each balloon and one channel each for aspirating the oesophagus and stomach. Some tubes only have three channels omitting the oesophageal aspiration channel. If such a tube has to be used, a nasogastric tube must be taped on, to aspirate the oesophagus above the oesophageal balloon.

Prior to intubation, both balloons should be filled with air to check for leaks and determine the pressure. The gastric balloon of a Minnesota tube should have 300–400 ml of air inserted and the pressure recorded by connecting it to a standard sphygmomanometer (pressure circa 60 mm Hg). The oesophageal balloon is then inflated until it is just beginning to distend and the pressure is recorded (about 120 ml of air and a pressure of 60–70 mm Hg). The channels should be checked to ensure that they are correctly labelled. Both balloons are then deflated and the channels clamped to keep them free of air.

The patient requires constant reassurance and encouragement as var/iceal bleeding and passing a tube are both frightening. Some sedation is often necessary and we currently use 5–10 mg of diazepam intravenously. Great care needs to be exercised with the use of sedatives in these patients as they metabolize these drugs slowly due to their liver impairment and have a danger of developing encephalopathy. Opiates should be avoided. Patients with chronic obstructive airways disease are particularly at risk; only minimal sedation can be used and blood gases must be monitored frequently. Some patients, particularly alcoholics, remain very agitated despite sedation. A heminevrin infusion has been recommended in this situation but we have found that this agent is required in large doses in these patients and takes some time to work. The patients may then suffer respiratory depression and take many hours to wake up. We favour the use of a gas anaesthetic given by an experienced anaesthetist in these agitated patients. If necessary, the patients are intubated and we often keep them ventilated and lightly anaesthetized until the tube can be removed. These anaesthetics have the advantage of being expired rapidly by the lungs and are not dependent on metabolism by the liver.

A lubricated teflon coated guide wire is passed down the gastric aspiration channel to aid the insertion of the tube. The tube is then well lubricated with jelly and passed through the mouth into the posterior pharynx. Most patients swallow the tube fairly easily. The tube is advanced until it is certain that the gastric balloon is in the stomach. Suction is applied to both aspiration channels to empty the oesophagus and stomach. The gastric balloon is filled with air to the previously determined volume. The tube is then withdrawn gently until the gastric balloon is felt to impact at the cardio-oesophageal junction. The pressure in the balloon is recorded and should be about 20 mm Hg greater than when recorded previously. The tube is taped to the patient's forehead with a wide band of elastoplast to ensure that there is sufficient traction on the tube to keep it gently impacted at the cardio-oesophageal junction. The reading in centimetres on the tube at the level of the patient's incisor teeth is noted. When used in this way the gastric balloon alone may control the haemorrhage and it is better not to inflate the oesophageal balloon unnecessarily. However, if fresh blood continues to be aspirated from the oesophageal aspiration channel then the oesophageal balloon should be inflated with the previously determined volume of air and the pressure checked. This pressure should be approximately 20 mm Hg more than that recorded previously and not greater than 30 mm Hg more.

The patient with a Sengstaken–Blakemore tube in place needs constant and experienced nursing and medical care. The oesophageal aspiration channel is placed on continuous low suction. The gastric aspiration channel is allowed to drain freely and be aspirated hourly. The volume of aspirated fluid, the pressures in the balloons, the addition of air to the balloons and the general monitoring of the patient must be recorded carefully. The balloons should only be inflated for the shortest time possible.

It is our practice to control the bleeding by oesophageal tamponade rather than by using vasopressin, as this method has a much greater success rate in skilled hands. The balloons are left inflated until the patient is stable. Subsequently, the varices are injected with ethanolamine oleate using either a rigid or flexible fibre-optic oesophagoscope. If there is any further sign of bleeding immediately after injection, it is worth re-inserting the Sengstaken–Blakemore tube for a few hours to recompress the varices. The balloons should not be inflated for more than twenty-four hours in total.

Other measures

In a few patients bleeding is not controlled by injection sclerotherapy. Transhepatic obliteration of varices with injection of gelatine foam and thrombin through a catheter has been advocated. This procedure is technically difficult and is not used in many centres. Normally, surgery is employed when scleropathy has failed. The operations favoured at the moment are oesophageal transection with a stapling gun and devascularization of the proximal stomach. Portasystemic shunts are now less often performed in the United Kingdom in patients with cirrhosis due to the high incidence of post-operative hepatic encephalopathy.

The use of propranolol has been advocated recently for the prevention of recurrent bleeding in patients with cirrhosis (Lebrec *et al.* 1981). However, other workers are questioning the value of beta-blocking agents in this condition (Walt *et al.* 1982). Indeed, these drugs may be harmful, because if a patient is receiving an adequate dose, he may not be able to mount a normal physiological response to a recurrent haemorrhage. Therefore, the current data suggests that these drugs should not be widely used in the prevention of recurrent variceal haemorrhage.

Conclusions

Much has still to be learned about the causes of the lesions resulting in upper gastro-intestinal haemorrhage. Moreover, although our techniques of diagnosis and management have become considerably more sophisticated, the overall mortality rate has not changed. There are many reasons for this lack of improvement and in many instances it is uncertain which type of management is best. Nevertheless, in each hospital admitting patients with upper gastro-intestinal haemorrhage, a well thought out policy of management should be followed with close cooperation with physicians and surgeons.

Further reading

Allen R.N. and Dykes P.W. (1976) A study of the factors influencing mortality rates in gastro-intestinal haemorrhage *Quarterly Journal of Medicine* **45**, 533–550.

Athanasoulis C.A., Baum S., Waltman A.C., Ring E.J., Imkembo A. and Salm T.J.V. (1974) Control of acute gastric mucosal haemorrhage. *New England Journal of Medicine* **290**, 597–603.

Avery Jones F. (1956) Haematemesis and melaena with special reference to causation and to the factors influencing the mortality from bleeding peptic ulcers. *Gastroenterology* **30**, 166–190.

Basso N., Bagarani M., Materia A., Leonardi P., Fiorani S., Bianchi E. and Sperazana V. (1979) Cimetidine and antacid prophylaxis of acute gastroduodenal mucosal lesions in high risk patients. *Gastroenterology* **76**, 1095.

Biggs J.C., Hugh T.B. and Dodds A.J. (1976) Tranexamic acid and upper gastro-intestinal haemorrhage—a double blind trial. *Gut* **17**, 729–734.

Conn H.O. and Blitzer B.L. (1974) Non-association of adreno-corticosteroid therapy and peptic ulcer. *New England Journal of Medicine* **294**, 473–479.

Cotton P.B. and Russel R.C. (1977) Disease of the alimentary system. Haematemesis and melaena. *British Medical Journal* **1**, 37–39.

Dawson J. and Cockel R. (1952) Ranitidine in acute upper gastro-intestinal haemorrhage. *British Medical Journal* **285**, 476–477.

Dronfield M.W. and Langman M.J.S. (1978) Acute upper gastro-intestinal bleeding. *British Journal of Hospital Medicine* **19**, 97–108.

Dykes P.W. and Keighley M.R.B. (1981) *Gastro-intestinal haemorrhage.* Bristol, Wright PSG.

Freeman J.G., Cobden I., Lishman A.H. and Record C.O. (1982) Controlled trial of terlipression ('Glypressin') versus vasopressin in the early treatment of oesophageal varices. *Lancet* **2**, 66–68.

Holcroft J.W. and Trunkey D.D. (1975) Pulmonary extravasation of albumin during and after haemorrhage shock in baboons. *Journal of Surgical Research* **18**, 91–97.

Hunt P.S., Hansky J. and Korman M.G. (1979) Mortality in patients with haematemesis and melaena; a prospective study. *British Medical Journal* **1**, 1238–1240.

Johnson W.C., Wildrich W.C., Ansell J.E., Robbins A.L. and Nabseth D.C. (1977) Control of bleeding varices by vasopressin. A prospective randomised study. *Annals of Surgery* **186**, 369–376.

Kayassen L., Keller U., Gyr K. and Stalder G.A. (1980) Somatostatin and cimetidine in peptic ulcer haemorrhage—a randomised controlled trial. *Lancet* **1**, 844–846.

Laurence B.H., Vallon A.G., Cotton P.B., Miro J.R.A., Oses J.C.S., Le Bodia L., Sudry P., Fruhmorgen P. and Boden F. (1980) Endoscopic laser photocoagulation for bleeding peptic ulcers. *Lancet* **1**, 124–125.

Lebrec D., Poynard T., Hillon P. and Behamou J.P. (1981) Propranolol for prevention of recurrent gastro-intestinal bleeding in patients with cirrhosis. A controlled study. *New England Journal of Medicine* **305**, 1371–1374.

Levy M. (1974) Aspirin use in patients with major gastro-intestinal bleeding and peptic ulcer disease. *New England Journal of Medicine* **290**, 1158–1162.

MacDougall B.R.D., Bailey R.J. and Williams R. (1977) H_2 receptor antagonists and antacids in the prevention of acute gastro-intestinal haemorrhage in fulminant hepatic failure. *Lancet* **1**, 617–618.

Mayberry J.F., Cousell B.R., Penny W.J. and Rhodes J. (1981) Mortality in acute gastro-intestinal haemorrhage, a six year survey from the University Hospital of Wales. *Postgraduate Medical Journal* **57**, 627–632.

Mitchell K., Theodossi A. and Williams R. (1982) Endoscopy on patients with portal hypertension and upper gastro-intestinal bleeding. In: *Variceal Bleeding.* eds. Westaby D., MacDougall B.R.D. and Williams P. Pp. 62–65. London, Pitman.

Nolan D.J. (1979) Rapid duodenal and jejunal intubation. *Clinical Radiology* **30**, 183–185.

Northfield T.C. and Smith T. (1970) Central venous pressure in the clinical management of acute gastro-intestinal bleeding. *Lancet* **2**, 584–586.

Pickard R.G., Sanderson I., South M., Kirkham J.S. and Northfield T.C. (1979) Controlled trial of Cimetidine in acute upper gastro-intestinal bleeding. *British Medical Journal* **1**, 661–662.

Salter R.H. (1968) Aspirin and gastro-intestinal bleeding. *American Journal of Digestive Diseases* **13**, 38–58.

Schiller K.F.R., Truelove S.C. and Gwyn Williams D. (1970) Haematemesis and melaena with special reference to factors influencing outcome. *British Medical Journal* **2**, 7–14.

Stevenson G.W., Cox P.R. and Roberts C.J.C. (1976) Prospective comparison of double contrast barium meal examination and fibreoptic endoscopy in acute upper gastro-intestinal haemorrhage. *British Medical Journal* **2**, 723–724.

Teres J., Cecilia A., Bordas J.M., Rimola M.B., Bru C. and Rodes J. (1978) Oesophageal tamponade for bleeding varices. *Gastroenterology* **75**, 566–569.

Thomas G.E., Cotton P.B., Clark C.G. and Boulus P.B. (1980) Survey of management in acute upper gastro-intestinal haemorrhage. *Journal of the Royal Society of Medicine* **73**, 90–95.

Tudhope G.R. (1958) The loss and replacement of red cells in patients with acute gastro-intestinal bleeding. *Quarterly Journal of Medicine* **27**, 543–560.

Virgillio R.W., Rice C.L., Smith D.E., James D.R., Zanns C.K., Hobelman C.F. and Peters R.M. (1979) Crystalloid versus colloid. *Surgery* **85**, 129–139.

Walt R.R., Burroughs A.K., Dubk A.A., Jenkins W.J. and Sherlock S. (1982) Propranolol for prevention of recurrent variceal bleeding in cirrhotic patients. *Gut* **23**, A908.

24 · Acute Diarrhoea

H. A. SHEPHERD

The hospital medical team will encounter acute diarrhoeal disease from community referrals of undiagnosed diarrhoea and less commonly by the referral of hospital in-patients who develop symptoms during admission. The potential range of aetiology is large and the definition of acute diarrhoea in itself influences the choice of pathology for discussion. Therefore, this chapter will concentrate upon the more common conditions that can present with the sudden onset of a diarrhoeal illness which has either developed during a stay in hospital or is of sufficient severity to have necessitated emergency admission to hospital from the community.

The major aetiological division lies between the infectious and non-infectious causes.

Infectious diarrhoea

Pathogenic mechanisms

Bacterial pathogenicity is mediated by three main mechanisms which may overlap within some species; toxin production without cell damage, (for example, *Vibrio cholerae*, *Shigellae* and *E. coli*), mucosal adherence and invasion, (for example, *Shigellae* and *Salmonella*) and cytotoxicity without invasion, (for example, *Clostridium* species and *Shigellae*). Those organisms which have the capacity to invade tissues are usually responsible for the production of copious amounts of pus, blood and mucus in the stool.

The colon may be attacked directly with impairment of water resorption and resultant diarrhoea, or it may be functionally over-loaded by hyper-secretory ileal disease.

The studies of cholera toxin have highlighted at least one biochemical mechanism for diarrhoea (Schafer *et al.* 1976). This mechanism is probably shared by other toxogenic bacteria. Activation of adenyl cyclase by cholera toxin leads to an increase in intracellular cyclic AMP. This toxic action is receptor mediated at the cell surface. However, the action of toxin from other organisms e.g. *Shigellae,* may involve local prostaglandin production rather than receptor binding (Flores *et al.* 1974). Cyclic AMP is known to inhibit the coupled influx of sodium and chloride into enterocytes and will cause active, sodium-dependent, chloride and bicarbonate secretion by crypt cells (Field 1976).

The clinical situation with cholera toxin is most profound because the combination of toxin with enterocyte surface receptor which requires only seconds of exposure, is permanent. Therefore, its toxic action probably only terminates when the cell is shed. However, not all transport mechanisms are affected and the coupling of glucose and sodium transport is one mechanism that can be recruited to overcome the effects of the toxin (Pierce *et al.* 1969).

The presence of normal gut flora is important in preventing colonization of the bowel by pathogenic bacteria, and treatment that influences these organisms is important (Meynell and Gubbaiah 1963).

Important infections seen in hospital practice (Table 24.1)

Shigellosis

The four *Shigellae* species listed in Table 24.1 cause disease in man. These non-motile Gram-negative bacilli are highly host adapted. The ingestion of small inocula (10 to 100 bacteria) are sufficient to cause disease. After an incubation period of between two and four days, symptoms of general malaise, anorexia, vomiting and headache, are often followed by bloody diarrhoea which may last up to two weeks. High fever with delirium and adominal tenderness are common. In the young and elderly the disease may be more severe with complicating dehydration, secondary renal failure and secondary pneumonia. However, *Shigella* bacteraemia is rare.

The organisms are found in the colonic lumen and invading the colonic wall. Toxin production may also have effects on modulating secretion of the ileum (Keusch *et al.* 1972). The organism may be recovered from the stool for up to four weeks following symptomatic recovery.

Salmonellosis

Salmonella is a large genus comprised of over 1000 Gram-negative species, which are characterized by their growth characteristics and antigenic structure. Smith (1972) categorized the *Salmonella* into three main groups according to clinical criteria; Group I: *Salmonella typhi* and *Salmonella paratyphi* A, B and C; Group II: includes *Salmonella typhimurium* and *Salmonella enteritidis* and Group III: the remainder. Group II and III organisms are those primarily responsible for causing gastro-enteritis and will be discussed.

Salmonella infections are common and, in the UK between 1969 and 1976, accounted for 88 per cent of the outbreaks of food poisoning (Turnbull 1979). Now, *Campylobacter* infections are equally common (Drake *et al.* 1981).

The infection is spread from animal reservoirs or human carriers via the

Table 24.1. The more common infections causing acute diarrhoeal illness

Cause	Diagnosis
Campylobacter sp. *fetus* sp. *jejuni*	Culture: stool blood Serology
Clostridium difficile (Pseudomembranous colitis)	Culture: stool Toxin assay: stool
Salmonellae sp. *typhimurium* *enteritis* *choleraesuis*	Culture: stool blood
Shigellae sp. *dysenteriae* *sonnei* *boydii* *flexneri*	Culture: stool blood (rarely isolated)
Yersinia sp. *enterocolitica* *pseudotuberculosis*	Culture: stool (difficult) blood Serology
Treponema sp. *syphillis*	Stool culture Tissue microscopy
Amoebae sp. *histolitica*	Stool microscopy Rectal biopsy
Giardiasis sp. *lamblia*	Stool microscopy Jejunal juice Jejunal biopsy Serology

Other organisms

Consider (especially in compromised host) Other *Clostridia*—e.g. perfringens *Staphylococci* sp. *aureus* Fungi, e.g. candida	Culture: stool faeces
Viruses, Herpes simplex Cytomegalovirus	Electron microscopy of faeces

faeco-oral route. Salmonella typhimurium is the most common isolate. The clinical syndrome follows ingestion of a minimal estimate of 10^7 organisms. The incubation period is between six and forty-eight hours. The general symptoms are usually followed by severe watery diarrhoea which will last between one and seven days. Patients with hypochlorhydria or previous gastric surgery are particularly at risk.

Septicaemia is not uncommon producing more profound clinical features. Occasionally, there are complicating metastatic *Salmonella* tissue infiltrates responsible for meningitis, osteomyelitis and endocarditis. However, these problems are more typical of the Group I organisms. *Salmonellae* primarily invade the ileum. Nevertheless, colonic salmonellosis is becoming increasingly recognized with clinical features resembling acute ulcerative colitis.

Campylobacter infection

The species *Campylobacter fetus* (sub-species *jejuni*) are Gram-negative, curved and motile bacilli which are now an important cause of infectious diarrhoea. Skirrow (1977) isolated these organisms from 7 per cent of adults and children with diarrhoea, but laboratories now report its more frequent isolation (up to 50 per cent in Oxford 1980). In the UK there is a trend for a higher incidence in the summer months. Infection spreads between people (especially children) or is obtained from animals (poultry) and contaminated food and water. The peak incidence of infection seems to be in early adult life (Grant *et al.* 1981).

The organism infects both the large and small bowel (Evans and Dadswell 1967). In 1979, colonic pathology resembling ulcerative colitis was reported for the first time (Lambert *et al.* 1979). The exact pathogenic mechanisms are unclear but toxin production and tissue invasion by the bacteria are probably involved (Butzler and Skirrow 1979). Although septicaemia occurs, organisms so far have not been demonstrated within either human ileal or colonic tissue (Longfield *et al.* 1979).

The typical incubation period is between three to five days, and diarrhoea is preceded for about two days by a 'flu-like' prodromal period. Fever to 40°C is common and may be associated with delirium. Abdominal pain increases as the diarrhoea begins. The diarrhoea is profuse, often blood-stained, watery and foul-smelling. Recovery begins after a further two days, organisms being excreted for up to five weeks in severe cases.

Pseudomembranous colitis

Infection with *Clostridium difficile*, a toxin-producing Gram-positive obligate anaerobe, produces a spectrum of clinical syndromes which are often but not invariably associated with administration of the broader-spectrum antibiotics (Lishmann *et al.* 1981). During active disease either the bacterium, or the toxin or both, are found in faeces and usually disappear upon recovery. The toxin consists of at least two components, a cytotoxin (molecular weight 240,000) which is toxic to cells in tissue culture and is the basis of the detection assay and also an enterotoxin which lacks cytotoxicity in tissue culture but which is damaging to mucosal cells *in vivo* (Taylor *et al.* 1980).

Short-lived attacks of antibiotic associated diarrhoea may not be associated with enterocolitis, and a much lower yield of positive isolates are made. Recent studies suggest that a third toxin may be present, which exerts an effect on gastro-intestinal motility and which may be present even when cytotoxin and enterotoxin levels are low (Justus *et al.* 1982). Furthermore, a carrier state may exist where the organism but no toxin can be isolated from asymptomatic adults (Viscidi *et al.* 1981).

Clostridium difficile is not a component of the normal human gut flora and it is likely that direct infection of the gut (rather than overgrowth) occurs as a result of antibiotics altering the normal protective flora of bacteria. This would explain why some attacks of colitis often follow the course of anti-biotics by several weeks and that *Clostridium difficile,* when isolated, is indeed sensitive to the antibiotic that was used originally (Bartlett *et al.* 1980).

Clinically, the watery diarrhoea (present in 90 per cent of patients) which is occasionally blood-stained, is preceded by cramping abdominal pains, low-grade fever and abdominal tenderness. Sigmoidoscopically, the charac-teristic raised yellow-white necrotic plaques can often be seen. Histo-logically, these plaques are found to consist of fibrin, polymorphs and slough covering the mucosa. Non-pseudomembranous forms exist. However, in these cases the pseudomembranes may be located more proximally in the colon and are missed at sigmoidoscopy (Tedesco 1979).

It has been observed that most patients improve quickly following the cessation of antibiotics. However, those who develop delayed symptoms in relation to the administration of antibiotics often become ill (Tedesco 1982).

Diarrhoea and the penicillin derivatives

There is no doubt that some patients develop a colitis in relation to the administration of penicillin and its derivatives but in whom *Clostridium difficile* or its toxin cannot be demonstrated (Toffler *et al.* 1978). The colitis causing a bloody diarrhoea characteristically affects the proximal colon, causing spasm, mucosal nodularity and punctate ulceration. This can be demonstrated by barium enema examination (Rimmer *et al.* 1982). It may be an allergic phenomenon which is probably a separate condition to pseudomembranous colitis (Toffler *et al.* 1978).

Yersinia enterocolitis

The *Yersinia* genus is a Gram-negative, rod-shaped class of bacteria. The species *Yersinia pestis, Yersinia pseudotuberculosis* and *Yersinia enterocolitica* are pathogenic for man. *Yersinia enterocolitica* is an uncommon cause of enterocolitis in adults. Infection is often associated with extra intestinal complications such as arthritis (including sacroileitis), erythema nodosum, and uveitis (Vantrappen *et al.* 1982). Infection probably originates from animal reservoirs (e.g. pigs), milk and infected water. Pathogenicity is attributable to: invasion of organisms, an enterotoxin causing a secretory diarrhoea and cytotoxin (Pai and Mors 1978; Maki *et al.* 1978).

Following an incubation period of between four and ten days, diarrhoea, fever and abdominal pain (often in the right iliac fossa) develop. General systemic symptoms are usually present when extra intestinal complications are found, which develop with the febrile disease. The course of the illness is variable and diarrhoea (bowels open up to ten times daily) may last up to twelve weeks and the syndrome can closely resemble inflammatory bowel disease clinically and radiologically. Perforation with peritonitis can occur.

Pathologically there is mesenteric adenitis with acute inflammation in the ileum (and appendix) and colon. Acute inflammatory cells with lymphoid aggregates are present in the mucosa and lamina propria, with superficial mucosal ulceration. The inflammation may be contiguous like that seen in ulcerative colitis, or resemble the 'skip' lesions of Crohn's disease.

The 'gay bowel'

Many of the organisms acquired by homosexual activities cause only local symptoms, e.g. proctitis due to gonorrhoea or *chlamydia*. However, *Campylobacter, Shigellae,* amoebae, *Giardia* and syphilis are also transmissible and can cause a diarrhoeal illness. Anorectal syphilis can present insidiously or with acute bloody diarrhoea, and should always be considered in cases of homosexual contact.

A severe watery diarrhoea may result from infection by the protozoan *Cryptosporidia.* This condition has been diagnosed by jejunal biopsy, the histology of which can demonstrate the organism and the associated mucosal damage. The colon can also be affected. Presence of this protozoan should prompt an assessment of the immune status of the patient in order to exclude Acquired Immune Deficiency Syndrome (AIDS) (Smith 1963; Artnak and Cerda 1984a,b).

Giardiasis

Ingestion of the cysts of *Giardia lamblia* from infected sources (particularly water) results in their maturation into trophozoites within the small bowel.

This infestation should be considered in patients returning from trips abroad, but infection can also occur within the United Kingdom. Hypochlorhydria and hypogammaglobulinaemia (particularly IgA deficiency) are thought to be important factors predisposing to infection by *Giardia*.

Symptoms usually take a few weeks to develop and patients often present with the sudden onset of explosive watery diarrhoea with systemic upset. The acute phase may subside within a few days or can develop with a chronic infection where symptoms are persistent but less severe (Wolfe 1978).

Amoebic colitis

Ingestion of the enterocysts of *Entamoeba histolytica* during travel within endemic areas promotes their maturation into trophozoites within the gut lumen and subsequent colonization of the colon. Further maturation of trophozoites to the adult amoebae in the colon is associated with the undermining invasion of the colonic mucosa producing the characteristic collar-stud ulcer appearance, associated with an intense acute inflammatory reaction (Krogstad *et al.* 1978).

The immunologically compromised patient

Immunodeficient patients, particularly those who are receiving chemotherapy for malignant disease, or those immunosuppressed following organ transplantation, are a special group of patients. They are not only susceptible to infection by common organisms, but may develop infections caused by the more obscure and less virulent organisms. Fungi (e.g. *Candida, Aspergillus* and *Cryptococcus*) and viruses (e.g. herpes simplex and cytomegalovirus), must be considered and can present with acute symptoms. A rare idiopathic necrotizing enterocolitis has also been reported in such patients (Perloff *et al.* 1976).

Non-infectious conditions (Table 24.2)

Acute inflammatory bowel disease

Crohn's colitis and ulcerative colitis can present as acute bloody diarrhoea and may progress rapidly to fulminant colitis with severe systemic symptoms.

The inflammatory process of ulcerative colitis involves the rectum and extends proximally. In the acute stages there is macroscopic mucosal swelling and hyperaemia, often with ulceration with blood and pus. Microscopically, the cellular infiltrate is largely limited to the mucosa, and there are crypt abscesses and glandular destruction with ulceration. Islands of

294 CHAPTER 24

Table 24.2. Non-infectious causes of acute diarrhoea

Cause	Diagnosis
Inflammatory bowel disease	Characteristic points: (i) Pyoderma gangrenosum (ii) Perianal disease (iii) Mouth ulcers Rectal biopsy Radiology
Ischaemic bowel disease	Radiology Common in the elderly patient
Faecal impaction	Radiology
(Compromised host) Idiopathic necrotizing enterocolitis	To be considered in the (i) Leukaemic (ii) Immunosuppressed
Other causes Drugs, e.g. Colchicine laxative abuse	History Melanosis coli on rectal biopsy (laxatives)

Tumours
(i) Large bowel neoplasia
(ii) Hormone secreting tumours, e.g.
    Vasoactive intestinal polypeptide
    (Verner–Morrison syndrome)
    Carcinoid syndrome
	Sigmoidoscopy, barium enema
	Hypochlorhydria
	Hypokalaemia
	Hypercalcaemia
	Elevated urinary 5 HIAA

surviving normal tissue surrounded by ulcerated sloughing mucosa are responsible for the characteristic 'pseudopolyp' appearance.

Crohn's disease differs in that the rectum may be macroscopically spared, with only patchy ulceration and inflammation seen more proximally. The perianal region is often involved. This is characterized by dusky red discoloration and fleshy skin tags in association with fissures and fistulae.

The terminal ileum is involved in about 85 per cent of patients, with variable amounts of colonic inflammation. Microscopy of the mucosa reveals the characteristic chronic inflammatory cell infiltrate involving all bowel wall layers in a patchy pattern. The presence of submucosal non-caseating histiocytic epithelioid granulomas in association with fissuring ulceration is characteristic of Crohn's colitis. However, there is often good preservation of mucosal glandular elements. There may be a superimposed acute inflammatory infiltrate.

Circulating immune complexes, in both diseases, may be responsible for some of the extra intestinal manifestations of ulcerative colitis and Crohn's disease (e.g. erythema nodosum, aphthous mouth ulceration, acute arthritis, uveitis and pyoderma gangrenosum), which usually remit as the bowel improves.

In the severely ill patients, toxic dilatation of the colon may develop (2–10 per cent of patients). The degree of colonic dilatation may fluctuate and can be segmental but represents an emergency situation. It is thought that transmural inflammation occurs with deep ulceration that paralyses the smooth muscle and leads to colonic dilatation (Fazio 1980). Hypokalaemia and hypo-albuminaemia may be aggravating factors.

Ischaemic disease of the colon

The gut demands at least 20 per cent of the cardiac output. Although within the mesenteric network of vessels there is a good collateral arcading supply, there is less overlap of the vascular supply at the distal transverse colon, the splenic flexure and in the recto-sigmoid colon (Marston *et al.* 1966). Ischaemic conditions localize to these areas.

Up to 50 per cent of mesenteric infarctions occur in patients with patent mesenteric vessels. This may reflect the presence of local shunting mechanisms resultant on small vessel disease (Edwards 1972). Large vessels may be stenosed or blocked by atheroma, thrombosis and emboli (e.g. from atrial fibrillation). The smaller vessels may be involved with arteritis. Interruption of the inferior mesenteric supply (arterial or venous) can present acutely with abdominal pain and bloody diarrhoea. This condition must always be considered in elderly patients presenting with these symptoms. The severity of the symptoms may depend upon the presence of gangrene (Marston 1980).

Faecal impaction

This condition may present with an acute diarrhoeal picture in the elderly and infirm.

Management

Clinical management of the patient is directed towards:
(1) Assessment of the patient.
(2) Making a firm diagnosis.
(3) Treatment, which includes general and specific measures. As a general precaution, patients should be barrier-nursed initially, in a side ward, until a contagious infectious diagnosis is excluded or treated. A scheme of management is shown in Fig. 24.1.

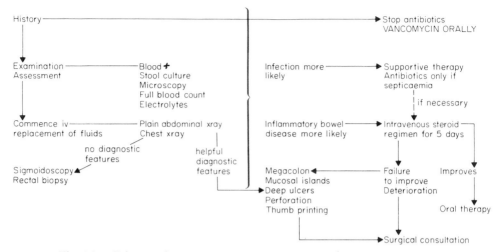

Fig. 24.1. Scheme of management and treatment of acute severe diarrhoea.

Assessment of the patient

Assessment includes the admission examination and regular monitoring thereafter in order to alert the physician to any deterioration.

During treatment, the pulse, blood pressure, temperature, abdominal tenderness and girth should be monitored. In addition, a central venous line should be inserted and central venous pressure monitored in shocked or toxic patients. Serum electrolytes should also be checked regularly. Stool charts are useful in order to record the frequency of diarrhoea and it is wise to record urine output. Routine urinary catheterization should be avoided in order to minimize the risk of introducing urinary infection.

It is essential to identify the toxic patient. If septicaemia is suspected it should be treated promptly (see below). The severity of a colitic attack may be judged in terms of stool frequency, temperature over 38°C, pulse in excess of 120/minute, leucocytosis greater than 10.5×10^9/litre, hypo-albuminaemia less than 3.0 g/dl, (NR 4–6 g/dl) and anaemia below 10.5 g/litre (Jalin *et al.* 1969). These parameters are for guidance and should not be regarded as rigid values; the documentation of change is also important. A rising pulse, abdominal distension and the loss of bowel sounds may herald the development of a toxic megacolon. Colonic dilatation and mucosal islands visible on an X-ray are bad diagnostic signs. Occasionally, linear strips of gas can be seen parallel to the colonic wall on plain abdominal X-ray. These represent extensive ulceration.

Diagnostic points and investigations

Not only is there symptomatic overlap between the conditions described but the superficial pathological picture can be such that no firm diagnosis can be made on clinical criteria alone. The sick patient with infective enterocolitis may have peripheral and local signs, including sigmoidoscopic appearances, indistinguishable from those found in severe acute inflammatory bowel disease. *Shigella, Salmonella, Yersinia, Clostridium difficile* and amoebic colitis often produce a contiguous colitic inflammation which involves the rectum and looks like ulcerative colitis. In addition, ulcerative skip lesions can be seen, with *Salmonella* and *Yersinia*, which resemble Crohn's colitis.

Toxic megacolon may develop in all of these conditions (Tedesco and Moore 1982; Fazio 1980). Clinical examination may be helpful. Inflammatory bowel disease may be diagnosed in the presence of those lesions particularly characteristic of inflammatory bowel disease, such as the perianal lesions of Crohn's disease, pyoderma gangrenosum and aphthoid mouth ulceration. The ultimate diagnosis may depend upon laboratory investigations alone although the most important guidelines are obtained from the history. Historically, a trip abroad, recent antibiotic administration, the ingestion of suspect food and identical features in close contacts strongly implicate infection. However, a past history of minor episodes of self-limiting bloody diarrhoea associated with aphthoid mouth ulceration favour inflammatory bowel disease. In the elderly, ischaemic episodes must be suspected, especially if atrial fibrillation or mitral valve disease are present, or if there is extensive peripheral atherosclerosis.

The discovery of impacted stool at rectal examination makes an overflow diarrhoea most likely. However, at an appropriate time, as with all cases of diarrhoea, sigmoidoscopy should be performed to exclude an underlying pathology. Sigmoidoscopy facilitates the collection of fresh stool and provides an opportunity for rectal biopsy to be taken. Blood-stained stool always implies that colitis is present. The plaque lesions of pseudomembranous colitis may be seen. Alternatively, obvious rectal sparing in the presence of severe bloody diarrhoea makes Crohn's disease more likely. Even in cases of known established inflammatory bowel disease, the possibility of superimposed infection, rather than relapse alone, must never be forgotten.

Investigations

Fresh stool should be examined microscopically in order to search for red cells, pus cells, parasites (or their cysts) and also cultured for all possible pathogens.

Bloods

Serum electrolytes and full blood count are of value in the assessment of the patient. The blood urea and packed red cell volume give an indication of the degree of dehydration. Serum potassium, sodium and albumin may also be low and require correction. However, the additional presence of an established iron deficiency anaemia favours inflammatory bowel disease.

As a guide, Caprilli *et al.* (1982) suggest that the presence of acidosis may have resulted from active fluid secretion particularly in infections, whereas alkalosis is more commonly found as a consequence of impaired water and electrolyte absorption. Therefore alkalosis is commonly due to colonic disease and found in association with bloody diarrhoea. Blood cultures should be taken routinely and blood also sent for *Yersinia* and *Campylobacter* serology. A mid-stream urine should be cultured.

Radiology

The plain abdominal radiograph is essential. It is valuable in the diagnosis and assessment of the patient. It should be performed before sigmoidoscopy to allow reliable interpretation of the bowel gas pattern. The mucosal pattern, if distorted, will aid the delineation of the extent of inflamed bowel. The distribution of faeces should be noted. Colon containing stool is unlikely to be involved in an inflammatory process and will therefore also indicate the extent of the disease (Bartram 1976). Faecal impaction may become immediately obvious. The characteristic mucosal thumbprinting of ischaemic colitis or evidence of the deep mucosal ulceration with mucosal islands seen in inflammatory bowel disease may be identifiable and aid diagnosis. The colonic mucosa in pseudomembranous colitis often has an oedematous shaggy appearance.

The diameter of the colon must be assessed and serially reassessed in order to detect the development of toxic megacolon. Megacolon is generally considered present if the colonic diameter exceeds 5 cm (Hywell Jones and Chapman 1969). Free gas, indicating a perforation which often can be silent in the very ill, should be further excluded by including a chest X-ray in the investigations.

The indications, if any, remain controversial for the use of an instant barium enema in those patients in whom inflammatory bowel disease is strongly suspected. This examination will demonstrate the full extent of the colitis and provide some help in the later management of the patient. However, some authors take the view that this investigation is dangerous and unnecessary and may even provoke toxic dilatation (Roth *et al.* 1975). There is no place for barium enema when colonic dilatation is present.

Treatment

General measures

Fluid and electrolytes should be replaced and anaemia corrected simultaneously. Normally, packed red blood cells should be used but whole blood must be used in the severely hypovolaemic patient.

When suspected, septicaemia must be promptly treated with intravenous antibiotics. The potentially nephrotoxic drugs should be avoided if there is a suspicion of renal failure. Ampicillin or cotrimoxazole and metronidazole can be used initially. These may be changed at a later stage when blood culture results are available.

In the toxic patient, it is wise to allow only clear fluids by mouth and to commence parenteral nutrition. This can be achieved by a peripheral line. Three thousand calories and fifteen grams of nitrogen can often be replaced every twenty-four hours without thrombophlebitis developing. The decision to continue parenteral feeding can always be reviewed depending upon the response of the patient to the first line treatment measures. However, any specific benefit from parenteral nutrition and bowel rest, has not been proven by controlled clinical trials in the case of inflammatory bowel disease (Driscoll and Rosenberg 1978).

Specific treatment

Inflammatory bowel disease

Consultation with surgical colleagues is desirable at an early stage if any adverse prognostic features are present. An intensive intravenous regimen for ulcerative colitis was first proposed by Truelove and Jewell (1974). This regimen is still used, although tetracycline has been replaced by metronidazole (Jewell 1982). The Oxford regimen consists of parenteral nutrition, intravenous prednisolone-21-phosphate (64 mg/24 hours), hydrocortisone rectal drip twice daily (100 mg in 100 ml of normal saline) and intravenous metronidazole 500 mg twice daily. The addition of an antibiotic to the steroid regimen is empirical and is not supported by controlled clinical trials. This therapy is continued for five days with an improvement being expected in about 70 per cent of patients with ulcerative colitis. Over 70 per cent of these patients will remain in remission and require only oral therapy.

Promptly treated, first attacks enjoy longer remission than cases where delayed treatment has been experienced (Truelove and Jewell 1974). If there is deterioration during treatment, or failure to improve after five days, then surgery probably will be necessary. In any case, these patients are more likely to have extensive colitis. Following improvement on the intravenous regimen, oral therapy with normal diet can be substituted, using prednisolone 40 mg daily and sulphasalazine 1 gram three times daily.

If there is doubt about the cause of the diarrhoea but the clinical features make inflammatory bowel disease the most likely diagnosis, it is wise to treat such patients with an intravenous steroid regimen. Our experience in Oxford has shown that no adverse effects result from the administration of steroids to cases of infective enterocolitis, or infective enterocolitis superimposed on pre-existing inflammatory bowel disease (which are often both retrospective diagnoses). Whereas, delay in treating genuine inflammatory bowel disease can have serious consequences.

Pseudomembranous colitis

If possible, any current antibiotic therapy should be discontinued. However, when the clinical situation dictates a recent study has suggested that it is safe to administer concurrent antibiotic therapy in some patients receiving vancomycin for antibiotic-associated colitis (Bolton and Losowsky 1982). Keighley and his colleagues (1978) recommended that vancomycin 500 mg four times a day should be given orally and continued for at least five days. Since that report it has been suggested that a smaller dose of vancomycin is sufficient; 125 mg four times daily is currently recommended (British National Formulary, 1984). This is important as the drug is expensive. Other therapies for this condition include cholestyramine (thought to bind *Clostridium* toxin, bacitracin (25,000 i.u. four times daily) and metroni-dazole (1.2 grams a day) (Kreutzer and Milligan 1978; Chang *et al.* 1980; Bolton 1979, respectively).

Steroids do not possess any major beneficial or harmful effects (Hober-man *et al.* 1976). This has relevance in cases of inflammatory bowel disease with *Clostridium difficile* infection (Keighley *et al.* 1982). The administration of anti-diarrhoeal anti-motility drugs in antibiotic colitis may be harmful (Pitman 1975).

Following vancomycin therapy, antibiotics can be safely used again— but in patients who only clear the toxin and not the organism from their stool, relapse is more likely. In this group, prophylactic vancomycin might be indicated during the administration of other antibiotics (Bolton and Losowsky 1982).

Infections

Isolation of organisms in the stool is not an indication for antibiotic therapy, which should only be used for specific reasons such as the treatment of septicaemia or in the immunologically compromised patient. Despite the severity of the symptoms at presentation, providing septicaemia is not present, gastro-enteritis is a self-limiting condition and only supportive therapy is necessary.

Some antibiotics, for example, neomycin, are of no value in the treat-ment of *Shigella* because they do not increase the clearance rate of the organism (W.H.O. 1980). Moreover, they do not shorten the duration of diarrhoea (Bengtsson *et al.* 1955). However, the absorbable antibiotics such as ampicillin and co-trimoxazole may influence *Shigellae* excretion and cause a more rapid clinical recovery (W.H.O. 1980).

In uncomplicated *Salmonella* gastro-enteritis, chemotherapy prolongs the faecal excretion of the organism. In addition, antibiotic therapy may encourage the development of plasmid mediated multiple drug resistance (Falkow 1975). When antibiotics must be used then ampicillin or co-trimoxazole are the drugs of first choice until sensitivities are available (Chang *et al.* 1977).

The situation with *Campylobacter* enterocolitis appears to be different in that antibiotics can reduce the faecal excretion time of organisms. However, it is still probably unwise to use them routinely in order to prevent development of antibiotic resistance (Butzler and Skirrow 1979). Erythromycin is the drug of first choice because of its narrow spectrum. The aminoglycosides, erythromycin, chloramphenicol and tetracycline are the most active drugs against *Campylobacter*. In the septicaemic patient, who is failing to improve with erythromycin, it is probably wise to substitute gentamicin as some strains of *Campylobacter* have become resistant to erythromycin. Cephalosporins are ineffective.

Giardiasis and amoebic colitis are treated with metronidazole and tinidazole.

The laboratory diagnosis of *Yersinia* infection is made by culture or serology. Isolation of the organism from blood in septicaemic patients is relatively easy. However, its isolation from faeces may take up to a week. The clinical syndrome responds dramatically to antibiotics. The aminoglycosides and tetracyclines are the recommended drugs.

Further investigation

Following improvement in the clinical condition of the patient, a formal double contrast barium enema examination should be performed both in those patients where a non-infectious course is suspected and when there is any doubt about the overall clinical picture, even if pathogens have been isolated. In this way, conditions such as inflammatory bowel disease, ischaemic colitis and occult neoplasia will not be overlooked.

Further reading

Artnak E.J. and Cerda J. (1984a) The gay bowel syndrome. 1. *Curr. Concepts in Gatroenterology* **2** (1), 2–9.

Artnak E.J. and Cerda J. (1984b) The gay bowel syndrome 2. *Curr. Concepts in Gastroenterology* **2** (2), 16–20.

Bartlett J.G., Taylor N.S., Chang T.W. and Dzink J.A. (1980) Clinical and laboratory observations in *Clostridium difficile* colitis. *American Journal of Clinical Nutrition* **33**, 2521–2526.

Bartram C.I. (1976) Plain abdominal X-ray in acute colitis. *Proceedings of the Royal Society of Medicine* **69**, 617–618.

Bengtsson E., Hedlundf P., Nisell A. and Nordenstum H. (1955) An epidemic due to *Salmonella typhimurium* occurring in Sweden in 1953; with special reference to the clinical complications, bacteriology, serology, antibiotic treatment and morbid anatomy. *Acta Medica Scandinavica* 153, 1–20.

Bolton R.P. and Losowsky M.S. (1982) When can antibiotics be used safely in patients with active or recently treated *Clostridium difficile* colitis? *Gut* 23, A891.

Bolton R.P. (1979) *Clostridium difficile* associated colitis after neomycin treated with metronidazole. *British Medical Journal* 2, 1479–1480.

Joint Formulary Committee (1984). *Vancomycin*. British National Formulary 8, 206. British Medical Association and Pharmaceutical Society of Great Britain, London.

Butzler J.P. and Skirrow M.B. (1979) Campylobacter enteritis. *Clinics in Gastroenterology*, 737–765. W.B. Saunders Company, London.

Caprilli R., Vernia P., Brancaleone C. and Santoro M.L. (1982) Arterial pH and stool blood as pathogenic markers for diarrhoea. *Gastroenterology* 82, 1029A.

Chang M., Dinkle L.M., Van Reken D., Anderson D., Wong M.L. and Feigin R.D. (1977) Trimethoprin-suphamethoxazole compared to ampicillin in the treatment of *Shigella. Paediatrics* 59, 726–729.

Chang T.W., Gorbach S.L., Bartlett J.G. and Sagimar R. (1980) Bacitracin treatment of antibiotic associated colitis and diarrhoea caused by *Clostridium difficile* toxin. *Gastroenterology* 78, 1584–1586.

Drake A., Gilchrist M., Washington J., Huizenga K. and Van Scoy R.E. (1981) Diarrhoea due to *Campylobacter fetus* sub-species jejeni. *Proceedings of the Mayo Clinic* 56, 414–423.

Driscoll R.H. and Rosenberg I.H. (1978) Total parenteral nutrition in inflammatory bowel disease. *Medical Clinics of North America* 62, 185–210. W.B. Saunders Co. Ltd., Philadelphia.

Edwards A. (1972) Ischaemia of the gut. *Medicine* 3, 233–237.

Evans R.G. and Dadswell J.V. (1967) Human vibriosis. *British Medical Journal* 3, 240.

Falkow S. (1975) *Infectious Multiple Drug Resistance.* Pion, London.

Fazio V.W. (1980) Toxic megacolon in ulcerative colitis and Crohns colitis. *Clinics in Gastroenterology*, 389–407.

Field M. (1976) Regulation of active ion transport in the small intestine. In: Acute diarrhoea in childhood. Ciba Foundation Symposium; Amsterdam; *Elsevier Excerpta Medica, North Holland* 42, 109–127.

Flores J., Grady G.F., McIver J., Witkin P., Beckman B. and Sharp G.W.G. (1974) Comparison of the effects of the enterotoxin of *Shigella dysenteriae* and *Vibrio cholerae* on the adenylate cyclase system of the rabbit intestine. *Journal of Infectious Disease* 130, 374–379.

Grant I.H., Richardson N.J. and Bokkenhauser V.D. (1981) Broiler chickens as a potential source of *Campylobacter* infections in humans. *Journal of Clinical Microbiology* 11, 508–510.

Hoberman L.J., Eigenbrodt E.H., Kihman W.J., Hughes L., Norgaard R. and Fordtran J. (1976) Colitis associated with oral clindamycin therapy. A study of sixteen cases. *Digestive Diseases and Science* 21, 1–17.

Hywell-Jones J. and Chapman M. (1969) Definition of megacolon in colitis. *Gut* 10, 562–564.

Jalin K.N., Sircus W., Card W.I., Falconer C.W., Bruce J., Crean G.P., McManus J.P.A., Small V.P. and Smith A.N. (1969) An experience of ulcerative colitis. 1. Toxic dilation in 55 cases. *Gastroenterology* **57**, 68–82.

Jewell D.P. (1982) Diagnosis and treatment of ulcerative colitis. *British Journal of Hospital Medicine* **27**, 456–462.

Justus P.G., Martin J.L., Goldberg D.A., Taylor N.S., Bartlett J.G., Alexander R.W. and Mathias J.R. (1982) Myo-electric effects of *Clostridium difficile:* Motility altering factors distinct from it's cytotoxin and enterotoxin in rabbits. *Gastroenterology* **83**, 836–884.

Keighley M.R., Burdon D., Arabi Y., Alexander-Williams J., Thompson H., Youngs D., Johnson M., Bentley S., George R. and Mogg G. (1978) Randomized controlled trial of vancomycin for pseudomembranous colitis and postoperative diarrhoea. *British Medical Journal* **2**, 1667–1668.

Keighley R.B., Youngs D., Johnson M., Allan R.N. and Burdon D.W. (1982) *Clostridium difficile* toxin in acute diarrhoea complicating inflammatory bowel disease. *Gut* **23**, 410–414.

Keusch G.T., Grady G.F., Mata L.J. and McIver J. (1972) The pathogenesis of *Shigella* diarrhoea. 1. Enterotoxin production by *Shigella dysenteriae*. *Journal of Clinical Investigation* **51**, 1212–1218.

Kreutzer E.W. and Milligan F.D. (1978) Treatment of antibiotic associated pseudomembranous colitis with cholestyramine resin. *John Hopkins Medical Journal* **143**, 67–72.

Krogstad D.J., Spencer H.C. and Healty G.R. (1978) Current concepts: Amoebiasis. *New England Journal of Medicine* **298**, 262–265.

Lambert M.E., Schofield P.F., Ironside A.G. and Mandal B.K. (1979) *Campylobacter* colitis. *British Medical Journal* **1**, 857–859.

Lishman A.H., Al-Jumaih I.J. and Record C.O. (1981) Spectrum of antibiotic associated diarrhoea. *Gut* **22**, 34–37.

Longfield R., O'Donnell J. and Yudt W. (1979) Acute colitis and bacteraemia due to *Campylobacter fetus*. *Digestive Diseases and Science* **24**, 950–953.

Maki M., Groroos P. and Vesikari T. (1978) In vitro invasiveness of *Yersinia enterocolitica* isolated from children with diarrhoea. *Journal of Infectious Diseases* **138**, 677–680.

Marston A., Pheib M.T., Thomas M.L. and Morson B.C. (1966) Ischaemic colitis. *Gut* **7**, 1–15.

Marston A. (1980) Ischaemic diseases of the colon. *Topics in Gastroenterology* **8**. Blackwell Scientific Publications, Oxford.

Meynell G.G. and Gubbaiah T.V. (1963) Antibacterial mechanisms in the mouse gut. 1. Kinetics in normal and streptomycin treated mice studied with abortive transductants. *British Journal of Experimental Pathology* **44**, 197–208.

Pai C.H. and Mors V. (1978) Production of enterotoxin by *Yersinia enterocolitica*. *Infection and Immunity* **19**, 908–915.

Perloff L.J., Chon H., Petrella E., Grossman R. and Barker C. (1976) Acute colitis in the renal allograft recipient. *Annals of Surgery* **183**, 77–83.

Pierce N.F. Sack R.B., Mitra R.C., Banwell J.G., Brigham K.L., Fedson D.S. and Mondal A. (1969) Replacement of water and electrolyte losses in cholera by an oral glucose electrolyte solution. *Annals of Internal Medicine* **70**, 1173–1181.

Pitman F.E. (1975) Lomotil and antibiotic colitis. *Annals of Internal Medicine* **83**, 124–125.

Rimmer M.J., Freeman A.H. and Low F.M. (1982) The barium enema diagnosis of penicillin associated colitis. *Clinical Radiology* **33**, 529–535.

Roth J.L., Stitcher J.E., Stein G.N. and Valdes-Dapena A. (1975) Toxic megacolon complicating ulcerative colitis. *The Systemic Manifestations of Inflammatory Bowel Disease* 133–175. Charles C. Thomas, Lukash W.M. and Johnson R.B. (eds). Springfield.

Schafer D.E., Lust W.D., Sircar B. and Goldberg N.D. (1976) Elevated concentration of adenosone 3', 5'-cyclic monophosphate in intestinal mucosa after treatment with cholera toxin. *Proceedings of the National Academy of Sciences USA* **67**, 671–679.

Skirrow M.B. (1977) *Campylobacter* enteritis—A 'new' disease. *British Medical Journal,* **2**, 9–11.

Smith D. (1963) Infectious syphilis of the anal canal. *Diseases of the colon and rectum* **6**, 7–14.

Smith H. (1972) *Antibiotics in Clinical Practice,* 2nd ed. Pitman Medical, London.

Taylor N.S., Thorne G.M. and Bartlett J.G. (1980) Separation of an enterotoxin from the cytotoxin of *Clostridium difficile. Clinical Research* **28**, 285A.

Tedesco F.J. and Moore S. (1982) Infectious diseases mimiking inflammatory bowel disease. *American Journal of Surgery* **48**, 243–249.

Tedesco F.J. (1979) Antibiotic associated pseudomembranous colitis with negative proctosigmoidoscopy examination. *Gastroenterology* **77**, 295–297.

Tedesco F.J. (1982) Pseudomembranous colitis: Pathogenesis and Therapy. *Medical Clinics of North America,* pp. 655–664. W.B. Saunders Co. Ltd, Philadelphia.

Toffler R.B., Pingould E.G. and Burrell M.I. (1978) Acute colitis related to penicillin derivatives. *Lancet* **2**, 707–709.

Truelove S.C. and Jewell D.P. (1974) Intensive intravenous regimen for severe attacks of ulcerative colitis. *Lancet* **1**, 1067–1070.

Turnball P.C.B. (1979) Food poisoning with special reference to salmonella—it's epidemiology, pathogenesis, and control. *Clinics in Gastroenterology* 663–714. W.B. Saunders Co. Ltd., London.

Vantrappen G., Agg H.O., Geboes K. and Ponette E. (1982) *Yersinia* enteritis. *Medical Clinics of North America* 639–653. W.B. Saunders Co. Ltd., Philadelphia.

Viscidi R., Willey S. and Bartlett J.G. (1981) Isolation rates and toxogenic potential of *Clostridium difficule* from various patient populations. *Gastroenterology* **81**, 5–9.

W.H.O. (1980) *Weekly Epidemiological Record* **55**, 393–400.

Wolfe M.S. (1978) Giardiasis. *New England Journal of Medicine* **298**, 319–320.

25 · Liver Failure and Alcohol Withdrawal Syndrome

JOAN TROWELL

Liver failure

Liver failure may occur as an acute illness in a previously healthy person or as the result of an acute deterioration in a patient with previously well compensated cirrhosis. The prognosis varies considerably with the underlying pathology but the presenting features of the illness and the practical management are similar in many respects. Because the liver is capable of regeneration, prompt appropriate action can reverse the outcome, even in patients with severe liver failure.

There is no effective artificial replacement for a failing liver but the management depends on identifying individual functions which are failing and supplementing these. Therefore, successful treatment depends on careful monitoring of the patient clinically, haematologically and biochemically, with attention to the details of an individual patient's response. Although general guides are possible, the treatment must be constantly reassessed in the knowledge of the patient's progress.

The management will be considered under the following headings:

1. Bleeding.
2. Infection.
3. Ascites.
4. Hypoglycaemia.
5. Encephalopathy.
6. Jaundice.
7. Artificial hepatic support systems.

A summary of the management is given in Table 25.1.

1. Bleeding

This may either be a generalized bleeding tendency resulting from abnormal coagulation, or it may be gastro-intestinal haemorrhage due to portal hypertension and the resulting oesophageal, gastric, and other varices, or it may be due to peptic ulceration. The diagnosis and management of haemorrhage from local lesions in the oesophagus, stomach and duodenum is discussed in Chapter 23.

Liver cell failure is associated with decreased synthesis of clotting factors (Tucker *et al.* 1973). Fibrinogen, factors II, V, VII, IX, X, XI, XII and XIII

Table 25.1. The management of liver failure

Clinical	Investigation	Treatment
Jaundice	Bilirubin	Relieve obstructed bile ducts
	Serum transaminase	If hepatocellular, none required
	Alkaline phosphatase	
	Exclude: bile duct obstruction	
	Ultrasound/cholangiograms	
Bleeding		
Signs of liver disease	Haemoglobin and indices	Vitamin K_1 IV
Bruising	Prothrombin time	Fresh blood transfusion
Petechiae	Clotting factors	Fresh frozen plasma
Meleana/occult bleeding	Platelet count	Clotting factors
Splenomegaly	Fibrin degradation products (blood and urine)	Platelet-rich infusions
Pulse	Endoscopy: oesophagus, stomach, duodenum	See Chapter 23
Blood pressure	Faecal occult blood	
Central nervous pressure peripheral perfusion		
Infection		
Localized site of infection	Blood film	Broad spectrum antibiotics, pending culture results
Lymphadenopathy	Differential white cell count	
Fever	Ascitic fluid: cells organisms	
	Culture: urine	
	blood	
	ascites	
	local sites	
	Cultures for pyogenic organisms including anaerobic	
	Also ZN stains	
	TB cultures	

Peripheral oedema	Diagnostic paracentesis for:	Sodium and water restriction
Skin turgor	cell count and culture (ZN)	Potassium chloride supplements
Lying/standing blood pressure	cytology for malignant cells	Diuretics: spironolactone
Weigh daily	protein/albumin level	frusemide
Measure girth	Blood urea and electrolytes	Consider: salt poor albumin
Record: fluid intake	Serum albumin	ultrafiltration
urine output	Urinary electrolytes	peritoneal—venous
		shunt
		Therapeutic paracentesis rarely
		justified
Hypoglycaemia	Blood glucose levels	Infusion of glucose
		Insulin/potassium as required
Encephalopathy		
Tremor	Exclude: infection	Routine nursing care
Fetor	bleeding	Routine physiotherapy
Impairment of intellect	hypokalaemia	Stop diuretics and sedative drugs
Handwriting	EEG	Purge/enema—magnesium
Constructional apraxia	Lumbar puncture if doubt of	sulphate
Respiration	diagnosis	Neomycin, lactulose
Liver size	Ammonia	Cut dietary protein
	Lactate	Correct hypokalaemia
	Acid/base balance	Treat infection/bleeding
		Consider: artificial liver support
		L-dopa or bromocryptine

are all predominantly synthesized in the liver. Factors II, VII, IX and X are dependent on vitamin K, and prolonged steatorrhoea and vitamin K malabsorption may contribute to the bleeding problems in chronic liver failure. In acute liver damage the factors with the shorter half lives disappear most rapidly from the circulation. Consequently, fibrinogen levels are relatively well preserved initially, although these may also fall with time in patients with severe liver damage (Green *et al.* 1976).

Disseminated intravascular coagulation (DIC) may occur in acute hepatic necrosis. This is characterized by a reduction of clotting factors and platelets and by the presence of fibrinogen degradation products (FDP) in the blood and urine (Rake *et al.* 1970). DIC in chronic liver disease is most often associated with infection, which should be sought and treated appropriately.

The platelet count may be low, especially in patients with cirrhosis and splenomegaly. Some hepatotoxins, such as alcohol, also affect platelet function.

Treatment

Vitamin K_1 is normally given by injection (intravenously if clotting is poor) as 10 mg daily for three to five days. This will have only limited benefit in liver failure and if bleeding is an active problem, fresh blood, fresh frozen plasma and clotting factors, and platelet-rich infusions are required (Mannucci *et al.* 1976; Green *et al.* 1975). DIC in liver failure rarely justifies heparin therapy but the associated sepsis should be treated energetically (Hillenbrand *et al.* 1974; Gazzard *et al.* 1974).

In the absence of active bleeding, the abnormal coagulation associated with liver failure may be treated with parenteral vitamin K. However, no benefit has been shown from prophylactic treatment with clotting factors and platelet infusions (Gazzard *et al.* 1974A), except in patients having surgery or other invasive procedures (Gazzard *et al.* 1975; Mannucci *et al.* 1976).

2. Infection

This is common in patients with liver failure and is often occult, presenting merely as a worsening of liver function, DIC, or the occurrence of ascites or encephalopathy. The primary source of infection should be sought and treated appropriately. In cirrhotics, septicaemia may occur without any obvious cause. Any patient with evidence of liver failure and deterioration should therefore have blood, ascitic fluid, urine and sputum cultures taken.

Treatment

When the clinical condition warrants it, treatment with a combination of broad spectrum antibiotics should be started pending the results of bacteriological studies (Conn 1964). Currently, we use a combination of gentamicin, flucloxacillin and metronidazole, given intravenously. If positive bacteriological cultures are obtained this regime is modified if necessary.

3. Ascites

Salt and water retention are characteristic of liver failure and if the patient has portal hypertension, the retained fluid accumulates as ascites. A low serum albumin contributes to this problem. However, it may occur even if the serum albumin is within the normal range, especially if the patient is overloaded with water and sodium. Local lesions, such as hepatic vein occlusion (Budd Chiari Syndrome) and tumours, especially primary hepatoma, may precipitate ascites in previously well compensated cirrhotic patients. These patients can often be distinguished by a rising serum alkaline phosphatase and a high protein content in the ascitic fluid. In addition, elevated serum α-fetoprotein levels and tumour cells in the ascitic fluid may be found in appropriate patients. Pain in a patient with ascites suggests tumour or hepatic vein occlusion if it is predominantly present over an enlarged liver. More generalized abdominal pain and ascites suggests infection of the ascitic fluid, which is most often due to coliforms, although other organisms may be responsible (Kerr *et al.* 1963; Conn 1976). Tuberculous peritonitis may present in this way. Infection may occur in ascitic fluid with very little to indicate this site of infection. Therefore, a diagnostic tap of ascites for a cell count and culture is mandatory in any patient deteriorating in any way with ascites and liver failure. Ascitic cell counts (predominantly polymorphonuclear leucocytes) of over 500 per cu mm, when combined with the characteristic clinical picture, should be taken as indicating infected ascites, even if organisms are not seen (Kline *et al.* 1976).

Constrictive pericarditis and congestive cardiomyopathy can cause ascites and must be excluded by carefully examining the cardiovascular system of the patient.

Treatment

Although diagnostic paracentesis is mandatory, therapeutic paracentesis is not recommended (Sherlock 1981).

Dietary sodium restriction and limitation of water intake should be employed in all patients with ascites. They should also be restricted in patients with compromised liver function and other stress, such as infection, gastro-intestinal haemorrhage, or after a surgical operation. Strict sodium restriction to between 20 to 30 mg of sodium per day should be undertaken where possible. This represents severe dietary sodium restriction, including substitution of milk and salt free bread. Few patients will adhere to such a regime out of hospital and it requires careful planning by an experienced dietitian. Such patients on intravenous infusions will rarely require any saline, as many drugs and clotting factor concentrates will provide an adequate sodium intake.

Water restriction is less obligatory unless the patient normally has an excessive fluid intake. Ideally an intake of 1.5 litres per day should suffice, but if the serum sodium falls the intake from all sources should be limited to under 1 litre per day. Such a fall in serum sodium occurs particularly during diuretic therapy and should not be treated with saline unless there is good clinical evidence of salt and water depletion.

Diuretics may be used in conjunction with dietary restriction to treat ascites. The secondary hyperaldosteronism associated with cirrhotic ascites requires an aldosterone antagonist such as spironolactone. This may be required in doses of up to 400 mg per day but should be started at 100 mg per day and increased after two days until a diuresis is achieved. If maximum doses of spironolactone do not achieve a diuresis, a loop diuretic, such as frusemide or bumetamide should be added. Accurate fluid balance, daily weights and blood urea and electrolyte levels must be measured and any sign of encephalopathy watched for. An ideal weight loss is 1 kg per day, as a more rapid diuresis leads to electrolyte imbalance and encephalopathy.

Serum potassium levels are frequently low in patients with liver failure and must be corrected with dietary supplements and potassium chloride, either orally or intravenously as appropriate.

In many patients, the diuresis resulting from this combined dietary and drug regime will effectively treat the ascites. However, in other patients— particularly the elderly, patients with severely compromised liver function and after surgical operation in cirrhotics—the salt and water restriction and diuretics lead only to a depletion of the intravascular compartment and a rising blood urea (Conn 1977). The renal blood flow in liver failure is already effectively reduced by shunting of blood from the renal cortex (Lieberman 1970). These patients can be improved with daily infusions of salt poor albumin which increases renal blood flow and may initiate a diuresis. This is effective treatment in the short term, but unsuitable for long-term treatment, both because of the need for constant intravenous infusions and because salt poor albumin, prepared from human blood, is in limited supply. Ultrafiltration of ascitic fluid and its reinfusion intravenously can be performed with the appropriate apparatus (Rhône–Poulenc). It is unsuitable for use in the presence of infection. Patients with cirrhosis, Budd Chiari syndrome and malignant ascites, have been treated successfully. Up to thirteen litres of ascites can be removed in twenty-four hours. High rates of filtration tend to block the filter, while lower rates predispose to pulmonary oedema (Lévy *et al.* 1975). Urine output also increases after ultrafiltration treatment, and the patient may become more responsive to diuretics (Moult *et al.* 1975). Moreover, the procedure can be repeated at intervals.

Peritoneal-venous shunts can be used for continuous treatment of ascites over many months. After making a small incision in the abdominal wall, the end of the plastic tube is inserted through the peritoneum into the pelvis. From there, it is passed out of the peritoneal cavity to a pressure sensitive valve. It is then tunnelled subcutaneously to drain into the internal jugular vein in the neck and thus to the superior vena cava (Le Veen *et al.* 1976). Patients with ascites from many causes have been treated successfully by this method. However, because it requires an initial surgical procedure, it is unsuitable for patients with very poor or deteriorating liver function. It is also contra-indicated if the patient has recently bled from oesophageal varices, as the increase in intravascular volume may contribute to recurrent haemorrhage (Le Veen *et al.* 1976).

4. Hypoglycaemia

This is a consequence of severe liver cell damage, with failure of normal mechanisms for maintaining blood glucose levels in the fasting state. It can cause sudden death (Samson *et al.* 1967).

Treatment

An intravenous infusion of glucose (or dextrose) maintains blood glucose levels. It is usual to use 5, 10 or 20 per cent solutions and occasionally some 50 per cent dextrose is required. Constant monitoring of the blood glucose and potassium levels is mandatory. The proper use of modern glucose 'stick' tests are very useful in this situation. Potassium supplements are usually required when dextrose solutions are infused into patients with liver failure because the additional glucose tends to cause potassium to move from the extracellular fluid into the cells. Insulin supplements may be required either when the patient is a latent or overt diabetic or when a high concentration of glucose is infused because fluid restriction is necessary.

5. Encephalopathy

This may present as insidious neuropsychiatric changes, sleep disorder, confusion, stupor or deep coma. It can occur either as the result of massive necrosis of liver cells in acute fulminating liver failure, or as the result of an additional stress such as constipation, bleeding, infection or electrolyte imbalance in a patient with chronic liver disease. It can also be precipitated either by drug therapy with sedatives or diuretics or by excessive dietary protein in susceptible patients. The prognosis and response to treatment varies with the underlying and precipitating causes. About 20 per cent of the patients with acute fulminating liver failure recover completely but the cirrhotic patients regain consciousness in over 70 per cent of instances (Sherlock 1981).

Treatment

Any precipitating cause such as an infection or electrolyte imbalance should be suspected and treated. Blood and other appropriate cultures should be taken. Diuretics and drugs which may have a sedative effect should be stopped. Any hypokalaemia should be treated with oral or intravenous potassium chloride. Dietary protein intake should be cut. The patient is purged with magnesium sulphate orally and a magnesium sulphate enema is given to empty the bowel. Lactulose (15–40 ml daily), neomycin (1–4 gm daily) and, more recently metronidazole (1.2–2.4 gm daily) have all been reported to be of value in the treatment of encephalopathy. Maintenance therapy with lactulose can reduce chronic encephalopathy (Conn *et al.* 1977). Levodopa, bromocriptine and intravenous infusions of sodium bicarbonate and albumin are among other treatments experimentally shown to improve hepatic encephalopathy. However, in practice there is little place for their use, other than in selected patients (Lunzer *et al.* 1974; Morgan *et al.* 1980).

6. Jaundice

When this is due to liver cell failure it is a guide to the duration and severity of the liver cell damage. It must be distinguished from the jaundice due to large bile duct obstruction. Normally the serum transaminase levels will be high; aspartate transaminase (AST or SGOT) and alanine transaminase (ALT or SGPT) are the two most commonly measured. Occasionally, the alkaline phosphatase is also elevated and in these patients, investigation of the extra-hepatic bile ducts must be performed. Ultrasound scans and computerized axial tomography (CAT) may demonstrate the dilated ducts but the more invasive techniques of percutaneous transhepatic cholangiogram (PTC) with a chiba needle or endoscopic retrograde cholangiopancreatogram (ERCP) will be necessary in some patients. The choice of examination depends largely on facilities and expertise available.

Treatment

If bile duct obstruction is demonstrated this must be relieved either at laparotomy or, if technically possible, the endoscopic techniques of sphincterotomy and gall stone removal may be more appropriate in patients with liver failure (Cotton 1980). If the extrahepatic bile ducts are healthy, no treatment is required for the jaundice of liver cell failure.

7. Artificial hepatic support systems

No artificial system has been shown to increase survival in acute fulminating liver failure. They are not appropriate for the treatment of hepatic coma in cirrhotic patients. Some are now of little practical importance but techniques which have been shown to alter conscious level and for which some success has been claimed are listed.

  (i) Exchange transfusion. This can be either with whole blood or by the use of plasmaphoresis (Trey *et al.* 1966; Lepore and Martel 1970).
 (ii) Cross circulation with a volunteer or donor, or with porcine, bovine, or baboon livers. These present ethical and technical problems which have prevented their widespread application (Burnell *et al.* 1967; Abouna *et al.* 1972; Condon *et al.* 1970).
(iii) Haemoperfusion with charcoal or resin. Charcoal haemoperfusion removes water soluble toxic metabolites, but not protein bound substances, and has caused problems with damage to the platelets in the blood and haemorrhage (Weston *et al.* 1974, 1977).
Modifications to this system and resins which can remove protein-bound toxins are possible developments. This technique is currently being used in several centres in Britain. However, its value has never been proven by a randomized control trial.
 (vi) Haemodialysis. This uses a highly permeable polyacrylonitrile membrane removing substances up to a molecular weight of 5000 (Rhône–Poulenc) (Silk *et al.* 1977).

Alcohol withdrawal syndrome

The majority of habitual heavy drinkers will show minor evidence of withdrawal after six to eight hours of abstaining from alcohol. Classically, if no drinking occurs during the night the patient develops morning shakes, a coarse rapid tremor accompanied by other evidence of autonomic overactivity, tachycardia, flushing and increased sweating. These symptoms are relieved by drinking further alcohol but if alcohol is withheld they continue for a few days and then gradually recede. However, in a minority of habitual heavy drinkers continuing abstinence leads to a major withdrawal syn-

Table 25.2. Clinical features and treatment of alcohol withdrawal

Features	Treatment
Tremor Sweating Tachycardia and pyrexia Insomnia and restlessness Convulsions Confusion Hallucinations	Chlormethiazole *orally* up to 4 capsules 3–4 hourly initial day followed by rapidly reducing doses or *intravenously* adjust infusion rate. If intolerant use diazepam

drome. This comes on insidiously after alcohol consumption ceases with the major features of convulsions and hallucinations (Table 25.2).

Convulsions

Twelve to thirty-six hours after the last drink the patient may have a convulsion, often grand mal and sometimes several fits may occur in succession and rarely status epilepticus may follow. Whether or not they have convulsions patients showing signs of alcohol withdrawal may develop delirium tremens (the D.T.s) after two to four days of abstinence.

The D.T.s

The D.T.s start insidiously with an increased restlessness, anxiety, agitation and insomnia. The tremor, sweating and tachycardia persist and increase. In addition, the patient is often pyrexial and may become increasingly confused and disorientated. They have illusions with gross misinterpretation of events occurring around them and misidentification of people with whom they are in contact. They may have visual, auditory and tactile hallucinations. Because of their illusions and hallucinations their environment becomes very hostile and frightening to them. They may behave irrationally and even endanger themselves in an attempt to escape from or protect themselves from these 'dangers' of which they alone are aware.

At this time, whether or not they show the more florid signs of delirium tremens, the patients often show jealousy, most characteristically coupled with the deluded view that their spouse is unfaithful.

The diagnosis of alcohol withdrawal should be considered in anyone who, with the onset of acute illness, hospital admission or other enforced abstinence becomes restless with tachycardia, sweating and tremor. The history of previous heavy drinking may not have been volunteered and the doctor should be alerted even in the absence of a volunteered history if

Table 25.3. Differential diagnosis of alcohol withdrawal

Differentiate from	Signs	Investigations
Thyrotoxicosis	Tremor, lid lag, thyroid bruit, tachycardia	Normal circulating thyroid hormone levels
Intoxication	Smell of alcohol Incoordination	Blood ethanol elevated
Wernicke/Korsakoff	Ophthalmoplegia	
Hepatic encephalopathy	Drowsy Flapping tremor	EEG shows increased slow wave activity
Cerebral haemorrhage	Fluctuating consciousness Localizing signs	CAT scan
Meningitis	Stiff neck	Lumbar puncture
Wilson's disease	Kayser–Fleischer rings	Caeruloplasmin reduced
Cerebral tumour	Focal neurological signs	CAT scan
Hypoglycaemia	Sweating, pale skin Look for evidence that patient may be diabetic on treatment, e.g. syringes, insulin, hypoglycaemic agents etc.	Blood glucose

the characteristic features occur. In a known heavy drinker, it should be anticipated that withdrawal symptoms will follow abstinence from alcohol. If the patient has, for example, undergone a major operation, the restlessness and irrational activity could have serious consequences. Appropriate and adequate sedation should be instituted early in the progression of symptoms.

The differential diagnosis of alcohol withdrawal ranges from thyrotoxicosis in patients who deny heavy consumption of alcohol (refuted by normal circulating levels of the thyroid hormone) to hypoglycaemia and to other alcohol and liver related neuropsychological syndromes in patients with chronic hepatic failure (Table 25.3).

Alcoholics may develop Wernicke and Korsakoff Syndromes with the characteristic ophthalmoplegia and confabulation. This may occur with features of alcohol withdrawal superimposed and the autonomic overactivity alerts the clinician to the dual problem.

Alcoholics may have severely damaged livers and, especially with infection or haemorrhage, may show signs of hepatic encephalopathy. The characteristic fetor and flapping tremor in a drowsy or comatosed patient distinguishes liver failure from the D.T.s. However, if sedation has already been given the differentiation may be less easy. An EEG with a predominance of slow wave activity or other biochemical tests indicating liver failure may help.

Alcoholics and other patients with liver disease have an increased incidence of intracranial haemorrhage, particularly subdural haematoma following minor and often forgotten head injury. They also have an increased susceptibility to infection including meningitis. These possibilities should always be considered in patients in whom the signs and symptoms are in any way atypical. Computerized axial tomography (CAT scan) and, if appropriate, lumbar puncture may be necessary to make the diagnosis clear.

Wilson's disease may present with liver disease and progressive neurological deterioration. Occasionally the diagnosis is not considered and the patient is seen undiagnosed in liver failure. In any young patient with chronic liver disease and even patients who are in their forties, the diagnosis of Wilson's disease should be considered and the characteristic Kayser–Fleischer rings and disordered copper metabolism will confirm this.

Treatment

The treatment of choice is chlormethiazole (Heminevrin). It can be taken orally as syrup or capsules and is available as an intravenous infusion. Ideally, if treatment is started early, the oral therapy will prevent the worst hallucinations and fits. The dose varies widely, depending on the rate of metabolism in the liver but up to four capsules every three to four hours may be required initially. This dose should only be used with experienced medical supervision in hospital. If less than this is given and the patient is still very agitated, supplementary doses should be given as the patient is much harder to control once frank hallucinations are occurring. The dose must be reduced after two days or earlier if the patient becomes drowsy. The aim is to continue sedation in reducing dose for about five days. If possible, more prolonged therapy should be avoided as addiction can develop. Confusion in the dose of orally prescribed chlormethiazole may occur as the chlormethiazole content of the capsule is 192 mg chlormethiazole *base* and the chlormethiazole content of 5 ml of syrup is 250 mg chlormethiazole *edisylate*. 10 ml of syrup are therapeutically equivalent to two capsules.

In patients who are unable to take oral medication (for example after an abdominal operation) the intravenous infusion should be used with the drip rate adjusted to maintain adequate sedation. This route may also be used to control patients in whom the diagnosis is only made late and when rapid control is required.

The occasional patient cannot tolerate chlormethiazole and they are usually sedated with diazepam. Chlorpromazine has also been used but is best avoided because of the risk of liver damage. There is now rarely any rationale for using paraldehyde injections which can cause serious problems especially in patients with a bleeding tendency.

Sometimes it is suggested that alcohol withdrawal should be treated with alcohol. This is a short-term expedient and usually bad practice as the alcoholic will require alcohol withdrawal at a future date especially if serious consequences and complications develop.

Further reading

Abouna G.M., Cook J.S., Fisher L.McA., Still W.J., Giovanni C. and Hume D.M. (1972) Treatment of acute hepatic coma by ex-vivo baboon and human liver perfusions. *Surgery* **71**, 537–46.

Burnell J.M., Dawborn J.K., Epstein R.B., Gutman R.A., Leinbach G.E., Thomas E.D., Volwiler W. (1967) Acute hepatitic coma treated by cross-circulation or exchange transfusion. *New England Journal of Medicine* **276**, 935–43.

Condon R.E., Bombeck C.T., Steigman F. (1970) Heterologous bovine liver perfusion therapy of acute hepatic failure. *American Journal of Surgery* **119**, 147–154.

Conn H.O. (1964) Spontaneous peritonitis and bacteremia in Laennec's cirrhosis caused by enteric organisms. *Annals of Internal Medicine* **60**, 568–569.

Conn H.O. (1976) Spontaneous bacterial peritonitis—multiple revisitations. *Gastroenterology* **70**, 455–457.

Conn H.O. (1977) Diuresis of ascites: fraught with or free from hazard. *Gastroenterology* **73**, 619–621.

Conn H.O., Leevy G.M., Vlahcevic Z.R., Rogers J.B., Maddray W.C., Seeff L., Levy L.L. (1977) Comparison of lactulose and neomycin in the treatment of chronic portal-systemic encephalopathy. *Gastroenterology* **72**, 573–585.

Cotton P.B. (1980) Non-operative removal of bile duct stones by duodenoscopic sphincterotomy. *British Journal of Survery* **67**, 1–5.

Gazzard B.G., Clark R., Borirakchanyavat V., Williams R. (1974) A controlled trial of heparin therapy in the coagulation defect of paracetamol induced hepatic necrosis. *Gut* **15**, 89–93.

Gazzard B.G., Lewis M.L., Ash G., Rizza C.R., Bidwell E., Williams R. (1974a) Coagulation factor concentrate in the treatment of the haemorrhagic diathesis of fulminant hepatic failure. *Gut* **15**, 993–998.

Gazzard B.G., Henderson S.M., Williams R. (1975) The use of fresh frozen plasma or a concentrate of factor IX as replacement therapy before liver biopsy. *Gut* **16**, 621–625.

Glat M. (1982) *Alcoholism* pp. 278–280. Hodder and Stoughton, London.

Green G., Dymock W., Poller L. and Thomson J.M. (1975) The use of factor VII rich prothrombin complex concentrates in liver disease *Lancet* **i**, 1311–1314.

Green G., Poller L., Thomson J.M. and Dymock I.W. (1976) Factor VII as a marker of hepato-cellular synthetic function in liver disease. *Journal of Clinical Pathology* **28**, 971–975.

Hillenbrand P., Parbhoo S.P., Jedrychowski A. and Sherlock S. (1974) Significance of intravascular coagulation and fibrinolysis in acute hepatic failure. *Gut,* **15**, 83–88.

Kerr D.N.S., Pearson D.T. and Read A.E. (1983) Infection of ascitic fluid in patients with hepatic cirrhosis. *Gut* **4**, 394–398.

Kline M.M., McCallum R.W. and Guth P.H. (1976) The clinical value of ascitic fluid culture and leucocyte count studies in alcoholic liver disease. *Gastroenterology* **70**, 408–412.

Lepore M.J., Martel A.J. (1970) Plasmapheresis with plasma exchange in hepatic coma. *Annals Internal Medicine* **72**, 165–170.

Le Veen H.H., Wapnick S., Grosberg S. (1976) Further experience with peritoneo-venous shunts for ascites. *Annals Surgery* **184**, 574–583.

Lévy V.G., Opolon P., Pauleau N., Capoli J. (1975) Treatment of ascites by re-infusion of concentrated peritoneal fluid *Postgraduate Medical Journal* **51**, 564–566.

Lieberman F.L. (1970) Functional renal failure in cirrhosis. *Gastroenterology* **58**, 108–110.

Lunzer M., James I.M., Weinman J. and Sherlock S. (1974) Treatment of chronic hepatic encephalopathy with Levodopa. *Gut* **15**, 555.

Mannucci P.M., Franchi F. and Dioguardi N. (1976) Correction of abnormal coagulation in chronic liver disease by combined use of fresh frozen plasma and prothrombin complex concentrates. *Lancet* **ii**, 542–545.

Morgan M.Y., Jakobovits A.M., James I.M. and Sherlock S. (1980) Successful use of bromocriptine in the treatment of chronic hepatic encephalopathy. *Gastroenterology* **78**, 663–670.

Moult P.J.A., Parbhoo S.P. and Sherlock S. (1975) Clinical experience with the Rhône-Poulenc ascites re-infusion apparatus. *Postgraduate Medical Journal* **51**, 574–576.

Rake M.O., Flute P.T., Pannell G. Williams R. (1970) Intravascular coagulation in acute hepatic necrosis *Lancet* **i**, 533–537.

Samson R.I., Trey C., Timne A.H. and Saunders S.J. (1967) Fulminating hepatitis, recurrent hypoglycaemia and haemorrhage. *Gastroenterology* **53**, 291–300.

Sherlock S. (1981) *Diseases of the liver and biliary system*, 6th edition, p. 91, p. 129. Blackwell Scientific Publications, Oxford.

Silk D.B.A., Hamid M.A., Trewby P.N., Davies M., Chase R.A., Langley P.G., Mellon P.J., Wheeler P.G. and Williams R. (1977) Treatment of fulminant hepatic failure by polyacrylonitrile membrane haemodialysis (Rhône-Poulenc) *Lancet* **ii**, 1–3.

Tray C., Burns D.G. and Saunders S.J. (1966) Treatment of hepatic coma by exchange blood transfusion. *New England Journal of Medicine* **274**, 473–475.

Tucker J.S., Woolf I.L., Boyes E.B., Thomson J.M., Poller L. and Dymock I.W. (1973) Coagulation studies in acute hepatic failure. *Gut* **14**, 418.

Weston M.J., Gazzard B.G., Buxton B.H., Winch J., Machado A.L., Flax H., Williams R. (1974) Effect of haemoperfusion through charcoal or XAD-2 resin on an animal model of fulminant liver failure. *Gut* **15**, 482.

Weston M.J., Langley P.G., Rubin M.H., Hamid M.A., Mellon P.J. and Williams R. (1977) Platelet function in fulminant hepatic failure and the effect of charcoal haemoperfusion. *Gut* **18**, 897–902.

26 · Acute Pancreatitis

R. W. G. CHAPMAN

Although often considered an acute surgical emergency, acute pancreatitis may present to the physician either on the general ward or in the intensive care unit.

There are few subjects in medicine as difficult or as controversial as the medical and surgical management of severe acute pancreatitis. It may give rise to a variety of complex respiratory and metabolic problems requiring a multidisciplinary approach, involving physician, surgeon and anaesthetist.

Aetiology

The main predisposing factors for acute pancreatitis in Great Britain are shown in Table 26.1. The commonest causes are biliary disease and alcohol abuse, which account for over 90 per cent of all patients with acute pancreatitis.

The incidence of acute pancreatitis in Great Britain has doubled in the last ten years, to over 200 new patients per million per annum (Imrie 1982). This probably reflects the increasing incidence of alcohol abuse in the community at large.

Table 26.1. Aetiological factors in acute pancreatitis in UK

Biliary disease ⎱ over 90 per cent of all cases
Alcohol ⎰
Viruses—Mumps
Coxsackie B
Hyperparathyroidism
Drugs—corticosteroids
azathioprine
Carcinoma of the pancreas
Carcinoma of the ampulla
Blunt trauma
Iatrogenic—post surgical operations
post ERCP/sphincterotomy
post translumbar aortography

Mortality tends to be higher in acute pancreatitis secondary to blunt trauma, endoscopic retrograde cholangio-pancreatography (ERCP), surgical operations and following translumbar aortography (Imrie 1982).

Clinical features

Acute pancreatitis is characterized by the sudden onset of severe abdominal pain, often associated with vomiting. The pain is usually in the epigastrium but may be generalized or localized to the left or right upper quadrants. It is persistent and may radiate through to the back.

Pyrexia, tachycardia and jaundice are often found on examination. Abdominal tenderness, rigidity and reduced bowel sounds are usually present. Bruising in the flanks (Grey Turner's sign) and in the periumbilical region (Cullen's sign) may appear after a few days and indicate fulminating haemorrhagic pancreatitis. Less than 5 per cent of patients with acute pancreatitis have fulminating pancreatitis. However, the mortality is high in these patients at between thirty to sixty per cent.

Diagnosis

The serum amylase is the most useful investigation and is usually elevated in patients with acute pancreatitis. A serum amylase level over 1200 iu/l (1000 somogyi units/100 ml) is diagnostic. However, increases in serum amylases may be found in several clinical conditions, including perforated peptic ulceration, mesenteric vascular occlusion, dissecting aortic aneurysm, small bowel obstruction, ectopic pregnancy, renal failure and macro-amylasaemia.

In patients with suspected acute pancreatitis but with elevations in serum amylase below the diagnostic level, it is important to measure the urinary amylase. The urinary amylase is usually elevated in excess of 3000 iu/l in acute pancreatitis. An increased amylase clearance in excess of 4 ml/minute and an amylase to creatinine ratio in excess of 5 per cent are also indicative of acute pancreatitis and may help in confirming the diagnosis in difficult cases. These diagnostic criteria are summarized in Table 26.2.

Rarely very severe acute pancreatitis may occur without elevated serum or urinary amylase levels, usually associated with complete pancreatic necrosis (Imrie 1982).

Haematological tests usually show a neutrophil leucocytosis and an elevated erythrocyte sedimentation rate (ESR). Disseminated intravascular coagulation (DIC) may complicate severe acute pancreatitis and in severe cases the platelet count, prothrombin time and fibrin degradation products should be measured.

The serum bilirubin, aspartate transaminase and alkaline phosphatase

Table 26.2. Diagnosis of acute pancreatitis

Acute upper abdominal pain ± vomiting
    ↓
    serum amylase > 1200 u/l*
               > 1000 somogyi units/dl*
    ↓ < 1200
    urine amylase > 3000 u/l*
    ↓
    amylase clearance > 4 ml/min*
    amylase to creatinine clearance ratio > 5 per cent*

---

*diagnostic of acute pancreatitis

are often mildly elevated. Hyperglycaemia often occurs although diabetic coma is very rarely observed.

In a minority of patients with hyperlipidaemia the serum is frankly lipaemic. Elevated triglyceride levels may cause analytical problems for the measurement of amylase, transaminase and lactic dehydrogenase. It is possible to dilute the serum sample with saline and reveal the binding effect which interferes with the amylase measurement (Fallat *et al.* 1973).

However, it is reasonable to assume that a patient with a compatible clinical presentation and marked hyperlipaemia is suffering from acute pancreatitis until proven otherwise (Cameron *et al.* 1973). Hyperlipaemia usually occurs in patients with alcoholic acute pancreatitis and is commonly transient, although primary hyperlipoproteinaemia may also predispose to acute pancreatitis (Cameron *et al.* 1973).

Hypocalcaemia is seen in over 70 per cent of patients with acute pancreatitis. Once thought to reflect extensive fat necrosis and precipitation of calcium salts, it is now realized that the hypocalcaemia is directly related to the low serum albumin which is commonly seen in severe cases (Allam and Imrie 1977).

Isoamylase, lipase and methaemalbumin assays take too long to be of value in the initial diagnosis of acute pancreatitis although methaem-albuminaemia is a useful sign of haemorrhagic pancreatitis (Lankisch *et al.* 1978).

Plain abdominal X-rays may be helpful in detecting radiopaque gall-stones and to exclude other causes of an acute abdomen. Occasionally a 'sentinel loop' of localized dilatation of small or large bowel can be seen in patients with acute pancreatitis. Chest X-ray may reveal a pleural effusion (usually left-sided) or left basal atelectasis.

Despite all the diagnostic techniques described, in some patients the diagnosis may remain uncertain and laparotomy may have to be undertaken as a diagnostic procedure. In such patients peritoneal aspiration should be performed before resorting to surgery. In the majority of patients with acute pancreatitis, a sterile 'prune juice' coloured aspirate with a high amylase concentration can be obtained. The presence of organisms in the aspirate is probably a reliable sign of a perforated viscus but false negatives may occur (Bradley *et al.* 1981).

Method for carrying out peritoneal aspiration with lavage (McMahon 1981)

A standard peritoneal dialysis cannula is used. After passing a nasogastric tube and ensuring that the bladder is empty the anterior abdominal wall, about two to three cm below the umbilicus, is anaesthetized down to the peritoneum with 20 ml of 2 per cent lignocaine containing 1:1000 adrenaline. Aspiration is then attempted with a syringe and thin needle. If liquid or gas with a faecal odour is obtained an alternative site is chosen (usually the left iliac fossa). A small (0.5 cm) skin stab is then made and the dialysis cannula inserted in the peritoneal space. The cannula is directed down into the pelvis. An attempt is then made to aspirate fluid, the volume, colour and odour of which is recorded. A litre of warmed normal saline is then run rapidly into the abdomen and the patient turned from side to side a few times. The colour of the fluid which returns is noted. Samples are sent to the laboratory for amylase assay and Gram stain. McMahon *et al.* (1981) have suggested that the presence of one or more of three features indicates that the attack is likely to be severe:

(1) Dark or prune juice coloured free fluid.
(2) More than 10 ml of free fluid irrespective of colour.
(3) Mid-straw coloured lavage return fluid.

This guide to severity of acute pancreatitis provides broadly similar results to the multiple criteria system described previously (McMahon, 1980). It has the advantage of providing a guide to severity within hours of admission as full biochemical grading is only possible at least twenty-four hours after admission. It has the disadvantage of the risk of unnecessarily introducing a peritoneal catheter in mild cases.

Treatment

The principles of treatment of acute pancreatitis are:

(1) adequate analgesia—usually pethidine (50–150 mg i.m. doses);
(2) i.v. replacement of fluid, electrolyte, protein and blood losses;
(3) 'resting' the pancreas by nasogastric suction and avoiding oral feeding;
(4) monitoring the hourly urine output.

Following the simple procedures outlined above, about two-thirds of patients with acute pancreatitis will improve within twenty-four hours and nasogastric suction and bladder catheterization can be discontinued.

Recent studies have shown that the mortality rate is approximately 8–10 per cent in patients with acute pancreatitis. Two studies have failed to show any improvement in survival with either intravenous glucagon or aprotinin (Trasylol) in the management of acute pancreatitis (MRC Multicentre Trial Study Group 1977, Imrie *et al.* 1978). Similarly, there is little evidence to support the routine use of antibiotics, anticholinergic drugs, calcitonin, corticosteroids or cimetidine.

Some workers advocate the use of anxiolytics, such as valium, in addition to analgesics. There is no controlled evidence of a beneficial effect of benzodiazepines. There are uncontrolled reports that somatostatin infusion produces a normalization of hyperamylasaemia and clinical improvement in acute pancreatitis (Raptis and Rosenthal 1977). Further controlled clinical studies are needed to fully evaluate the effects of somatostatin.

Table 26.3. Prognostic factors in patients with acute pancreatitis*

1. Age > 55 years
2. WBC $> 15\times10^9$/l
3. Glucose > 10 mmol/l (no diabetic history)
4. Urea > 16 mmol/l (no response to i.v. fluids)
5. PaO$_2$ < 8.0 kPa
6. Calcium < 2.0 mmol/l
7. Albumin < 32 g/l
8. LDH > 600 i.u./l
9. SGOT > 100 i.u./l
If three or more factors are present within 48 hours of
  hospitalization = severe acute pancreatitis

*After Imrie *et al.* 1978

The art of managing acute pancreatitis lies in the early identification of severe cases which will require intensive monitoring and therapy. Studies from the United States and Great Britain have shown that an objective grading of disease severity in terms of mortality is possible using relatively simple clinical and laboratory data (Ranson *et al.* 1976, Imrie *et al.* 1978). The grading system proposed by Imrie *et al.* (1978) is shown in Table 26.3. Using this system the mortality of severe pancreatitis was shown to be 22 per cent, whereas that of mild pancreatitis was only 0.6 per cent.

Treatment of severe pancreatitis

The management of acute pancreatitis is outlined in Fig. 26.1. Management is largely concerned with the early identification and treatment of respiratory, renal, cardiac, infective and metabolic complications.

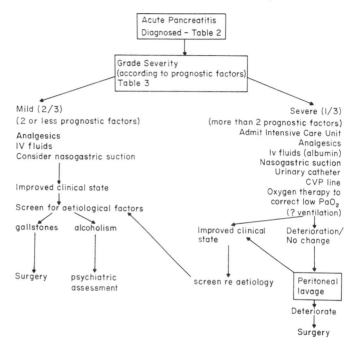

Fig. 26.1. The management of acute pancreatitis.

Respiratory insufficiency

It is important to monitor arterial blood gases routinely on a regular basis. Approximately half of all patients show a PaO_2 level below 60 mm Hg within the first few days of the illness. The mechanism of the arterial hypoxaemia has not been fully elucidated. If the hypoxaemia does not respond to humidified oxygen then mechanical ventilation should be considered.

Cardiac failure

It has been shown that a high proportion of patients dying of acute pancreatitis have suffered a myocardial infarct. The mechanism of coronary insufficiency remains unclear. In view of this, some authorities recommend the routine digitalization of older patients with acute pancreatitis (Imrie

1982). There is no controlled evidence available regarding the use of cardiac glycosides in acute pancreatitis.

Renal failure

Adequate fluid replacement usually maintains urinary output. Central venous pressure monitoring is helpful in maintaining a normal plasma volume. Up to ten litres of fluid may be required in the first twenty-four hours of treatment. Rarely, despite a normal central venous pressure, urine output falls and high doses of intravenous frusemide or bumetamide are then indicated. In a small number of severely ill patients, dialysis may be indicated. Nevertheless, the mortality in this group of patients is high.

Peritoneal lavage

The diagnostic role of peritoneal lavage has been discussed earlier in this chapter. Animal experiments have suggested that peritoneal lavage may also be a useful therapeutic manoeuvre.

The principle is that kinins, polypeptides and other toxins which would be absorbed across the peritoneum into the systemic circulation are removed. Although there is a lack of well controlled clinical studies in human patients, most studies have shown clinical improvement following lavage in patients with severe acute pancreatitis (McMahon 1981). However, there is no convincing evidence that mortality in severe acute pancreatitis is reduced by peritoneal lavage. It appears that peritoneal lavage does not influence the progression of disease in the pancreas itself, in either animals or man, irrespective of this benefit on systemic complications.

At the present time, in the absence of a controlled clinical trial, therapeutic peritoneal lavage should only be considered in patients with severe acute pancreatitis who are responding poorly to conservative medical therapy.

Surgical treatment

The majority of patients with severe acute pancreatitis will recover with the medical measures outlined previously. In patients who are not responding, controversy exists as to the timing, the selection of patients and the benefits of surgical intervention (Gauthier *et al.* 1981).

In patients selected for emergency surgery, the whole of the pancreas is exposed at laparotomy. The aims of surgery are to remove any necrotic pancreatic tissue, to drain the pancreas and to provide a feeding jejunostomy for later use (Imrie 1982). However, the mortality of early surgical resection is very high (10 to 57 per cent) and well controlled clinical studies are needed to confirm the role of radical surgery in patients not responding to medical treatment (Gauthier *et al.* 1981).

The role of endoscopic sphincterotomy in patients with gallstone related pancreatitis remains controversial. Provisional reports suggest that this procedure may be helpful in selected patients (Safrany and Cotton 1981).

Late complications of acute pancreatitis

Pseudocysts, pancreatic abscesses, main duct strictures and fistula formation may occur as late complications of acute pancreatitis.

Approximately 15–20 per cent of patients with acute alcoholic pancreatitis and 3 per cent of those with gallstones develop pseudocysts. 50 per cent regress spontaneously. The course of pancreatic pseudocysts can be accurately monitored by the use of ultrasonography or computed tomography. These techniques can also be used to aspirate non-resolving pseudocysts. Surgery should be reserved for those patients in whom the pseudocyst becomes infected.

Pancreatic abscesses are less common than pseudocysts; they are found in 3–5 per cent of patients. Abscesses should be confirmed with ultrasonography and drained surgically. Pancreatic fistulae are uncommon; when present they usually communicate with the colon around the splenic flexure. Most will close spontaneously without resort to surgery.

The timing of biliary surgery following a severe attack of acute pancreatitis in patients is controversial. It should probably be deferred until the attack of acute pancreatitis has completely resolved. Biliary surgery can be safely performed in mild cases within two weeks after the onset of symptoms of acute pancreatitis (Osborne *et al.* 1981).

Further reading

Allam B.F. and Imrie C.W. (1977) Serum ionised calcium in acute pancreatitis. *British Journal of Surgery* **64**, 665–668.

Bradley J.A., Bradley P. and McMahon M.J. (1981) Diagnostic peritoneal lavage in acute pancreatitis—the value of microscopy of the lavage fluid. *British Journal of Surgery* **68**, 245–246.

Cameron J.L., Capuzzi D.M., Zuidema G.D. and Margolis S. (1973) Acute pancreatitis with hyperlipemia. *Annals of Surgery* **177**, 483–489.

Fallat R.W., Vester J.W. and Gluck C.J. (1973) Suppression of amylase activity by hypertriglyceridemia. *Journal of the American Medical Association* **225**, 1331–1334.

Gauthier A., Escoffier J.M., Camatte R. and Sarles G. (1981) Acute pancreatitis. *Clinics in Gastroenterology* **10**, 209–224.

Imrie C.W. (1982) The treatment of acute pancreatitis. In: *Topics in Gastroenterology* 9, eds. Jewell D.P. and Lee E. pp. 245–262. Blackwell Scientific Publications, Oxford.

Imrie C.W., Benjamin I.S., Ferguson J.C., McKay A.J., MacKenzie I., O'Neill J. and Blumgart L.H. (1978) A single centre double blind trial of trasylol therapy in primary acute pancreatitis. *British Journal of Surgery* **65**, 337–341.

Lankisch P.G., Koop H. and Otto J. (1978) Evaluation of methaemalbumin in acute pancreatitis. *Scandinavian Journal of Gastroenterology* **13**, 975–978.

McMahon M.J. (1981) Acute pancreatitis: The role of peritoneal lavage. In: *Pancreatic Disease in Clinical Practice*, eds. Mitchell C.J. and Kellehar. pp. 321–345. Pitman, London.

McMahon M.J., Playforth M.J. and Pickford I.R. (1980) A comparative study of methods for the prediction of severity of attacks of acute pancreatitis. *British Journal of Surgery* **67**, 22–25.

MRC Multicentre Trial of Glucagon and Aprotinin (1977) *Lancet* **ii**, 632–634.

Osborne D.H., Imrie C.W. and Carter D.C. (1981) Biliary surgery in the same admission for gallstone-associated acute pancreatitis. *British Journal of Surgery* **68**, 758–761.

Ranson J.H.C., Rifkind K.M. and Turner J.W. (1976) Prognostic signs and non-operative peritoneal lavage in acute pancreatitis. *Surgery, Gynecology and Obstetrics* **143**, 209–219.

Raptis S. and Rosenthal J. (1977) Somatostatin: potential diagnostic and therapeutic value. *Acta Hepato-Gastroenterologica* **24**, 61–63.

Safrany L. and Cotton P.B. (1981) Preliminary report: urgent sphincterotomy for acute gallstone pancreatitis. *Surgery* **89**, 424–428.

27 · Acute Renal Failure

A. E. G. RAINE

Acute renal failure is a relatively rare medical emergency. In contrast to many other acute problems in medicine, its presentation may be virtually silent and yet its complications, such as hyperkalaemia, can be rapidly life-threatening. For these reasons it is vital to understand clearly, the combination of clinical assessment and essential investigations which are needed together to treat acute renal failure correctly. This chapter aims to outline the problems encountered in acute renal disease and their management. Emergency renal *presentation* will be discussed; although acute and chronic renal failure usually have a different aetiology, time course and prognosis, the distinction may become blurred when treating an emergency problem of uraemia.

Acute renal failure is usually defined as a sudden reduction in urine output to less than 400 ml in twenty-four hours, together with accumulation in the blood of urea, creatinine and other nitrogenous waste products. This definition does not distinguish between pre-renal failure, which may respond immediately to appropriate treatment, and established acute renal failure with a clinical course lasting perhaps for several weeks. In addition, in up to 50 per cent of cases of acute renal failure, oliguria does not occur with daily urine volumes over 400 ml and up to two litres (Anderson *et al.* 1977). Histological changes are only of limited help in definition. Acute tubular necrosis is often used as a pseudonym for acute renal failure but the classical histological appearances of necrosis of tubular epithelial cells and interstitial inflammatory change are often not identified at biopsy (Finckh *et al.* 1962). The pathogenesis of acute renal failure remains unclear despite much research; the competing theories are compared in detail elsewhere (Schrier and Conger 1980).

Acute renal problems in the general hospital present in one of a few characteristic ways. These are poor urine output (oliguria), uraemia as an unexpected biochemical finding and acute renal failure occurring secondary to shock, surgery or trauma or as part of systemic disease. In a one-year survey, sixty cases of acute renal failure were diagnosed (most due to acute tubular necrosis), compared with 1500 with pre-renal failure, 150 with obstructive post-renal failure, and 200 with chronic renal failure (Dombey *et al.* 1975). Hence, a sense of perspective must always be maintained with any apparently renal problem.

Oliguria

Oliguria is seldom volunteered as a symptom and is usually detected in hospital by the nursing staff. Uraemia is present in only a small proportion of patients who develop oliguria. It is essential at first to exclude simple causes, such as dehydration or obstruction. Typically, such patients are post-operative or have had a diagnostic procedure such as endoscopy or angiography. As a result, they have received little or nothing by mouth for some hours, resulting in physiological oliguria. Equally, difficulty in passing urine is common after surgery and is often exacerbated by anticholinergic agents. The previous twenty-four-hour intake of fluid should be determined and obvious signs of outflow obstruction excluded by careful physical examination, including palpation of the bladder and rectal examination. The state of hydration must be accurately assessed. The traditional clinical signs of reduced skin turgor and ocular tension occur relatively late, may be misleading in the elderly and inaccurate in inexperienced hands. The presence of postural hypotension with a tachycardia is more helpful and indicates that there is already a fluid deficit of 2–3 litres or more. Simple dehydration is corrected by oral or, if necessary, intravenous fluid replacement (0.9 per cent sodium chloride, normal saline) and urinary retention by catheterization. If the problem is not solved by these measures then it must be suspected that acute renal failure has developed.

Differentiation of acute and chronic renal failure

Uraemia is quite often an unexpected biochemical finding in patients presenting to their general practitioner or to hospital. Usually, it is possible to decide whether this is recent or long-standing using simple guidelines.

History

In patients with chronic renal failure there is a gradual onset over months of the typical symptoms of thirst, nocturia, polyuria, pruritis and leg cramps. These are followed later by increasing malaise, fatigue, dyspnoea, anorexia, and morning nausea. The latter symptoms arise only when the glomerular filtration rate (GFR) is very low (around 10 ml/min) in chronic disease and may occur in relatively less uraemic patients with acute renal failure. Polyuria and nocturia particularly suggest long-standing disease.

Examination

Hypertension is present in some 80 per cent of patients with chronic renal failure (Curtis *et al.* 1969) and the optic fundi will usually show changes of long established elevation in pressure. In contrast, hypertension is *not* usual in acute tubular necrosis, and if present in acute uraemia, suggests that it is due to a primary renal glomerular disease. Marked uraemic pigmentation and the presence of peripheral neuropathy suggest chronic rather than acute disease. Anaemia is almost universal in chronic renal failure, due to suppression of erythropoiesis, but its presence or absence may be misleading for several reasons. Haemoglobin concentration is well-maintained in polycystic kidney disease and it may be spuriously high in hypovolaemic states superimposed on chronic renal disease. Moreover, anaemia may develop rapidly after the onset of acute renal failure and is aggravated by haemolysis (Stewart 1967). The clinical consequences of extreme uraemia, such as pericarditis, asterixis, fits and metabolic coma will occur in both severe, acute and chronic renal failure and do not help distinguish the two.

Investigations

A number of clues may suggest the existence of long-standing disease. Left ventricular hypertrophy seen on the electrocardiogram (ECG) or echocardiogram indicates established hypertension. The radiological signs of secondary hyperparathyroidism (especially clavicular and phalangeal erosions) suggest renal osteodystrophy; they are very common in chronic renal failure but are not seen in acute disease. Small kidneys demonstrated by abdominal X-ray or intravenous urography will confirm the existence of chronic renal failure. However, kidneys may be normal-sized or enlarged in chronic uraemia caused by polycystic disease, amyloidosis, diabetes mellitus, scleroderma or renal vein thrombosis.

Differential diagnosis of acute renal failure

There are a vast number of potential causes of acute renal failure and those encountered commonly as emergencies are shown in Table 27.1. The time-honoured division into pre-renal, post-renal and intrinsic renal failure is imprecise, but remains useful, not least because principles of management for the three are clearly separated. Pre-renal and post-renal causes of uraemia *must* be diagnosed as early as possible, since they may be immediately reversed by correct treatment, if it is given early enough.

Pre-renal failure

Pre-renal failure is by far the commonest cause of uraemia in general hospitals. It occurs when a fall in renal perfusion pressure lowers glomerular filtration to such an extent that the daily load of nitrogenous waste cannot be

Table 27.1. Major causes of acute renal failure

Renal Ischaemia
  Haemorrhage
  Trauma
  Septicaemia
  Postoperative
  Aortic dissection
  Rhabdomyolysis
  Hypovolaemia (pancreatitis, gastro-enteritis)
  Cardiogenic shock
  Pulmonary embolism
  Renal artery embolism

Haemolysis
  Transfusion reaction
  Falciparum malaria
  Intravascular haemolysis

Nephrotoxins
  X-ray contrast media
  Paraquat
  Heavy metals
  Organic solvents
  Drugs; aminoglycosides, tetracycline, cephaloridine (toxicity) penicillins,
          anti-inflammatory agents (interstitial nephritis)

Primary Renal Disease
  Acute glomerulonephritis
  Vasculitis
  Systemic lupus erythematosis
  Polyarteritis nodosa
  Infectious endocarditis
  Goodpasture's syndrome
  Infection, especially leptospirosis
  Malignant hypertension
  Obstetric accident
  Thrombotic micro-angiopathy

Obstruction
  Tubules; myeloma
              uric acid
  Outflow tract; calculi, renal debris
                      retroperitoneal fibrosis
                      pelvic malignancy
                      prostate

---

excreted and therefore accumulates in the blood. Hypovolaemia or renal hypotension from any cause may do this and unless the renal ischaemia is reversed, acute tubular necrosis ensues. The commonest serious causes are major traumatic or gastro-intestinal haemorrhage, burns, septicaemic or cardiogenic shock, abdominal surgery, dissecting aortic aneurysm and pancreatitis (Clarkson 1980). Volume depletion from over-treatment with diuretics, for example, may cause dramatic elevations in plasma urea to 20 mM/l or more, with relatively little rise in plasma creatinine. A plasma creatinine concentration of more than 250 μmol/l has a 90 per cent probability of being associated with renal impairment (Morgan *et al.* 1977). Similar disproportionate increases in plasma urea occur when protein catabolism is increased, as in infection, trauma, or steroid therapy. The clinical features in pre-renal failure are those of hypovolaemia, tachycardia, hypotension with a further postural drop, dehydration and poor peripheral perfusion. Since these signs will also be present after progression to acute tubular necrosis, criteria to distinguish the two are needed.

(i) *Urine microscopy*

In pre-renal failure the urine is typically free of cells, casts or protein. An exception is severe congestive heart failure, where pre-renal failure and proteinuria of 3 g/24 hours or more may occur. Once acute tubular necrosis has set in, the urinary sediment shows evidence of tubular damage: tubular cell casts, epithelial cells, moderate proteinuria, and occasional red cells and leucocytes.

(ii) *Urine composition*

In pre-renal uraemia the kidney retains the ability to re-absorb sodium (and thus water) and does so avidly in response to renal under-perfusion. Therefore, a small volume of urine is excreted with a low sodium concentration, high concentration of urea which is not re-absorbed and high osmolality. If

Table 27.2. Differentiation of pre-renal and established renal failure (adapted from Miller *et al.* 1978).

Investigation	Pre-renal uraemia	Acute renal failure (oliguric and non-oliguric)
Urine sodium mmol/l	< 20	> 40
Urine osmolality mosm/kg	> 500	< 400
Urine: plasma urea	> 15:1	< 10:1
Urine: plasma creatinine	> 40:1	< 20:1

established renal failure supervenes, renal concentrating capacity is abolished, urinary sodium concentration rises, that of urea falls and urine osmolality approaches that of plasma. Guidelines have been derived on this basis to distinguish pre-renal uraemia from acute tubular necrosis, though none are perfect. Those shown in Table 27.2 are derived from a study by Miller *et al.* (1978) and apply for both oliguric and non-oliguric acute renal failure. These indices will be obscured if mannitol or a diuretic has been given, as this will increase sodium concentration and reduce urine osmolality. In acute glomerulonephritis the electrolyte pattern may mimic pre-renal uraemia but urine microscopy will show many red cells and red cell casts (Miller *et al.* 1978).

Post-renal uraemia

Post-renal uraemia, although less common, must never be overlooked. It is immediately reversible, may indicate the presence of an unsuspected under-lying disease process, and if not diagnosed, an unnecessary renal biopsy may be performed. Post-renal uraemia is likely if there is complete anuria; the only other cause of this being bilateral renal arterial occlusion. Ureteric obstruction must be bilateral in order to cause post-renal failure. This happens relatively rarely with renal calculi and a single extra-ureteric disorder such as retroperitoneal fibrosis or endometriosis may be present. Haemorrhage from polycystic kidneys and debris from papillary necrosis may lead to obstruction. In addition, uric acid crystallization must be suspected in patients who obstruct following chemotherapy for tumours. The history may thus include symptoms of renal colic, prostatic disease in men, pelvic malignancy in women, or of back-ache typical of retroperitoneal fibrosis. In post-renal failure the urine is usually free of protein or cells, and it may show crystals or traces of papillary tissue.

Radiology

Radiological investigation is essential in acute renal failure, especially in excluding obstruction. The simplest way of doing this is by ultrasound examination for pelvicalyceal dilatation. This procedure should be performed first and followed only if necessary by a high dose intravenous pyelogram with tomography, the standard procedure (Fry and Cattell 1979). This will show kidney size, reveal the site of obstruction if present and suggests acute tubular necrosis if an immediate nephrogram but no excretory phase is seen. It must not be forgotten that high-dose pyelography may precipitate fluid overload and pulmonary oedema. There is now also good evidence of the development of contrast-induced oliguric acute renal failure in patients with diabetes, myeloma, or pre-existing renal failure, especially if dehydrated (Editorial, 1979).

Immediate management of pre-renal and post-renal failure

Pre-renal uraemia

As soon as this has been confirmed, renal perfusion must be restored urgently. By far the safest way, both to assess hypovolaemia and to correct it rapidly, is by means of a central venous pressure (CVP) line. The CVP will be low in pre-renal uraemia (unless due to cardiogenic shock) and should be maintained at 5–8 cm H_2O. This is achieved by infusion of 0.9 per cent sodium chloride with an initial challenge of 500 ml in thirty minutes, which is then increased or decreased as necessary: 2–3 litres may be required over a few hours. Once volume deficits are corrected, it is worth giving a loop diuretic (frusemide, bumetanide, or ethacrynic acid). These drugs increase renal cortical blood flow and there is some evidence, although not confirmed, that they may halt the onset of acute tubular necrosis (Tiller and Mudge 1980). An increase in urine volume to 40–50 ml/hour after administration of frusemide 80–120 mg i.v. supports the diagnosis of pre-renal uraemia. Hypertonic mannitol is also used in this context but has no advantages over frusemide and carries a risk of precipitating fluid overload. If urine output does not improve after volume repletion and diuretics, acute tubular necrosis may be assumed to be established. Even so, administration of high dose frusemide (250–500 mg i.v. six hourly for 24–48 hours) is recommended by some. This is relatively risk-free apart from ototoxicity and in some retrospective analyses (Cantarovitch et al. 1973) has shortened the time course of acute renal failure, although this is disputed. It is better established that high-dose frusemide administration may convert oliguric to non-oliguric acute renal failure (Anderson et al. 1977), which simplifies management. When pre-renal uraemia is a consequence of low cardiac output, inotropic support will be required rather than volume expansion; CVP and if possible left atrial pressure measurements using a Swann–Ganz catheter are essential to make this distinction. In such cases a dopamine infusion should be given (Henderson et al. 1980). In low doses (1–2 µg/kg/min) dopamine increases renal blood flow by direct renal dopaminergic vasodilatation and in higher doses (5–10 µg/kg/min) it increases cardiac output by activation of myocardial beta-adrenergic mechanisms. High doses (greater than 15 µg/kg/min) must be avoided; these cause hypertension through peripheral alpha-adrenergic vasoconstriction, reducing both cardiac output and renal perfusion. However, there may be benefit in using a combination of both frusemide and low-dose dopamine at the onset of acute oliguric renal failure (Lindner 1983). Clearly, acute tubular necrosis following on pre-renal failure is often only one consequence of serious trauma or systemic disease and such patients require full intensive care unit management.

Post-renal uraemia

If complete anuria is present and no evidence of post-renal obstruction is obtained radiographically, renal vascular occlusion must be suspected and immediate renal arteriography is required, especially in the context of arterial embolism or aortic disease or surgery. When obstruction has been confirmed as the cause of anuria, it must be relieved by the appropriate means. That is, bladder catheterization when the urethra is obstructed or in the case of ureteric obstruction, antegrade pyelography leading to percutaneous nephrostomy or alternatively, retrograde insertion of ureteric catheters at cystoscopy. Both procedures require urgent collaboration with radiological and urological colleagues. A marked natriuresis should be anticipated after relief of obstruction and very accurate replacement of daily fluid and electrolyte losses is needed.

Renal causes of acute uraemia

These are encountered less frequently than pre-renal or post-renal causes of renal failure. A careful history and clinical examination may point to the underlying disease and, here again, simple investigations are invaluable. In acute glomerulonephritis there may be a history of recent streptococcal infection and oedema is usually present, together with hypertension. The urine contains red cells and red cell casts, the anti-streptolysin O titre is usually raised and serum complement levels are reduced. A similar clinical picture with uraemia, oliguria, hypertension together with red cells and red cell casts in the urine may occur in rapidly progressive glomerulonephritis associated with systemic diseases, especially those exhibiting necrotizing vasculitis. These include polyarteritis nodosa, SLE and other collagen diseases. There will usually be extra-renal symptoms, such as fever, arthralgia, myalgia or abdominal pain. In these cases, urgent renal biopsy should be performed. Renal angiography is a diagnostic alternative in polyarteritis as it demonstrates arterial micro-aneurysms.

Renal function may deteriorate dramatically in rapidly progressive nephritis. It is important to establish the underlying diagnosis because several of these diseases may respond to specific therapy. For example, even advanced polyarteritis nodosa may regress on treatment with high doses of prednisolone and cyclophosphamide (Fauci *et al.* 1976). Goodpasture's syndrome is the likely diagnosis when a combination of dyspnoea, haemoptysis, haematuria and uraemia are all present. The diagnosis can be made rapidly by demonstrating anti-glomerular basement membrane antibodies in the serum (biopsy can thus be avoided) and treatment here is with urgent plasmapheresis and immunosuppression.

Renal biopsy should, in general, be performed if pre- and post-renal causes of acute uraemia have been excluded, the kidneys are not contracted in size and there are no contra-indications, such as one non-functioning kidney, thrombocytopaenia, or excessive bleeding tendency (McGonigle and Sharpstone 1980). If essential, the prolonged bleeding time present in uraemia may be temporarily shortened by infusion of cryoprecipitate (Janson *et al.* 1980).

Acute interstitial nephritis may also be diagnosed by renal biopsy. Recognition of this disorder is increasing. Usually, it develops as a result of a hypersensitivity reaction to drugs such as antibiotics (especially penicillins and sulphonamides) thiazides and non-steroidal anti-inflammatory agents (van Ypersele de Strihou 1979). Patients with this condition usually present with acute oliguric renal failure, sometimes with associated fever, poly-arthralgia and skin rash. Plasma and urinary eosinophilia may be present, together with an increase in plasma IgE levels. It is important not to miss this cause of uraemia, because a course of high-dose prednisolone therapy may produce a dramatic return of renal function.

Myoglobinuria caused by rhabdomyolysis secondary to trauma, viral infections or severe exercise may lead to acute oliguric renal failure (Koffler *et al.* 1976). However, the mechanism is unclear. Myoglobin is present in the urine and the plasma levels of creatine kinase and aldolase are very high as they are released from damaged muscles. Similarly, intravascular coagulation or haemolysis, from any cause, may rapidly lead to renal failure. If this is suspected, urgent haematological advice is required. Uraemia also often occurs late in the course of liver failure (hepatorenal syndrome). Furthermore, the co-existence of jaundice and uraemia should also suggest lepto-spirosis which must be excluded.

Management of established acute renal failure

Progressive uraemia is invariably fatal. Therefore, the first principle of management is to contact the nearest Renal Unit and, if necessary, transfer patients for dialysis well before the need for this becomes an emergency. Before this stage, good conservative management of acute renal failure centres on meticulous attention to several factors.

Potassium

Hyperkalaemia is an early, silent and very serious complication of acute oliguric renal failure; it may be unsuspected until asystole occurs. Plasma potassium levels must be measured at least daily and more frequently if the level is above 6 mmol/1. Dietary potassium should be limited to 30 mmol/day or less and no potassium supplements, or potassium-retaining diuretics (spironolactone, amiloride, triamterene) should be given in acute renal failure. Cardiac monitoring is essential but is *not* a substitue for plasma potassium measurements, as the absolute correlation between the two is poor. The ECG changes of hyperkalaemia are illustrated in Figure 27.1, together with the response to treatment. If the ECG shows QRS widening, indicating slowing of intraventricular conduction, or loss of P waves, emergency treatment of hyperkalaemia (Kunis and Lowenstein 1981) should be as follows:

(i) Calcium gluconate 1–2 g (10–20 ml 10 per cent solution) given as an i.v. bolus. This immediately counteracts the cardiac effects of potassium without lowering the plasma levels, although the mechanism is unclear.

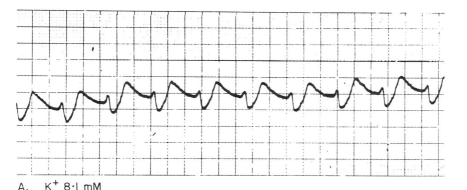

A.   K$^+$ 8·1 mM

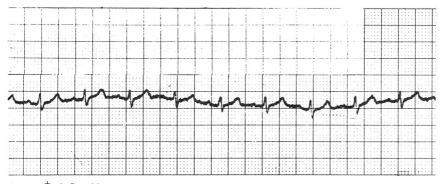

B.   K$^+$ 4·2 mM

Fig. 27.1. ECG changes (lead I) of acute hyperkalaemia in a forty year old woman with acute-on-chronic renal failure.
(A) At presentation. Note absent p waves, gross widening of QRS complex fusing with T wave.
(B) 30 min later, after immediate i.v. administration of 10 g calcium gluconate, 50 mmol sodium bicarbonate, 20 units insulin +25 g dextrose.

(ii) 50–100 ml of 4.2 per cent sodium bicarbonate given by rapid i.v. infusion. This produces a transient alkalosis which will, within minutes, move potassium from the extracellular to the intracellular compartment and lower potassium concentration significantly. This intracellular shift of potassium is augmented by the

(iii) administration of soluble insulin 20 units i.v. covered by the intravenous injection of 25–50 g dextrose (50–100 ml of 50 per cent solution). The effect of insulin and glucose commences after fifteen to twenty minutes and lasts for two to three hours. It is thus useful holding therapy but *not* the first treatment to give.

Ion exchange resins, e.g. calcium resonium 15–30 g t.d.s., orally or rectally, increase faecal excretion of potassium. They take several hours to act and should therefore be used prophylactically when plasma potassium approaches 6 mmol/l. After immediate control has been achieved, using the above measures, dialysis must be commenced as soon as possible.

Fluid and electrolyte balance

Together with hyperkalaemia, hypervolaemia leading to pulmonary oedema is the most serious immediate complication of acute oliguric renal failure. It must be avoided, since it can only be reversed by urgent dialysis. Once correct hydration is established, judged clinically and by CVP measurements, daily weights provide the simplest and safest guide for maintaining fluid balance; fluid charts are notoriously unreliable. The standard rule is to allow a fluid input (oral plus i.v.) of the previous twenty-four-hour measured output, urinary and gastro-intestinal, plus 500 ml to replace insensible loss. This approach is usually satisfactory but the input may need to be increased if the patient is pyrexial or has extensive burns. Daily intake of sodium is also regulated by the previous twenty-four hour output and usually should be less than 30 mmol/day. The presence of non-oliguric acute renal failure may complicate fluid and sodium intake; up to two litres daily of urine may be passed, with correspondingly higher fluid, sodium and even potassium requirements. There is no substitute for meticulous daily monitoring of all three.

Nutrition

Protein restriction to 30–40 g daily is needed in acute renal failure. This slows the development of uraemia. In addition, an intake of carbohydrate to provide 2000 calories daily is usually given to minimize the rate of endogenous protein catabolism. If necessary, these calories may be given by the parenteral route. There are exceptions to this rule. Profound negative nitrogen balance may delay wound healing and increase the risk of infection. If this is suspected, protein intake should be increased, especially if the patient is severely catabolic. In these cases it is usually best to begin dialysis, which allows a normal protein intake.

Infection

Septicaemia remains a major cause of death in acute renal failure (Kerr 1979). For this reason, indwelling intravenous lines and urinary catheters should be used only when essential. Scrupulous attention needs to be paid to these lines and catheters and to any superficial trauma, with frequent cultures from these sites and regular blood cultures. Any proven infection must of course be treated promptly with the appropriate antibiotic. Nevertheless, the cautions applying to antibiotic therapy that are outlined below should be noted.

Dialysis

Immediate dialysis may be required as an emergency if there are clinical indications such as pulmonary oedema or hyperkalaemia or complications of severe uraemia such as pericarditis or pre-coma. However, these usually occur only with blood urea concentrations of 50–80 mmol/l. Current practice is for dialysis to be commenced prophylactically well before this, with the aim of keeping blood urea concentrations below 30–35 mmol/l. Peritoneal dialysis is more widely available than haemodialysis but may not control uraemia in hypercatabolic patients. In addition, it is often complicated by peritonitis and it also elevates the diaphragm which increases the risk of respiratory complications. On the other hand, haemodialysis may not be possible if the blood pressure is too low and the need for heparinization will exacerbate any bleeding tendencies. Dialysis may be required even before pre-renal and post-renal causes of uraemia have been excluded. It is impossible to predict for how long it may be needed. The duration of the oliguric phase in acute renal failure is very variable, ranging from a few days to ten weeks or more (Kerr 1979).

Drugs

Many of the drugs required in patients with acute renal failure are excreted by the kidneys. They will inevitably accumulate, often with nephrotoxic or other serious side effects, unless both their dose and frequency of administration are reduced (Evans, 1980). In general, only drugs whose pharmacokinetics in renal failure are known should be used. The nephrotoxicity of the aminoglycosides, for example, is dose-related. Gentamicin is often needed in the treatment of septicaemia associated with acute renal failure and so its dosage regime must be carefully adjusted using frequent plasma levels. Cephaloridine should not be used as it may produce proximal tubular damage, especially in combinations with aminoglycosides or frusemide. Tetracyclines (except doxycycline) must not be used in any patient with impaired renal function, as they increase protein catabolism.

To conclude, the emergency treatment of acute renal failure requires sound diagnostic acumen both to identify reversible factors and to recognize the serious clinical and biochemical consequences of acute uraemia which may be present. The principles of conservative management may readily be applied in any clinical setting, but this must not obscure the need to seek specialist advice and if necessary to transfer patients for haemodialysis before the problems of severe uraemia arise.

Further reading

Anderson R.J., Linas S.L., Berns A.S., Henrich W.L., Miller T.R., Gabow P.A. and Schrier R.W. (1977) Non-oliguric acute renal failure. *New England Journal of Medicine* **296**, 1134–1138.

Cantarovitch F., Galli C., Benedetti L., Chena C., Castro L., Correa C., Loredo J.P., Fernandez J.C., Locatelli A. and Tizado J. (1973) High-dose frusemide in established acute renal failure. *British Medical Journal* **4**, 449–451.

Clarkson A.R. (1980) Acute renal failure. *Medicine* (Third Series) **25**, 1279–1284.

Curtis J.R., Eastwood J.B., Smith E.K.M., Storey J.M., Verroust P.J., de Wardener H.E., Wing A.J. and Wolfson E.M. (1969) Maintenance haemodialysis. *Quarterly Journal of Medicine* **38**, 49–89.

Dombey S.L., Sagar D. and Knapp M.S. (1975) Chronic renal failure in Nottingham and requirements for dialysis and transplant facilities. *British Medical Journal* **2**, 484–485.

Editorial. (1979) Radiocontrast-induced renal failure. *Lancet* **2**, 835.

Evans D.B. (1980) Drugs and the kidney. *British Journal of Hospital Medicine* **24**, 244–251.

Fauci A.S., Doppman J.L. and Wolff S.M. (1978) Cyclophosphamide-induced remissions in advanced polyarteritis nodosa. *American Journal of Medicine* **64**, 890–894.

Finckh E.S., Jeremy D. and Whyte H.M. (1962) Structural renal damage and its relation to clinical features in acute oliguric renal failure. *Quarterly Journal of Medicine* **31**, 429–446.

Fry I.K. and Cattell W.R. (1979) Radiological investigation of renal Disease. In Black, Sir Douglas and Jones, F.N. (eds). *Renal Disease*, pp. 219–269. Blackwell Scientific Publications, Oxford.

Henderson I.S., Beattie T.J. and Kennedy A.C. (1980) Dopamine hydrochloride in oliguric states. *Lancet* **2**, 827–828.

Janson P.A., Jubelirer S.J., Weinstein M.J. and Deykin D. (1980) Treatment of the bleeding tendency in uraemia with cryoprecipitate. *New England Journal of Medicine* **303**, 1318–1322.

Kerr D.N.S. (1979) Acute renal failure. In Black, Sir Douglas and Jones F.N. (eds). *Renal Disease*, pp. 437–493. Blackwell Scientific Publications, Oxford.

Koffler A., Friedler R.M. and Massry S.E. (1976) Acute renal failure due to non-traumatic rhabdomyolysis. *Annals of Internal Medicine* **85**, 23–28.

Kunis C.L. and Lowenstein J. (1981) The emergency treatment of hyperkalaemia. *The Medical Clinics of North America* **65**, 165–176.

Lindner A. (1983). Synergism of dopamine and furosemide in diuretic–resistant oliguric acute renal failure. *Nephron* **33**, 121–126.

McGonigle R. and Sharpstone P. (1980) Procedures in practice: kidney biopsy. *British Medical Journal* **1**, 547–549.

Miller T.R., Anderson R.J., Linas S.L., Henrich W.L., Berns A.S., Gabow P.A. and Schrier R.W. (1978) Urinary diagnostic indices in acute renal failure. *Annals of Internal Medicine* **89**, 47–50.

Morgan D.B., Carver M.E. and Payne R.B. (1977) Plasma creatinine and urea: creatinine ratio in patients with raised plasma urea. *British Medical Journal* **2**, 929–932.

Schrier R.W. and Conger J.D. (1980) Acute renal failure: pathogenesis, diagnosis and management. In Schrier, R.W. (ed). *Renal and Electrolyte Disorders*, pp. 375–408. Little Brown and Company, Boston.

Stewart J.H. (1967) Haemolytic anaemia in acute and chronic renal failure. *Quarterly Journal of Medicine* **36**, 85–105.

Tiller D.J. and Mudge G.H. (1980) Pharmacologic agents used in the management of acute renal failure. *Kidney International* **18**, 700–711.

van Ypersele de Strihou C. (1979) Acute oliguric interstitial nephritis. *Kidney International* **16**, 751–765.

28 · Diabetic Emergencies

ROBERT TURNER

Hyperglycaemic coma with ketosis

Diabetic keto-acidosis, in spite of modern therapy, can still have a consider-able mortality, particularly in the aged. Deaths are usually due to compli-cations, e.g. overwhelming infection, stroke, myocardial infarct, rather than to the primary metabolic disturbance. Nevertheless, unless patients receive vigilant care, unnecessary deaths can occur from electrolyte disturbances, hypoglycaemia, shock or induced heart failure.

Clinical diagnosis

An inexperienced doctor can be worried that it is difficult to discern hypo-glycaemia from hyperglycaemic coma. In reality, there is little difficulty, because although both have a tachycardia and coma, the former patient is perspiring and has a bounding pulse, whereas a diabetic coma patient is markedly dehydrated, has a tendency to have low blood pressure with thready pulse, and may have acidotic (Kussmaul) breathing. The ready availability of an immediate blood glucose assay with a glucose oxidase strip removes any lingering doubt (as long as one ensures the strip was correctly stored in an air-tight bottle, and if a meter is used that it is functioning correctly).

The term 'diabetic coma' is a misnomer, because most patients, although very sick, are not in coma and are only drowsy. Once a patient is in true coma, with no response to painful stimuli, the patient is unusually severely affected.

Clinical history

It is important to try to get details of the patient's insulin therapy if they are established diabetics. Most patients will carry details on a card or in their diary, but further information may be needed from a relative, friend or phone call to the patient's doctor. The duration of the current illness and specific symptoms are important. One particularly needs to find out if there have been any symptoms suggestive of infection, or other serious illness such as a heart attack or stroke which might have precipitated the 'coma'.

Previous diuretics may alert one to a greater need for potassium therapy than usual.

Clinical examination

A full examination is essential, including:

1. The *degree of dehydration* is particularly important, examining for a dry tongue and loss of skin turgor ('lift' a fold of skin on the neck, and see if it remains elevated). Once dehydration (in practice salt and water deficit) is apparent, the patient will have lost at least three litres of fluid. Marked dehydration signifies six or seven litres of fluid loss.

2. The *pulse rate, blood pressure* and the *temperature of the limbs* will indicate the severity of the cardiovascular disturbance. A low blood pressure and marked dehydration indicate a need for even more vigorous intravenous therapy than is usual. In old age, or a patient with a history of cardiac abnormality, *signs of heart failure* should be sought in spite of dehydration (raised jugular venous pressure, basal crepitations).

3. The *abdomen* needs to be examined to determine if the *bladder* is enlarged, as often occurs partly because of electrolyte disturbance. Most ill patients will have *absent bowel sounds* and an ileus.

4. *Evidence for infection,* including examination of the *chest,* inspection of the *pharynx* and *ear drums,* and if feasible obtaining *urine* for microscopy for white cells (as well as being sent to the laboratory for culture).

5. *Other causes of coma?* Even though the patient has obvious ketosis and dehydration of hyperglycaemic coma, it is prudent to ascertain if there might be a further cause for coma, such as *neck stiffness* indicating meningitis or subarachnoid haemorrhage, or the possibility of an overdose of drugs.

A *tender abdomen* is likely to be secondary to the 'ketosis', which can mimic 'peritonitis'. However, the possibility of intra-abdominal infection or acute pancreatitis needs to be considered. The patient will be too ill to operate on immediately, and signs of 'peritonism' usually disappear as the patient recovers from ketosis.

Investigations

(i) *Plasma glucose* concentration should be measured by the laboratory in addition to a rapid glucose oxidase 'stick' determination.

(ii) *Plasma potassium* is probably the most important investigation as untreated hypokalaemia, or over replacement leading to hyperkalaemia, can be lethal. The presenting potassium value is usually high, even in the presence of total body deficit, because of the acidosis *(vide infra)*.

These are easily the two most important investigations, and others, whilst advisable, are not so essential.

(iii) An arterial puncture for *blood gases* can be taken for measurement of pH, PO_2 and PCO_2. A pH down to 7.1 causes little anxiety, but if the pH is 6.8 or 6.9, it may be dangerous *(vide infra)*.

(iv) A raised *blood urea* can be due to pre-renal rather than renal failure. A plasma creatinine will give slightly better indication as to whether there may be long-standing renal failure.

(v) A *plasma sodium* is usually normal or low, but may be raised with severe 'dehydration' from a prolonged presentation.

Potential causes of death

The major disasters one needs to avoid are:

1. *Insufficient intravenous (i.v.) fluid* to replace deficit, so hypotension is prolonged (although care needs to be taken not to over-transfuse to provoke heart failure).

2. *Inadequate care of unconscious patient,* and inhalation of vomit.

3. Too much insulin therapy leading to *hypoglycaemia* (it is unusual to have difficulty in lowering the blood glucose).

4. Insufficient potassium therapy, leading to *hypokalaemia.*

5. Non-recognition of *renal-failure,* and need to modify fluid therapy.

6. *Inadequate therapy of infection* which precipitated the coma.

Therapy

Intravenous fluids

The immediate threat to the patient is usually 'shock' because of the grossly depleted circulating volume from a prolonged osmotic diuresis, possibly aided by vomiting. Therefore, the most important therapy is *prompt replacement* by intravenous fluids. If a patient is markedly 'dehydrated', and in the order of six litres in deficit, one can aim to give three litres in the first hour. Some doctors feel that giving 500 ml in one hour is rapid replacement, compared with the usual 500 ml in four hours in a surgical ward. This is inappropriately slow if the patient is hypotensive. It may be necessary to have two infusions to give sufficient intravenous fluid. If the blood pressure is virtually unmeasurable, initial treatment with a plasma expander, such as 'Haemaccel', helps to keep the initial fluid replacement in the vascular volume rather than releasing it into the intracellular tissues and the cells.

Intravenous saline

This constitutes the major therapy. The plasma sodium can be either less than normal, normal or raised, the latter being unusual. 'Normal saline' contains 154 mmol/l sodium, and as some of the water enters the cells the plasma sodium is bound to rise on therapy. It probably does not matter if this increases even to 160 mmol/l, as it may be advantageous in preventing cerebral oedema *(vide infra)* and is probably not harmful.

If a patient is nearly fully conscious but hyperglycaemic and dehydrated, there can be a temptation to try to give oral fluids. This should be avoided, as it is difficult to replete the lost sodium and potassium orally, and vomiting is often induced. Prompt i.v. fluids allows the patient to recover faster than with oral therapy.

Potassium

Following the osmotic diuresis, the patient is inevitably potassium-deficient. However, because of the concomitant acidosis, the plasma potassium is often normal, or even high, at presentation. The treatment with insulin lowers the plasma potassium, and treatment with alkali *(vide infra)*, correcting an acid-base disturbance, will also tend to lower the plasma potassium. As a general rule it is probably not necessary to give potassium in the first hour, unless the ECG happens to show marked hypokalaemia changes (usually due to previous diuretic therapy).

By the first hour the plasma potassium will have been measured, and if it is normal or only slightly high (e.g. less than 6 mmol/l) potassium therapy can be started with 20 mmol potassium chloride per litre. This rate of potassium can usually be continued throughout the period of intravenous fluid therapy. If the plasma potassium is low (less than 4 mmol/l) then 40 mmol per litre potassium should be given.

Insulin

Therapy with insulin, to prevent even more marked hyperglycaemia and more marked ketosis, is instituted after setting up intravenous fluids. Give a pure form of soluble insulin, human or pork, e.g. Humulin S, Actrapid, Velosulin, as one does not wish to unnecessarily stimulate anti-insulin antibody production with a beef insulin. The insulin can be given in several ways:

1. Constant intravenous infusion

This is the most reliable method of insulin therapy and is best given by a syringe pump. It is usually stated that the insulin should be dissolved in a protein containing buffer such as a gelatin solution usually available as a plasma expander (e.g. Haemaccel), to prevent the insulin sticking to the glass or plastic tubing. In practice, the amount of insulin stuck to tubing is small, and as one is in any case going to adjust the insulin infusion rate to the plasma glucose response, any insulin that is lost will be compensated for. Nevertheless, if a gelatin solution is available, it is prudent to use it.

The average patient will need six units/hour to lower the plasma glucose concentration to normal. The normal basal insulin production rate is in the order 1–1.5 u/h. The 6 u/h virtually completely inhibits new glucose production from the liver, but has little effect on increasing glucose uptake by the periphery. Because of this, the plasma glucose tends to fall very predictably at approximately 4 mmol/l per hour, this being due to the normal glucose uptake by the periphery. If a patient has been very dehydrated, and large amounts of intravenous fluids have been given, the plasma glucose can initially fall at a greater rate than this. This simple prediction of the rate of glucose response allows one, in most patients, to delay taking a further sample for laboratory estimation of plasma glucose concentration for two hours, to check that the response is as expected. In practice, it is optimal to ask the nurse to take a finger tip capillary blood sample every hour (obtained with an Autolet or similar device) to measure the glucose concentration with a glucose oxidase 'strip' at the same time as she measures the pulse and blood pressure. This assists in assessing response to therapy, and the laboratory sample is a check on the ward measurement.

2. Intramuscular insulin

If a syringe pump is not available, and the patient is not 'shocked', adequate insulin delivery is obtained by giving 20 u soluble insulin intramuscularly (i.m.), followed by 6 u i.m. every hour. It is advisable to check that the nurse realizes that intramuscular injections, with an approx. 3 cm needle are intended, rather than the usual subcutaneous route with a short needle. The muscles are fairly well perfused with moderate 'dehydration', and the insulin absorbed even though the skin is 'shut-down'. If the patient initially has a moderately low blood pressure, an initial intravenous bolus of 10 u soluble insulin can also be given, to act whilst the intramuscular insulin is being absorbed.

3. Intravenous insulin to intravenous fluids

Insulin is sometimes put into the i.v. saline being infused to treat dehydration. This has a disadvantage that changing rates of fluid requirement also change the dose of insulin delivered. In addition, insulin diluted into a large volume of fluid tends to stick to the plastic container to a greater extent than in a small fluid volume in a syringe pump. Whilst many patients have been treated by this method, a better alternative is probably to give i.v. insulin boluses hourly into the drip set to the patient. The short plasma half-life of insulin (four minutes) makes this unphysiological, but in practice insulin has an effect on insulin receptors for at least thirty minutes, and this form of therapy is remarkably effective. However, steady infusion of insulin or the intramuscular route is preferred.

Arterial pH

This is the least important of the initial investigations because of the uncertainty of the desirability of treating acidosis unless the pH is very low (i.e. less than seven). The insulin therapy prevents further efflux of free fatty acids from adipose tissue for oxidation to ketone bodies in the liver, and in any case the acidosis will improve as the muscles and brain utilize the ketone bodies.

There are three possible disadvantages of giving bicarbonate therapy unless it is essential:

(i) Rapid restoration of a normal pH causes an influx of potassium into cells, and can temporarily induce marked plasma hypokalaemia leading to cardiac dysfunction.

(ii) The oxygen-dissociation curve of haemoglobin is more or less in a normal position when the patient presents in diabetic coma, as it is affected by two conflicting influences, being moved to the right by acidosis and to the left by reduced 2,3-diphosphoglycerate (2,3 DPG) which is a marked feature of red cells in diabetic keto-acidosis. Treatment of acidosis thus causes the curve to shift to the left under the influence of the still reduced 2,3 DPG. This means that the haemoglobin has greater affinity for oxygen and will tend to release less oxygen to hypoxic tissues. If there is markedly reduced perfusion of an organ, this increased haemoglobin affinity may become critical in the supply of oxygen to that organ.

(iii) The infused bicarbonate does not cross the blood–brain barrier, but diffused $P\mathrm{CO}_2$ can paradoxically decrease the pH of the CSF. This is not known to affect cerebral function, although it has been wondered if it might in some patients lead to cerebral oedema. No causal link has been demonstrated and this is the least important reason for withholding bicarbonate.

In practice, one only needs to treat a low pH if

(i) the patient is obviously distressed by over-breathing, or

(ii) the pH is less than seven, in which case the buffering capacity of plasma proteins is nearly exhausted and any sudden disturbance of circulation, e.g. by cardiac dysrrhythmia or temporary hypotension, may cause excessive acidosis and death. In addition, cardiac contractability may be less good with a pH of < 7, although cardiac muscle metabolizes ketone bodies preferentially to glucose. The blood pressure does not obviously rise in patients with acidosis who are given bicarbonate therapy.

If the pH is less than seven, 50–100 mmol sodium bicarbonate can be given by i.v. infusion over twenty minutes. In view of the effect of lowering the plasma potassium, 20 mmol potassium chloride can be added to the infusion. The pH can be rechecked, and the infusion repeated if the pH is less than seven.

Care of unconscious patient

When a patient initially presents, it is difficult not to have him lying on his back whilst blood samples are being taken and intravenous drips set up. If the patient is unconscious, care must be taken to ensure that an *airway is maintained* at all times. At the earliest opportunity the patient must be put into a *lateral position.*

A major cause of concern is the possibility of the patient vomiting, as the electrolyte disturbance often leads to an ileus. The stomach usually contains a litre of stale fluid, which often has the appearance of altered blood. This fluid can be suddenly and catastrophically vomited and inhaled. Thus, if the patient is unconscious, particularly if there is an absent gag reflex, it is important that a *naso-gastric tube* is inserted at an early opportunity, so that the gastric contents can be aspirated before the patient has an opportunity to vomit.

Monitoring urine output, and risk of renal 'shut-down'

Patients present dehydrated and therefore pass little urine during the first two hours of admission. However, the electrolyte disturbances sometimes induce a large atonic bladder in the absence of bladder neck obstruction or prostatic disease.

If the patient is conscious, there is usually no need to insert a urinary catheter. The patient will soon start to urinate following repletion of the fluid deficit.

If the patient is unconscious, particularly if there is an atonic bladder, it is advantageous to pass a catheter at an early stage to monitor the urine output. In practice, it is unusual for a patient to be sufficiently ill that catheterization is indicated.

If after three hours, a semi-conscious patient is not passing urine, then he needs to be catheterized to determine if there is *renal 'shut-down'*. It is important to determine this because:

(i) If there is renal shut-down, particular caution needs to be taken that the correct amount of fluid is given and the patient is not 'over-transfused'.

(ii) Care needs to be taken that hyperkalaemia does not develop.
Patients in diabetic coma have hyperaldesteronism because of the fluid depletion and excrete large amounts of urine potassium even as lost fluid volume is being repleted. If a patient does not pass urine, there is an increased risk that the potassium will either not fall or will even rise with usual replacement doses, possibly leading to dangerously high plasma potassium concentrations. Thus, if there is 'renal shut-down' the amount of potassium in the intravenous fluid needs to be either reduced or stopped, and repeated plasma potassium measurements must be made.

Control of intravenous fluids—central venous line

In a fit young person, even if excess intravenous fluid is given, it will be excreted in the urine without any problem. However, if the patient is elderly, if there has been a history of heart failure, or if there has been 'renal shut-down', over-transfusion can lead to marked heart failure. This can, to a certain extent, be prevented by putting up a central venous manometer to assess the right heart filling pressure. It is usually safe to transfuse a patient until the central venous pressure (CVP) is approximately 10–12 cm water above the mid-axillary line. This will not exclude the risk of left heart failure, as this can occur from a dysfunctioning left ventricle even though the right heart filling pressures are normal. However, measurement of the CVP does prevent over-filling of the circulation and excessive increase of the right heart pressures, so that patients are not unnecessarily put into left heart failure.

Treatment of occult infection

A large proportion, approximately 50 per cent, of patients who present in diabetic 'coma' have no obvious reason for their metabolic deterioration. In some of these it may have been induced by virus infection, in others by an occult bacterial infection. The normal variables by which bacterial infection is detected are not appropriate in diabetic coma. The metabolic disturbance means that most patients become hypothermic, even if they have marked septicaemia. The patients become febrile as their fluid is repleted. The metabolic disturbance itself causes a raised white count, even up to 30,000 neutrophils $\times 10^6$, in the absence of infection.

If a cause of the loss of diabetes control is not apparent, it is important to search for infection including the inspection of the throat and eardrums in children. In addition, it is prudent to do three blood cultures and take a urine sample for microscopy and culture. If an obvious infection is apparent, then the appropriate antibiotic should be given. If none is apparent, patients should probably receive an antibiotic, such as amoxycillin, with or without flucloxacillin or erythromycin. Some physicians say this is not necessary.

Phosphate or magnesium

Patients presenting with diabetic coma always have a low plasma phosphate and a low plasma magnesium. It has been suggested that the patient should receive intravenous phosphate, partly to replete the 2,3 DPG to make normal the haemoglobin oxygen dissociation curve. It has also been suggested that repletion of the magnesium may similarly help. However, controlled studies of these additions have not shown any clinical benefit. Whilst one can make an academic case for including them, this adds an extra complexity to the management of the patient. It is probably more important to concentrate on the important facets of the disease rather than spend time thinking about these factors.

Risk of thrombosis

A proportion of patients, particularly the elderly, either develop a stroke or heart attack, or occasionally have peripheral gangrene. The marked dehydration and blood hyperviscosity, together with increased platelet stickiness associated with the poorly controlled diabetes, makes it likely that these are secondary events (although in some patients one wonders if an occult infarct might have precipitated the metabolic disturbance). It is sometimes wondered if a seriously ill patient should receive full anticoagulant therapy with intravenous heparin to prevent such complications. However, some patients do bleed with this therapy, and a controlled study of the benefits and risks is needed.

Cerebral oedema

This is characterized by a patient who was unconscious, then wakes up and subsequently has a deteriorating conscious level. A possible mechanism is that the brain still has high glucose and sorbitol concentrations following the hyperglycaemia, and that a lower circulating plasma glucose causes an osmotic shift of fluid into the brain. It is thus probably prudent to lower the plasma glucose to beneath the urine threshold, but not down to normal (*vide infra*). Similarly, an elevation of the plasma sodium to 160 mmol/l by infusing 0.9 g/dl saline (154 mmol/l) is probably advantageous rather than disadvantageous. If the level is above this, 'half strength' saline can be given to prevent marked hypernatraemia.

Therapy after 4–6 hours

Usually the blood glucose concentration comes down to about 12 mmol/l at the same time as the patient's fluid depletion has been treated.

One aims to lower the plasma glucose concentration to approximately 10–12 mmol/l, and not right down to a normal 4 or 5 mmol/l. Thus, there is little risk of inducing hypoglycaemia, which can be difficult to recognize in an unconscious patient. In addition, it is conceivable that this moderate therapy lessens the risk of developing cerebral oedema.

Once the plasma glucose has been lowered to 10–12 mmol/l, the insulin infusion can be reduced to 1.5 or 2 u/h, and the dose altered according to two-hourly then four-hourly blood glucose measurements. At the same time the infusion of normal saline can usually be reduced to 500 ml every four hours, as the patient's fluid loss has been repleted. The infusion can be changed to '4 per cent dextrose with 1/5 normal saline' to provide some calories regularly and some sodium chloride. The potassium should be continued, usually at 20 mmol/l, as it can take days to replete the intracellular potassium reserves. Once intravenous fluids have been stopped, oral potassium, e.g. Slow K 2 tablets four times daily) can be continued.

If the insulin was given intramuscularly, once the plasma glucose has reduced to 10–12 mmol/l, insulin can be changed to 6 u subcutaneously (s.c.) four-hourly. This is less than the above dose recommended for i.v. infusion, as the muscles will still contain a reservoir of insulin which will be released over the next few hours. The dose can be altered according to two-hourly blood glucose measurements using glucose-oxidase strips.

Subsequent therapy and insulin requirements

If the patient presented with ketosis, this signified little or no insulin secretion. Thus, the patient will need full insulin replacement therapy, at least initially. A newly-presenting patient will have some beta cell reserve which will recover over the next four weeks as the plasma glucose is lowered, and the 'honeymoon period' of moderately low insulin requirements is entered.

If the patient is being treated by subcutaneous injections, for a man of normal weight one would anticipate initially 32–36 u/day as a basal requirement (which can be provided by ultralente insulin) and in the order of 16–24 u soluble insulin for breakfast and 12–18 u soluble for dinner (although less may be needed initially if small meals are taken). In a previously treated person, the normal insulin requirement will indicate how much insulin might be needed. An obese person may need more than a non-obese person. If no long-acting insulin had previously been used, and one wishes to provide the basal requirement with ultralente, an initial loading dose of three times the estimated dose will be needed for the first dose only.

For all regimens, blood glucose levels before each meal (breakfast, lunch, dinner and before bed) and preferably also at three a.m. will be needed to assess control, and doses altered according to the response. When a newly-presenting patient is sent home, instructions concerning reducing the dose as the 'honeymoon period', is entered can be given.

Re-education

Admission of a known-diabetic in ketotic coma signifies a lack of proper education and diabetes care, as such gross episodes should be avoidable. The patient should be taught how to monitor blood glucose levels when ill and how to appropriately increase insulin therapy if needed. If a patient is too ill to eat, he usually needs more basal insulin requirement even if insulin is not needed to cover a meal. If he is vomiting and cannot take food, early advice should be sought, particularly if the patient has ketonuria. If needed, early admision to hospital can be arranged before the patient enters ketotic coma.

The management of diabetic coma is summarized in Table 28.1.

Hyperglycaemic non-ketotic coma

This type of coma usually occurs in elderly patients who have type II, non-insulin-dependent diabetes. This is usually not previously diagnosed and an intercurrent infection often precipitates the illness. The patients are always dehydrated and have usually taken several days to become ill. However, patients with renal disease, who cannot excrete glucose easily and who early in the course of the disease have renal 'shut-down', can develop the syndrome in two days.

The syndrome's main difference from classical ketotic coma is the lack of ketosis, which is probably because the gross hyperglycaemia maintains a moderate insulin output sufficient to prevent ketone body formation. The term 'hyper-osmolar' which is often used, is equally appropriate to ketotic and non-ketotic coma. In both, the raised glucose (and often urea) makes them 'hyper-osmolar'. Patients with non-ketotic coma more frequently present with hypernatraemia, but this can happen in both types of coma.

The management is identical to 'ketotic coma', except that the patients tend to be more insulin-sensitive, and with prompt rehydration the plasma glucose can fall at 8 mmol/l per hour rather than the usual 4 mmol/l per hour. The patients are more likely to have renal 'shut-down', are more likely to be provoked into heart failure (and thus need to have a prophylactic central venous catheter inserted) and to have a thrombotic complication such as peripheral gangrene. Elderly patients can remain semi-comatose or confused for a week. After insulin therapy for a few days or weeks, the patients can usually be managed by diet or tablet therapy.

Table 28.1. Summary of management of diabetic coma

History—including previous insulin therapy, any indication of an intercurrent illness or infection which precipitated the illness.

Examination—particularly degree of 'dehydration', blood pressure, pulse, abdomen. Look at chest, throat, ears for source of infection.

If diagnosis suspected—confirm with finger-prick glucose-oxidase strip.

Blood tests for laboratory
  —glucose
  —potassium (also urea, sodium, creatinine—but not urgent)
  —blood count (W.B.C. always raised!)
  —blood cultures if infection suspected (even if hypothermic—as hyperglycaemia inhibits fever)
  —arterial blood for pH, PCO_2, PO_2.
If available—*urine* for microscopy and culture.

Therapy
1. *i.v. fluids*—154 mmol/l saline—up to 3 litres in first hour.
   After first hour, add 20 mmol/l potassium chloride (as long as plasma potassium less than 6 or no hyperkalaemia on ECG).
   Increase to 40 mmol/l if plasma potassium less than 3.5 mmol/l.
   Put up *C.V.P.* to monitor i.v. fluids if history of heart failure or patient aged.
   If hypotension a problem, infuse a plasma expander, e.g. Haemaccel, and put up a second drip to replace lost fluid more quickly.
2. *Insulin*—either (i) 6 u/hour human or pork purified soluble insulin dissolved in 'Haemaccel'.
   or (ii) 20 u intramuscular stat followed by 6 u every hour i.m. (add 10 u i.v. at start if blood pressure low).
3. *Sodium bicarbonate*—only if pH less than 7. Infuse 50 or 100 mmol $NaHCO_3$, with added 20 mmol potassium chloride i.v. over 20 minutes. Then repeat pH, and repeat if pH still less than 7.
4. **Take care of unconscious patient**
   (a) Put in left lateral position.
   (b) If semiconscious, put in nasogastric tube to aspirate stomach at earliest opportunity.
5. If no urine by 4 hours, *catheterize bladder*.
6. Treat for bacterial infection (or for Q fever, mycoplasma etc.) with erythromycin if an occult infection is possible. Take 3 blood cultures first.

Subsequent therapy
Ask nurse *hourly* to measure blood pressure, pulse, finger-prick glucose-oxidase blood glucose.
Check laboratory plasma glucose and potassium at 2 hours and usually at 4 hours.
Blood glucose will usually have fallen at 4 mmol/l per hour. Once 10–12 mmol/l, reduce i.v. insulin to 2 u/hour, or stop i.m. insulin and change to 6 u 4-hourly s.c. When patient is eating, change i.v. insulin to subcutaneous infusion or injections.
At the same time the patient's fluid loss has usually been repleted, and change to '4 per cent dextrose and 1/5 normal saline' if available, otherwise give 5 per cent dextrose and i.v. saline as needed for 'dehydration'. Continue 20 mmol KCl to every litre altering amount according to plasma potassium. Continue oral potassium for 5 days.

Hypoglycaemia

A patient with suspected hypoglycaemia should have an immediate finger-prick blood glucose estimated to confirm the diagnosis. 30 ml of 50 per cent glucose can be injected intravenously. It is very important that the needle should be kept in place, afterwards for a minute or two, to allow blood to infuse through the vein to wash the glucose into the circulation. Indeed, if available, it is advantageous to follow the glucose by 20 ml 0.154 M saline. These precautions are needed to prevent venous thrombosis, which can occur if the needle-syringe are immediately withdrawn, as pressure on the vein then keeps the irritative glucose in the vein.

If the patient fails to become conscious, the finger-prick blood glucose assay should be repeated and more intravenous glucose given if required. If the patient fails to recover in spite of hyperglycaemia, secondary cerebral oedema is a possibility, and intravenous dexamethasone 4 mg can be given.

If a suitable vein for i.v. glucose cannot be obtained, 1 mg of glucagon i.m. will usually cause sufficient plasma glucose rise after ten to fifteen minutes for oral glucose to be given.

A patient who has been unconscious for several hours may take some time to return to full consciousness. The longer the prolongation of coma, the greater the chance there is for some cerebral deficit to have occurred.

Further reading

Hosker J.P. and Turner R.C. (1982) Insulin treatment of newly-presenting ketotic diabetic patients into the honeymoon period. *Lancet* **ii**, 633–635.

Johnston D.G. and Alberti K.G.M.M. (1980) Diabetic emergencies: practical aspects of the management of diabetic keto-acidosis and diabetes during surgery. *Clinics in Endocrinology and Metabolism* **9**, 437–460.

Kreisberg R.A., Kitabchi A.E., Burhen G.E., Carroll H.J. and Ol M.S. (1982) *Diabetes Mellitus and Obesity*. Eds. Brodoff B.N. and Bleicher S.J. Williams and Wilkins. pp. 56–551.

Schade D.S., Eaton P.R., Alberti K.G.M.M. and Johnston D.G. (1981) *Diabetic coma: keto-acidotic and hyperosmolar*. University of Mexico Press, Albuquerque.

29 · Commoner Endocrine Emergencies

C. W. BURKE

Acute cortisol insufficiency

The clinical setting

Acute cortisol insufficiency may be the cause of, or a complication of, a presenting emergency. The clinical features of cortisol insufficiency are consistent but non-specific; so that the diagnosis of this life-threatening but eminently treatable condition depends on disentangling the pattern from clinical 'red herrings'. As a result, the diagnosis is more often suspected than confirmed, yet it regularly fails to be recognized with fatal results.

The clinical settings in which it occurs may be divided into three. The most obvious is pituitary suppression by pharmacological doses of steroids; either the patient's steroid therapy has been interrupted or the patient is being overwhelmed by intercurrent illness without the necessary increase in the steroid dose being made. This state of affairs should be obvious from the history. However, there are some patients who cannot communicate their steroid-dependence and may not be carrying a warning card. Therefore, positive enquiry should always be made if there are features consistent with steroid insufficiency in any urgent case, medical or surgical. Steroid therapy does not always disable hypothalamic-pituitary adrenocorticotrophic hormone (ACTH) function: alternate-day steroid therapy causes little suppression (Burke 1978). Any subject with healthy function to start with will show a prompt recovery of ACTH function within a couple of days after a short (less than three weeks) course of even daily steroids, whatever the dose. The effect on the pituitary depends on the combination of daily dose and duration of administration, as well as upon the susceptibility of the individual: approximate guidelines are given in Table 29.1.

A second clinical setting in which acute steroid insufficiency occurs is as a complication of another acute illness by adrenal infarction or sepsis. Infarction is classically associated with meningococcal septicaemia, especially in children (Waterhouse–Friedrichsen syndrome, 'adrenal apoplexy'). It is also seen in several other conditions of shock such as fulminant infections, burns, trauma and so on (*Lancet* 1976). The importance of this may be over-emphasized as infarction found at necropsy may be an agonal event rather than be functionally important ante-mortem. Where ante-mortem plasma cortisol levels have been measured in cases of adrenal infarction they

Table 29.1. Approximate guidelines for duration of pituitary ACTH suppression after steroid therapy

Steroid dose and duration (mg/day of prednisolone)	Likely duration of ACTH suppression	
	Total suppression	Limited stress response
Alternate day therapy, any dose	Little suppression	In occasional patients only, for few weeks only
Less than 3 weeks, any dose	2–3 days	3–5 days
6 weeks, replacement dose (7.5 mg/d or less)	2 days	Up to 5 days
3 months, replacement dose (7.5 mg/day or less)	Up to 1 week	Up to 1½ weeks
3 months, 20 mg/day or more	Up to 1 month	Up to 3 months
6 months; 10 mg/day or more	Up to 3 months	Up to 6 months
over 6 months, 10 mg/day or more	Up to 6 months	Up to 12 months

have surprisingly often been 'normal' (that is appropriately elevated). Septic infarcts and micro-abscesses may contribute to steroid insufficiency in severe septicaemias, especially in those due to staphylococcal infections and occasionally also in septicaemia due to bacterial endocarditis. Whether or not steroid insufficiency commonly results from such causes, the possibility of it certainly occurs commonly and requires appropriate action.

Infarction of the pituitary with resulting cortisol insufficiency is not common and is virtually confined to two situations. First, infarction of the hyperplastic pituitary of pregnancy may occur due to shock as a result of post-partum haemorrhage (Sheehan's syndrome, very rare). Secondly, it may occur in the presence of pre-existing (if unrecognized) pituitary disease. In the latter situation, 'pituitary apoplexy' occasionally presents, usually with meningeal symptoms or at least headache, resembling subarachnoid haemorrhage or meningitis. If steroid deficiency develops, the patient then becomes shocked and may be misdiagnosed as having meningitis with septicaemia. However, this is an uncommon problem.

The third clinical setting in which acute cortisol insufficiency is seen is when some crisis overtakes a patient with subacute or chronic destruction of the adrenals or pituitary. It is most unusual for primary cortisol insufficiency due to either cause to present acutely without some clue in the history. In cases of primary adrenal disease, there is nearly always a background of symptoms such as weakness, weight loss and unexplained gastro-intestinal disturbance. In pituitary disease, there is usually a background of reproductive failure. However, occasionally insidious panhypopituitarism may advance to the point where it is misdiagnosed as primary hypothyroidism, when incautious thyroxine substitution may precipitate acute adrenal insufficiency. In addition, sudden thyroxine therapy in severe primary hypothyroidism may rarely unmask the hypothyroidism of the adrenals. The acute crisis in patients with chronic cortisol insufficiency is most commonly precipitated by infection, trauma or dehydration.

In Britain, most cases of subacute or chronic adrenal failure are due to auto-immune 'adrenalitis'. Bayliss (1980) quotes the proportion as being two-thirds, but bases this on a study now fifteen years old (Mason 1968) and the figure should probably now be put much higher (Irvine and Barnes 1972). Most British endocrinologists would have difficulty in remembering more than a couple of recent cases of Addison's disease due to other causes. As well as infarction, these causes include tumour metastases (especially from lung, breast and ovary) and any kind of disseminated fungal, protozoal or granulomatous disease. (The latter are much less rare causes in countries where such infections occur more regularly.) Nowadays, acute cortisol insufficiency in the United Kingdom seldom occurs as a complication of undiagnosed Addison's disease due to tuberculosis. However, the possibility is always there.

Clinical features

Hypoglycaemia

Hypoglycaemia is a regular feature of acute cortisol insufficiency and it is especially common when (as in hypopituitarism) there is growth hormone deficiency in addition. Children (especially babies, as in those with congenital adrenal hyperplasia) and alcoholics are particularly liable to hypoglycaemia when steroid-deficient.

Gastro-intestinal symptoms

Gastro-intestinal symptoms are a dominant feature of cortisol insufficiency, whether it is acute or chronic. Acutely, the order of frequency of these symptoms is: anorexia, nausea, vomiting, diarrhoea and abdominal pain.

Hypotension, hypovolaemia and shock

Postural hypotension, often asymptomatic, is a frequent sign. After taking a lying blood pressure, the patient should (if possible) be standing for two minutes before the standing reading is made, as in mild steroid insufficiency the fall in blood pressure may not be immediate. As acute steroid insufficiency progresses, with its associated circulatory and electrolyte changes, many patients develop non-postural hypotension and later frank clinical shock and tachycardia. The onset of dehydration and shock will occur sooner if salt is lost either due to vomiting or in the urine. However, like Bayliss (1980), I have been caught out by a 'normal' blood pressure in a steroid-deficient patient who had essential hypertension.

Fever

Fever is regularly a sign in cortisol insufficiency even in the absence of infection. The mechanism is unknown.

Myalgia and cramps

Myalgia and cramps are features of acute cortisol insufficiency.

Vitiligo

Vitiligo is associated with auto-immune Addison's disease only, and will not usually be present in other forms of adrenal failure.

Pigmentation

Pigmentation due to pituitary peptides that are released with ACTH is found in patients who have had an adrenalectomy for Cushing's syndrome and in a few cases of Addison's disease. Older books give an impression of patients with Addison's disease as showing a progressive illness of weakness and pigmentation, punctuated by gastro-intestinal episodes and culminating in Addisonian crisis. Pigmentation in the Addisonian patients that I have seen in recent years has been trivial or absent; indeed some have shown a translucent-skinned appearance like that of hypopituitarism. In any case, pigmentation implies chronicity and will not be seen in acute adrenal destruction. When present, pituitary pigmentation is unmistakable, affecting the palmar creases, other skin creases, the buccal mucosa, exposed areas and scars.

Pseudohypo-adrenalism

'Pseudohypo-adrenalism' refers to patients with wasting disorders, pigmentation, hypotension and hyponatraemia not due to Addison's disease. Examples of these are tuberculosis, lung tumours especially with vasopressin excess, steatorrhoea and chronic renal failure. This subject is reviewed by Burke (1978) and Irvine and Barnes (1972).

Laboratory findings

Plasma cortisol

A sample of blood for cortisol assay should always be drawn from any patient suspected of having cortisol insufficiency, regardless of the circumstances and before any treatment is given. If the result comes back higher than 600 nmol/l or so, it shows that the original suspicion was incorrect. However, that is the only place of cortisol assays in the casualty department, for the following reasons:

(i) The normal range is from as low as 80 nmol/l at night rising to 700 in the early morning and up to 1000 or more in acutely ill people.

(ii) Steroid-deficient patients may have plasma cortisol levels up to 400 and rarely 500 nmol/l.

(iii) The result will not be available in time to save the steroid-deficient patient, who must receive immediate treatment based on clinical suspicion.

When the diagnosis of Addison's disease is likely, it can be confirmed by drawing simultaneous blood samples for cortisol and ACTH in the casualty department before treating the patient. The later demonstration that the ACTH was inappropriately high in relation to a normal or low cortisol level then requires only the measurement of adrenal antibodies to establish that the patient has auto-immune Addison's disease.

Clearly, when a steroid-deficient patient has recovered, cortisol assays will be required to confirm the diagnosis; under tetracosactrin stimulation to prove primary adrenal disease and in response to insulin hypoglycaemia to prove ACTH deficiency.

The commonest laboratory abnormality

The commonest laboratory abnormality in acute cortisol insufficiency is a moderate elevation of blood urea (e.g. 8–15 mmol/l).

Electrolytes

Electrolytes change late: hyperkalaemia combined with hyponatraemia is more suggestive than either alone. In acute cases there will not be time to show sodium loss in the urine which is inappropriate to the low serum sodium. In any case, this is also a feature of other conditions that may clinically resemble steroid insufficiency, for example ectopic vasopressin production and salt-losing renal disease.

The importance of not overlooking azotaemia is great; a boy recently admitted with weight loss and hyponatraemia was misdiagnosed as having chronic renal failure, until sudden collapse with hypotension and vomiting some days later in the ward led to the correct diagnosis of Addison's disease.

Blood count

A variety of haematological changes occur in steroid-deficient patients: normochromic or iron deficient anaemias, neutrophilia, raised ESR and eosinophilia. Lack of depression of the eosinophils in response to exogenous ACTH was the basis of the Thorn test for Addison's disease in former days.

Other biochemical changes

Raised serum enzymes (transaminases, alkaline phosphatase) may be found in steroid deficient patients, as may hyperprolactinaemia and raised thyroid stimulating hormone (TSH) with low thyroxine levels. Hypercalcaemia is confined to the Addisonian form of steroid deficiency.

The only specific feature of these haematological and biochemical abnormalities is that they revert to normal with steroid replacement.

Electrocardiograph

This often shows non-specific low voltage and S-T segment changes, as does the ECG in hypothyroidism. The specific feature is that the changes disappear within a few hours of steroid therapy; this manoeuvre may sometimes be diagnostically useful.

Treatment

There are three essentials of treatment: administration of hydrocortisone, replacement of salt loss, and search for and treatment of any cause such as septicaemia, tumours and so forth. A conventional approach to steroid and electrolyte replacement is shown in Table 29.2.

Hydrocortisone (cortisol) hemisuccinate or sodium phosphate salts are the steroids of choice in acute cortisol insufficiency, and are given intramuscularly. In theory, a very shocked patient with poor muscle perfusion might do better with an intravenous dose, but there is no evidence that this is necessary in practice. The intramuscular dose is 100 mg given six hourly. The plasma half-life of cortisol is of the order of two hours, though receptor occupancy is somewhat longer. Cortisol itself is preferred to synthetic steroids such as dexamethasone or prednisolone because they have little salt-retaining action. Insoluble steroid acetates should never be used, especially cortisone acetate which is very slowly absorbed from muscle, has to be converted to cortisol to act and should now be of historical interest only. As the patient improves, the cortisol dose can be reduced and in a day or two simple replacement therapy should be possible. In ACTH-deficient patients with normal aldosterone function this can be with prednisolone 2.5 mg three times a day. However, appropriate therapy for patients with adrenal destruction is hydrocortisone 30 mg/day in divided doses together with fludrocortisone 0.05 to 1.0 mg/day as a source of mineralocorticoid.

Once the patient is on replacement therapy the requisite endocrine assays can be carried out to confirm the diagnosis. Adrenal stimulation tests can be carried out by temporarily changing the steroid to dexamethasone which does not interfere in cortisol assays, but replacement must be interrupted for three to five days to carry out pituitary stimulation tests of ACTH function.

The reader is reminded that ACTH administration has no therapeutic role in steroid insufficiency due to pituitary suppression by exogenous steroids. ACTH will always 'wake' the suppressed adrenal in a few days, but does not of course provide any assistance to the suppressed pituitary.

The need for salt replacement varies from case to case but in severe cortisol deficiency it is at least as great as the need for cortisol. It should not be forgotten that until the advent of cortisol, patients with Addisonian crisis were regularly resuscitated by skilled physicians using saline alone. The saline replacement shown in Table 29.2 is the maximum likely to be required

Table 29.2. Urgent therapy of suspected severe cortisol deficiency

Immediate action on presentation:
(i) Draw plasma cortisol; perform ECG; serum electrolytes.
(ii) Infuse 1 litre 0.9 per cent NaCl in 1 hour.
(iii) Inject 100 mg hydrocortisone hemissuccinate or 100 mg hydrocortisone sodium phosphate intramuscularly.

Subsequent 24 hours
(i) 3–4 litres 0.9 per cent NaCl i.v.
(ii) Hydrocortisone 50 mg 6-hourly i.m.
(iii) Serum electrolytes (×1 only).
(iv) Check reversal of ECG changes if any.

Second 24 hours
(i) Saline as required by condition and serum Na.
(ii) Hydrocortisone 50 mg bd or tds, oral or i.m.

Third 24 hours
100 mg hydrocortisone in divided doses.

Subsequently
Replacement steroid therapy (see text).
Take steps to confirm diagnosis (see text).

but most cases will require three litres or more in the first twenty-four hours. Thereafter, smaller amounts can be given as required.

Plasma, rather than dopamine, is advised where shock is profound.

The ectopic ACTH syndrome

This results in patients being admitted as an emergency sufficiently often to warrant comment.

Clinical features

Ectopic ACTH production by relatively benign or slow-growing tumours may present with the classical features of Cushing' syndrome; this is not an emergency and is not discussed further. More commonly, the speed of tumour growth and the rate of ACTH release are so great that the patient is overcome by the metabolic consequences, and presents as an emergency before there is time for the features of Cushing's syndrome to develop. The cardinal features then are sudden and recent onset of diabetes, sudden onset of hypertension, gross muscle weakness and hypokalaemic alkalosis. To these may be added any features due to the tumour itself.

The diabetes presents typical features of thirst, polyuria and polydipsia, cramps and sometimes confusion. Keto-acidosis is however uncommon, as it is in other forms of purely steroid-induced diabetes: the patient will have high insulin levels. Typically, these symptoms will have been present for a few days or weeks at the most.

The myopathy is usually very striking, both the direct muscle effects of cortisol excess and the hypokalaemia contribute to it. While the patient has often become unable to walk, climb stairs or even get out of bed, standard 'neurological examination' tests of distal muscle may reveal little. These symptoms usually develop over a few days or weeks. The myopathy is proximal and easily shown by clinical tests of girdle and trunk muscles, such as inability to raise the trunk off the bed, to rise from a chair without assistance or inability to rise from a squatting position. It occasionally is severe enough to cause dyspnoea.

Hypertension is also usual; it is of recent onset and ranges in severity from mild to quite severe, e.g. 220/140 mm Hg.

Features such as skin atrophy, purpura, hirsutes and pigmentation that are so helpful in diagnosing the presence of chronic Cushing's syndrome are minimal or absent in these acute cases. The exception is that the combination of acute-onset cortisol excess with gross hirsuties is suggestive of primary adrenal carcinoma, a rare disease.

The primary tumour in ectopic ACTH production may or may not be obvious. Up to 75 per cent are small-celled lung tumours; so the first search should be for signs of lung cancer. Next commonest is an endocrine pan-creatic tumour, which may not be obvious. A variety of other tumours such as medullary thyroid tumour, carcinoids and others complete the list. There may be other signs of tumour endocrine activity, such as gastrin excess with diarrhoea, malignant hypercalcaemia and gynaecomastia due to gonado-trophin excess.

Laboratory findings

Hypokalaemic alkalosis

The serum potassium is commonly 2 mmol/l or lower, while plasma bicar-bonate is in the thirties. Other electrolytes show relatively little disturbance.

Glucose

Glucose levels are usually in the range 10–30 mmol/l; ketonaemia and ketonuria are slight or absent as a rule.

Cortisol levels

Cortisol levels are massive: as high as 5000 nmol/l or more in plasma, and 10,000 nmol/day in urine. Results from such assays may not be available for some time and it may be necessary to start treatment in their absence. However, two or more plasma samples and two or more timed urine collec-tions should be made if possible before steroid production is inhibited.

ACTH levels

ACTH levels are also massive. While some patients with more chronic or mild ectopic ACTH production may resemble pituitary-dependent Cushing's disease cases in having ACTH levels in the range 40–250 ng/l, ACTH levels over 250 ng/l, in the clinical setting under discussion, are pathognomonic of ectopic ACTH production. Whether ACTH samples should be drawn initially (with the necessary precautions for ACTH sampling) will depend on the level of clinical suspicion; if this is only moderate it may be best to reserve this difficult and expensive assay until the cortisol excess is confirmed.

Other investigations

Other investigations will be made as appropriate. In the kind of case under discussion, the hazard of radiological invisibility of some hormone-produc-ing lung tumours is less likely as they are usually sizeable.

Treatment

The most urgent requirement is to give the patient some potassium; this may provide time in which to get steroid assays performed. The diabetes usually requires insulin treatment initially but the hypertension usually resolves when the steroid overproduction is controlled.

Patients with this syndrome commonly excrete up to 100 mmol/day of potassium in the urine, and the giving of smaller amounts is likely to be ineffective. Table 29.3 gives some recommendations.

In desperate cases, adrenolytic therapy can be started as soon as the steroid samples have been taken; in less urgent cases it can wait for a few days. When adrenolytic therapy is started, several things can happen quite suddenly. First, the patient's insulin requirement will fall abruptly or even disappear, with resulting hypoglycaemia unless a careful frequent watch is made. Second, the patient's hypertension may disappear abruptly and if blood pressure lowering drugs have been used this may be a problem. Third, the patient's potassium excretion will fall abruptly and after a lag period as short as a few days in which K repletion takes place, serum levels will suddenly rise and the amount of replacement must be reduced.

For the non-expert, the easiest method of adrenal inhibition is with the reversible enzyme inhibitor metyrapone. This inhibits the addition of the last hydroxyl group (11-β-hydroxylase) in cortisol synthesis, causing a fall in cortisol production and a rise in precursor production. Steroid assays are thus likely to be uninterpretable in patients on metyrapone. The inhibition is

Table 29.3. Urgent therapy in ectopic ACTH syndrome

Day 1 and if possible day 2 also	Potassium (K) replacement 100 mmol Sliding scale insulin Urine collection for cortisol Plasma cortisol samples
Day 3 + day 4	Continue K replacement, reducing to 50 mMol/day if serum K is normal Metyrapone 750 mg 4 hourly in milk Watch falling insulin requirement
Day 5 onward	Further reduce or stop K and insulin Continue Metyrapone 750 mg 4 hourly If ineffective may try combination adrenolytic therapy: Metyrapone 500 mg 4 hourly Aminoglutethimide 250 mg bd Dexamethasone 0.5 mg bd Fludrocortisone 0.1 mg daily

incomplete and provision of steroid replacement is only rarely necessary. A suitable dose, if metyrapone is used on its own, is 750 mg four-hourly; the drug has a short duration of action. It may cause nausea if given on an empty stomach and should be given in milk. Very high ACTH levels can overcome the drug's action and may be only temporarily effective on its own.

The combination of aminoglutethimide which inhibits a different adrenal enzyme, together with metyrapone does reliably reduce cortisol production to near zero (Child *et al.* 1976). Patients on the combination may become steroid deficient unless given replacement dexamethasone (enabling steroid assays on therapy) and fludrocortisone (to replace aldosterone whose production aminoglutethimide inhibits). Aminoglutethimide is toxic; more than 750 mg/day maximum should not be used. The fall in cortisol production caused by the combination is precipitous. For these reasons, its use is a matter for the expert.

Effective adrenolytic therapy produces remarkable clinical improvement, bed-bound patients becoming ambulant within forty-eight hours while as stated above their diabetes and hypertension are rapidly alleviated.

Urgent thyrotoxicosis

The clinical setting

Urgent thyrotoxicosis may arise in one of two ways. First, a recognizably thyrotoxic patient may develop a complication (e.g. intractable cardiac dysfunction) or an intercurrent illness that demands urgent control of the thyrotoxicosis. For example, a patient may require urgent surgery for some other condition, with the likelihood of thyroid storm if surgery is carried out in uncontrolled thyrotoxicosis. Secondly, a patient may be admitted as an emergency, perhaps because of a septicaemia, and have unrecognized thyrotoxicosis. Here too, the possibility of thyroid storm exists. Apart from these situations, thyroid storm is now almost unknown (Hoffenberg, 1980). However, in these circumstances urgent thyrotoxicosis is regularly encountered and failure to recognize it may result in the death of the patient.

Complications of recognizable thyrotoxicosis that demand immediate reduction of thyroid hormone levels are few. Uncontrollable atrial fibrillation, especially if combined with intractable heart failure or pulmonary emboli, is one. On occasion, intractable thyrotoxic vomiting is another. A third group consists of severe psychiatric complications such as mania or other psychoses. Much more often the thyrotoxicosis is incidental to, or unmasked by, something else. Important clinical features then include failure of tachycardia or fever to resolve upon treatment of the primary condition; pulse rates above 120 in sinus rhythm should not usually be ascribed to infections. Fever over 40°C with such a tachycardia is a particularly dangerous sign in thyrotoxicosis. Particularly difficult to interpret are the neurological manifestations of acute or accelerating thyrotoxicosis. Agitation and excitement may give way to clouded consciousness, with extensor plantor responses. The usual clinical features of thyrotoxicosis, which may or may not be apparent, will not be described here.

Laboratory findings

The usual fall in the peripheral conversion of thyroxine (T4) to triiodo-thyronine (T3) that is seen in severely ill patients still occurs when they also happen to be thyrotoxic. Septicaemic or post-surgical patients with gross thyrotoxicosis may thus have normal circulating levels of T3. Therefore, a case can be made for the prohibition of serum T3 assays on hospital in-patients as they may be so misleading. In the acutely ill, assays of free thyroxine concentration or free thyroxine index are to be preferred as acute changes in thyroid-binding prealbumin (TBPA) and thyroid-binding globulin (TBG) in severely ill patients may affect total T4 levels. However, very few hospitals provide a same-day service for T4 assays (although modern radio-immunoassays can give a result within an hour) and so treatment must be instituted after blood has been drawn without further delay. Two- or four-hourly radio-iodine uptakes can be performed but in such seriously ill patients these may be impracticable, or even misleading.

Treatment

Where the circumstances allow, for example in psychotic patients, a week of propranolol 20–40 mg tds followed by partial thyroidectomy is a certain and effective method of control of the thyrotoxicosis. Radio-iodine may take many weeks to be effective and has no place in acute treatment, while anti-thyroid drugs by themselves also take some weeks to reduce thyroid levels.

Where the need for reduction of thyroid hormone levels is more urgent, the management becomes the same as that of thyroid storm, and depends on the use of iodide or the recently-discovered effect of some contrast media in reducing T3 levels. Iodide sharply but temporarily inhibits the thyroid even in thyrotoxicosis but it should never be given without antithyroid drugs to take over from it. This is because iodide in the thyrotoxic patient may later provoke a sharp burst of hormone release (Jod–Basedow effect). It is highly desirable to give the first dose of antithyroid drug an hour before the iodide. Therefore, a suitable regimen is to give propylthiouracil (PTU) 150 mg (which unlike carbimazole inhibits T4 to T3 conversion), or carbimazole 15 mg, at once and eight-hourly thereafter, with potassium iodide 60 mg one hour after the first dose of PTU and repeated once more within the next twenty-four hours, with 60 mg daily for one week only thereafter.

The outlook in severe thyrotoxicosis has been much improved by propranolol. Though thyrotoxic patients metabolize the drug more rapidly, there is no need in practice to give more than 40 mg tds and this should be started at once. It is not contra-indicated in thyrotoxic heart failure; on the contrary it is of great benefit. Some units add prednisolone in a daily dose of 20–40 mg to the above regimen for two reasons; first to counter 'adrenal exhaustion' and second because steroids reduce thyroid hormone production and T4 to T3 conversion in thyrotoxicosis. While the need for this measure may be doubtful, if other circumstances permit the use of steroids they will be more beneficial than harmful.

The latest treatment substitutes iopanoic acid or sodium ipodate for iodide. These X-ray contrast media contain iodide but in addition bear chemical resemblances to thyroxine and are competitive inhibitors of 5′-deiodinase. By this property they produce remarkably rapid falls in circulating T3 (Fig. 29.1; also Wu *et al.* 1978). They release their iodide slowly, so they should be given with antithyroid drugs to prevent iodide-induced exacerbation. This treatment is as effective and safer than iodide. On my own unit, the current treatment of urgent thyrotoxicosis is therefore: sodium ipodate (Solu-Biloptin) 3 g at once and at three-day intervals thereafter, with carbimazole 15 mg eight-hourly and propranolol. This treatment will

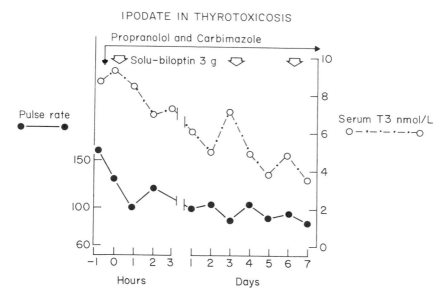

Fig. 29.1. The use of ipodate in thyrotoxicosis.

render a patient ready for surgery to an acute abdomen, for example, in two to three days. If the surgery must be done more urgently, the treatment can nevertheless be continued for it is sure to prevent thyroid storm.

Adequate fluid replacement is essential throughout and standard therapy for heart failure with diuretics is appropriate.

Urgent aspects of hypothyroidism

Myxoedema coma is so rare that a lengthy description is not justified here. Much more commonly, hypothyroidism has to be considered in a (usually elderly) patient presenting with hypothermia, bradycardia, slow reflexes and a puffy appearance. Hypothyroidism is very unlikely to be the cause but in many cases it is wise to proceed at the outset as if it were. Another relatively common need for urgent consideration of hypothyroidism is in the patient with previously undiagnosed, if only moderately severe, myxoedema who requires urgent surgery for some other condition. The reader is referred to standard texts for the clinical features.

Laboratory tests

There is no certain biochemical means of confirming hypothyroidism in hypothermic patients. The protein-binding of thyroid hormones is altered at low temperatures, and there will probably be severe changes in acute-phase reactive proteins such as TBPA that bind thyroxine; so assays of serum total T4 are unreliable. Free T4 can be assayed but may be temporarily depressed by acute non-thyroidal illness. In addition, cold is the only external stimulus to TSH release in man.

The ECG is often abnormal in hypothermia and the ECG changes in myxoedema are non-specific. Tests such as the measurement of plasma cholesterol are of little use.

The best plan in any patient in whom it seems desirable to rectify possible hypothyroidism urgently is to start treatment on clinical grounds, after drawing blood for free thyroxine and thyroid antibodies. Negative results received later will enable withdrawal of therapy without further investigations but apparently positive results should be confirmed after recovery by withdrawing thyroid hormone and performing appropriate tests after four to six weeks without T4 therapy or two to three weeks without T3 therapy.

Treatment

Choice of thyroid hormone

The possible need to withdraw therapy makes it desirable to use a short-acting hormone. This is especially true where undesirable effects, such as exacerbation of cardiac ischaemia, may occur. The plasma half-life of T4 is seven days and its fractional turnover only about 10 per cent per day; the half-life of T3 is one to two days and its fractional turnover 50 per cent per day. The speed of action of T3 is more rapid (depending on the action being tested) than that of T4: although both hormones in fact cause changes in systolic time intervals within twenty-four hours of administration to hypothyroid persons. Injectable T4 has to be imported, whereas T3 for injection is readily available. For all these reasons, T3 is the treatment of choice in urgent hypothyroidism.

Should thyroid hormone be given at all? Attempts to instantly reverse such a severe biochemical change affecting every cell may be considered unwise. However, patients with hypothyroidism are very bad anaesthetic risks and the combination of hypothermia with hypothyroidism is often fatal. The decision must rest solely on the level of clinical suspicion at the bedside.

If T3 is to be given, a single starting dose of 20 micrograms (approximately a quarter of the normal daily production rate) is appropriate. Its effect should be assessed over thirty-six hours or more before the next dose is given; if there is more benefit than harm (e.g. no cardiac problems) the dose can be slowly increased over seven to ten days to 20 μg three times a day, which is adequate short-term replacement. Untoward effects should be managed by returning to a dose level at which they were not present.

Oral administration is preferred where absorption is satisfactory. If injection is required, it must be remembered that T4 and T3 are soluble in water only at extreme acid or alkaline pH and that they are absorbed to glass and plastic surfaces. Severe local reactions can occur from alkaline T3 injection into muscle. Parenteral administration is best by injection into the side arm of a fast-running i.v. infusion—only 100 ml of fluid need be used. Adverse effects will be delayed, not immediate.

It is customary to give corticosteroid support. The main reason is that occasionally, the pituitary or adrenals may be very hypothyroid and temporarily unable to mount an appropriate stress response. 50 to 100 mg of cortisol hemisuccinate or cortisol sodium phosphate per day for three to five days is ample.

Severely hypothyroid patients commonly have profound hyponatraemia, often due to vasopressin excess (thought in turn to be due to hypothyroidism of the hypothalamus or of baro- or osmo-receptors). This should be managed by fluid restriction, rather than salt administration or salt-retaining steroids such as fludrocortisone, especially as cardiac failure is likely to be present.

It is rare for pericardial effusions to be large enough to compromise the circulation in hypothyroidism but this possibility should be assessed.

Hypercalcaemia

There are many excellent review articles on the causes and management of hypercalcaemias (for example Heath 1980; Fisken *et al.* 1980; Goodwin 1982) and only the emergency aspects will be considered here.

What level of serum calcium constitutes an emergency?

The first thing to do is to correct the serum calcium for serum protein changes, which are likely to be present in severely ill patients. The correction can be based on serum albumin: for every g/l by which albumin exceeds 40 g/l subtract 0.025 mmol/l from the calcium, and vice versa. This may not be helpful in myeloma, where albumin may be low but other calcium-binding proteins increased.

Serum calcium levels below 4 mmol/l after correction are not likely to be life-threatening, unless they rise further, and serum calcium levels below 3.5 mmol/l are not likely to be the cause of serious illness. It must be remembered that there are plenty of people with asymptomatic hyperparathyroidism who are found accidentally to have serum calcium levels between 3 and 3.5. Further, a calcium level over 4 mmol/l can be converted quickly to one below 3.5 in many cases by the simple measure of rehydration (Hosking *et al.* 1981). Until this measure has been carried out, the severity of hypercalcaemia cannot be properly assessed. Other emergency measures will only rarely be required at the outset and should be deferred whenever possible.

Treatment

Fluid

This is required in large quantities and saline produces a satisfactory diuresis which helps relieve the body of its calcium burden. At least five litres of normal saline, even up to eight or ten, should be given in twenty-four hours and intake and output watched over twelve hour periods. If output lags or pulmonary congestion develops, frusemide should be injected as required. Frusemide has the advantage of causing hypercalciuria. Some care is required because the intravenous fluids are being given for two purposes: induction of diuresis and volume replacement. Care must be taken to keep the balance on the 'wet' side. This treatment commonly results in hypo-kalaemia, which should be monitored by frequent ECG and serum levels as necessary. Quite large amounts of potassium may be required: 50 mmol/day or more.

Other treatments

These should be delayed until the serum calcium has stabilized in response to fluid therapy, when a decision can be taken whether continuation therapy with steroids, oral phosphate or intermittent mithramycin is required to retain control.

However, in occasional patients in whom the serum calcium remains dangerously high despite fluid therapy other measures may be required after a few hours. There is a wide range of these but only a few can be recommended: a critique of their value is made by Heath (1980).

Steroids can be relied on to reduce serum calcium in sarcoidosis, myeloma and vitamin D intoxication only. Nowadays, they should not be used as 'front-line' treatment unless the diagnosis is already known—which in the circumstances being discussed is unlikely. Intravenous phosphate should be discarded from the armamentarium in my opinion. Heath (1980) states it is 'the most effective therapeutic agent available for control of hypercalcaemia. Its use carries unequivocal dangers and therefore it should be restricted to the very rare patient with life-threatening hypercalcaemia who cannot be controlled by other means'. In this context, by 'life-threatening' hypercalcaemia he means a calcium so high as to be likely to cause death forthwith—say 5–6 mmol/l. This would appear to be the only indication for intravenous phosphate and will hardly ever be encountered. Indomethacin and also calcitonin, after enthusiastic early reports, are being increasingly found to be poorly effective.

Where the effect of really adequate saline-frusemide therapy is judged inadequate after twelve hours, my own recommendation is low-dose mithramycin, 1–1.5 mg infused over four hours, not more often than every three days. The effect is seen over the following twenty-four to forty-eight hours.

Further reading

Bayliss R.I.H. (1980) Adrenal cortex. In: Sonksen P.H. and Lowy C. (eds) Endocrine and metabolic emergencies. *Clinics in Endocrinology and Metabolism* **9**, 477. W.B. Saunders, London.

Burke C.W. (1978) Disorders of cortisol production: diagnostic and therapeutic progress. In: O'Riordan J.L.H. (ed.) *Recent Advances in Endocrinology and Metabolism*, p. 61. Churchill Livingstone, London.

Child D.C., Burke C.W., Burley D.M., Rees L.H. and Fraser T.R. (1976) Drug control of Cushing's syndrome. *Acta Endocrinologica* **82**, 330.

Fisken R.A., Heath D.A. and Bold A.M. (1980) Hypercalcaemia—a hospital survey. *Quarterly Journal of Medicine* **49**, 405–418.

Heath, D.A. (1980) The emergency management of disorders of calcium and magnesium. In: Sonksen P.H. and Lowy C. (eds) Endocrine and metabolic emergencies. *Clinics in Endocrinology and Metabolism* **9**, 487–502. W.B. Saunders, London.

Hoffenberg R. (1980) Thyroid emergencies. *Ibid*, Pp. 503–512.

Hosking D.J., Cowley A. and Bucknall C.A. (1981) Rehydration in the treatment of severe hypercalcaemias. *Quarterly Journal of Medicine* **50**, 473.

Goodwin F.J. (1982) Symptomless abnormalities: hypercalcaemia. *British Journal of Hospital Medicine* **281**, 50–58.

Irvine W.J. and Barnes E.W. (1972) Adrenocortical insufficiency. In: Mason A.S. (ed.) Diseases of the adrenal cortex. *Clinics in Endocrinology and Metabolism* **1**, 549–594. W.B. Saunders, London.

Lancet (1976) Adrenal haemorrhage, apoplexy and infarction. *Lancet* **2**, 295.

Mason A.S., Meade T.W., Lee J.A.H., and Morris J.N. (1968) Epidemiological and clinical picture of Addison's disease. *Lancet* **2**, 744.

Wu S-Y., Chopra I.J., Solomon D.H. and Johnson D.E. (1978) The effect of repeated administration of ipodate (Orografin) in hyperthyroidism. *Journal of Clinical Endocrinology* **47**, 1358.

30 · Haematological Emergencies

JOHN BELL & DAVID WEATHERALL

Anaemia

Profound anaemia requiring urgent intervention may result from either inadequate erythropoiesis or excessive intravascular or extravascular loss of red cells. Defective red cell production may be due to bone marrow failure or deficiencies of necessary substances for normal haemopoiesis. Intravascular blood loss is the result of haemolysis while extravascular loss may be due to haemorrhage or hypersplenism .

Haemolytic anaemias

The haemolytic anaemias may be due to auto-immune phenomena, disturbances of the red cell membrane, altered red cell metabolism, haemoglobinopathies, micro-angiopathic damage to red cells or to the invasion of the red cells by parasites.

Immune haemolytic anaemia

One of the most important forms of anaemia to be diagnosed and treated promptly is auto-immune haemolytic anaemia. It may be diagnosed by the presence of altered red cell morphology on the blood film (polychromatophilia, anisocytosis and regenerative macrocytosis), an elevated reticulocyte count and a positive direct antiglobulin test (Coombs' test). The haptoglobin level is often depressed.

Severe acute auto-immune haemolysis may be due to drug therapy with agents such as penicillin or methyl-dopa. These should be stopped immediately. Idiopathic auto-immune haemolysis may be treated with corticosteroids, given as 100 mg hydrocortisone four-hourly intravenously, or oral prednisolone 60 mg daily. Immune haemolytic anaemias related to lymphoproliferative diseases such as lymphomas or chronic lymphatic leukaemia often respond to reduction of the tumour mass together with corticosteroid therapy.

If corticosteroids fail to check severe haemolysis with a rapidly falling haemoglobin, patients may require emergency splenectomy. Chronically, immunosuppression with cyclophosphamide or azathioprine may be required.

Blood transfusion is very difficult in the face of immune haemolysis because cross-matching is impossible to interpret. For this reason, blood replacement should be reserved for extremely severe cases.

Membrane abnormalities

Congenital abnormalities of the red cell membrane are thought to be responsible for the chronic haemolysis seen in conditions such as hereditary spherocytosis and elliptocytosis. Affected patients may develop aplastic crises following intercurrent viral infection; they become rapidly anaemic and reticulocytopenic. The bone marrow shows a paucity of red cell precursors. Urgent transfusion is required.

Glucose-6-phosphate (G6PD) deficiency

Intracorpuscular metabolic defects may lead to haemolysis. The most common is G6PD deficiency, an X-linked condition which is found in Negro, Oriental and Mediterranean races. Patients with this deficiency are likely to develop acute haemolysis when given drugs such as primaquine or sulphonamides, or foods such as fava beans. Withdrawal of the triggering agent will stop the haemolysis but transfusion may be required.

Sickle cell disease

The haemoglobinopathy most frequently requiring emergency management is sickle cell anaemia, the homozygous state for haemoglobin S. Deoxyhaemoglobin S has a tendency to form long fibrils which deform the red cells which then occlude small vessels and are rapidly destroyed resulting in a haemolytic anaemia. Negroes, persons of Mediterranean origin and some Arabs and Indians may be affected.

An acute exacerbation of sickle cell anaemia is referred to as a sickle crisis and may take several forms (Table 30.1), the most common of which is the vaso-occlusive thrombotic crisis. Patients present with severe pain in the limbs, back, chest or abdomen. Fits or other acute cerebrovascular events

Table 30.1. Sickle crisis

1. Thrombotic	2. Haemolytic
(a) bone	3. Aplastic
(b) abdominal	4. Sequestrian
(c) Pulmonary	
(d) CNS	

may occur. The diagnosis has usually been established since infancy but can be confirmed by characteristic morphological changes on the blood film. Treatment should include rehydration with saline and 5 per cent dextrose and adequate analgesia. Despite the risk of addiction it is essential to provide adequate analgesia; pethidine or related agents should be used for severe bone pain but changed to a milder analgesic as soon as possible. An underlying precipitating factor such as infection, cold or dehydration must be searched for and treated appropriately.

In severe sickle crises, supportive care may be inadequate and exchange transfusion, if the presenting haemoglobin level is above 6–7 g/dl, may be required in an attempt to reduce the level of sickle cells to less than 30 per cent. Further transfusions will suppress the marrow and keep the proportion of sickle cells low. Most patients have steady-state haemoglobin levels of 8–10 g/dl and should not be transfused at this level as this simply increases blood viscosity and tends to precipitate further crises.

Haematological crises are less common but may be life-threatening. With infection, a patient may fail to maintain a hyperactive bone marrow, the reticulocyte count will fall and haemolysis will lead to a dramatic fall in the haemoglobin level. Transfusion is always required in such aplastic crises. In very young children, the spleen may sequester most of the circulating red cells and produce severe anaemia; the organ may become noticeably larger over a period of hours. Again, transfusion is required. Similar sequestration episodes may involve the liver in older people. Pleuritic pain, haemoptysis or infiltrates on a chest X-ray, particularly if associated with a falling haemoglobin level, are all features which suggest the diagnosis of pulmonary infarction due to sequestration of sickled erythrocytes in the pulmonary circulation. This complication should be treated with oxygen therapy, transfusion or exchange transfusion depending on the presenting haemoglobin level, together with careful monitoring of the blood gas levels.

Patients with any form of sickle cell crisis require meticulous examination of the chest, abdomen for liver or spleen size, together with a twice daily haemoglobin or PCV level and reticulocyte count. It is essential to instigate the simple measures outlined above early.

Deficiency anaemias

Anaemias due to deficient intake or absorption of iron, vitamin B_{12} or folate may present as acute haematological emergencies. Particularly in the case of vitamin B_{12} deficiency, patients may present with profound anaemia and cardiac failure. A blood film and a full blood count will often help to establish the diagnosis. Microcytic hypochromic changes accompany iron deficiency anaemia while macrocytes and multilobular granulocytes are characteristic of a megaloblastic anaemia. Blood samples for folate and vitamin B_{12} levels should be obtained and a bone marrow performed before treatment of a megaloblastic anaemia.

The iron deficiency anaemias are most often encountered in association with malnutrition or chronic blood loss from the gastro-intestinal tract. During the diagnosis and management of the underlying cause, treatment should be started with oral iron supplements. Parenteral iron is virtually never required except in cases of malabsorption. If blood transfusion is required, it should be administered as packed cells and be accompanied by a diuretic, such as frusemide 40 mg, with alternate units. This is particularly important in the elderly with impending heart failure.

While the mortality from iron deficiency anaemia is low, that associated with severe megaloblastic anaemia may be as high as 14 per cent when the packed cell volume (PCV) at presentation is less than 25 per cent. The major causes of death are left ventricular failure and myocardial infarction. Therapy should consist of parenteral vitamin B_{12} (1000 μg/day for one week then monthly for life) and folic acid (5 mg daily) until blood tests establish the cause of the anaemia. It has been suggested that the early mortality may be partly due to the hypokalaemia that accompanies a reticulocyte response and potassium supplementation has been recommended. In patients with profound anaemia and heart failure it may be necessary to raise the haemoglobin by the slow infusion of packed cells with diuretic cover (see above). Where possible, progress should be monitored with a central venous pressure line. In extreme cases, exchange transfusion, replacing two to three units of the patient's blood with whole blood, may be life-saving.

Emergencies related to the spleen

Splenomegaly is associated with a number of acute medical emergencies. These are more likely to occur in patients with massive splenomegaly, particularly those with myelofibrosis, chronic granulocytic leukaemia, lymphomas and chronic malaria.

Splenic infarction is accompanied by severe pain over the spleen or radiating to the left shoulder. There may be an associated rub over the spleen. It is most commonly seen in myelosclerosis or chronic myeloid leukaemia. Analgesia is the only treatment required. In patients with large spleens, splenic rupture may follow even minor trauma. It is characterized by left upper quadrant pain, a falling haemoglobin level and the signs of haemorrhage and shock. The shock should be managed with volume replacement; surgical intervention is almost always necessary.

There are hazards associated with splenectomy that require urgent therapy. A marked thrombocytosis may occur post-splenectomy, with platelet counts rising to levels greater than 1.0×10^{12}/l. Above this level, there is a risk of thrombotic complications and aspirin (300 mg/day) and dipyridamole (50 mg tds) is often given; the efficacy of this treatment is not certain.

Splenectomy produces a marked susceptibility to overwhelming septicaemia, particularly by *Streptococcus pneumoniae*. A splenectomized patient with septicaemia may become moribund in a few hours and requires immediate aggressive treatment with antimicrobial agents, including large intravenous doses of penicillin. The use of the multivalent pneumococcal vaccine to prevent this complication is, as yet, of unproven value. The overwhelming malaria due to *P. falciparum* that occurs in splenectomized patients can be prevented only by meticulous use of the appropriate prophylactic drug.

Bone marrow failure

Patients with inadequate haematopoiesis present clinical problems of management. The bone marrow may fail because of aplasia or replacement by an abnormal cell line as in leukaemia. The commonest causes of marrow hypoplasia are drug reactions, response to cytotoxic agents and virus infection, particularly hepatitis. The diagnosis is made from a blood film and a bone marrow examination. Presentation is with the symptoms and signs due to deficiencies of any or all of the formed blood elements. Fatigue and dyspnoea may reflect anaemia, localized or disseminated infection granulocytopenia, and purpura or haemorrhage thrombocytopenia.

Patients with bone marrow failure should have certain routine investigations. Blood cultures, perineal, axillary and nasal swabs should be obtained for bacteriological investigation. A chest X-ray and electrocardiogram (ECG) should be performed and plasma levels of urea, electrolytes, calcium and uric acid should be obtained. Specific complications should be managed as described below.

Infection

Patients with bone marrow failure must be considered to be immunosuppressed. They are susceptible to a wide spectrum of infective illnesses not normally seen in hospital practice. They should receive regular (four-hourly) oral toilet with an antiseptic mouth wash and amphotericin lozenges. Their stools should be kept soft and rectal examination should be avoided. Full barrier nursing regimes are probably not effective but simple precautions such as exclusion of staff with infections and isolation from patients with infections should be instituted. Since most infections are from endogenous organisms it may be worth decontaminating the gastrointestinal tract by using the FRAMCON regime (framycetin sulphate 500 mg six hourly, colistin sulphate 1.5×10^6 units six-hourly and nystatin 0.5×10^6 units six hourly). Scrupulous care of drip sites are vital and intravenous lines must be changed regularly.

A pyrexia must be carefully investigated and 'blind' antibiotic therapy must be used on occasion. In the presence of a pyrexia of more than 37.5°C, blood cultures, urine cultures and a chest X-ray are mandatory. An appropriate 'blind' intravenous antibiotic regime is:

Gentamicin 2 mg/kg loading dose
                    1.5 mg/kg 8 hourly
Ticarcillin   3 gm 4 hourly

Gentamicin levels should be carefully monitored, particularly in the face of impaired renal function. Such a regime covers most bacterial infections but may require modification should the bacteriological screen identify resistant organisms.

Atypical organisms must be considered in every infection in an immunosuppressed patient. Viral illnesses are common. They can be identified by electron microscopy of virus obtained from skin or oral lesions or from urine, or retrospectively by changes in viral titres. The commonest pathogens are the DNA viruses; herpes simplex, herpes zoster, Epstein–Barr (EB) virus and cytomegalovirus (CMV). Management of these infections has, in the past, been supportive but the recently introduced antiviral agent acycloguanasine (Acyclovir) may be of benefit. It should be given in a dose of 5 mg/kg 8-hourly intravenously (i.v.) for herpes simplex infections and 10 mg/kg 8-hourly i.v. for herpes zoster.

Protozoal infections can also be a serious problem in patients with bone marrow failure. *Toxoplasmosis* can present as fever, lymphadenopathy, rash, pneumonitis or most seriously as a necrotizing encephalitis. It may be easily confused with viral infections, particularly those due to CMV. The diagnosis is based on increasing antibody titres, identification of the organism in the cerebrospinal fluid (CSF) or aspirates, or from typical lymph node histology. Treatment should be instituted with pyrimethamine (100–200 mg loading dose and 25 mg daily) and a sulphonamide (100–150 mg/kg/day) for one month.

Pneumocystitis carini is the other major protozoal pathogen in immunosuppressed patients. It produces a pneumonitis and seems to remain localized in the lung. The diagnosis should be suspected in patients with coarse crepitations, arterial hypoxaemia and a chest X-ray which shows diffuse pulmonary infiltrates, in whom a pyrexia has failed to settle on conventional broad spectrum antibiotics. Open lung biopsy or transbronchial biopsy will establish the presence of the organism. Trimethoprin and sulphamethoxazole in high dose (20 mg/kg/day trimethoprin, 100 mg/kg/day sulphamethoxazole in four divided doses) is the treatment of choice and should usually be administered intravenously. In the presence of thrombocytopenia, the hazards of a lung biopsy may be too great and blind therapy may be necessary. Pentamidine isethionate is an alternative therapeutic agent.

Persistent pyrexia despite adequate antibiotic treatment may be due to fungal infection. Cultures are often negative and it may be necessary to biopsy involved organs such as the lung to demonstrate infection. Early and aggressive treatment is necessary for survival and hence a decision between blind therapy and aggressive investigation must often be made. Once a diagnosis has been established, amphotericin B (0.3 mg/kg/day) is the drug of choice. 5-Fluorocytosine may be synergistic, particularly for cryptococcal and candida infections. Even with early therapy, the results of treatment for systemic fungal infections are not good.

One of the most common fungal pathogens is candida which may be localized to the mucous membranes of the mouth or may become widely disseminated. The use of scrupulous oral toilet reduces the likelihood of this complication (see above). Established oral candidiasis should be treated with amphotericin lozenges, hydrogen peroxide mouth washes and a full oral toilet regime as described earlier. Aspergillus is usually associated with a pneumonia in immunosuppressed patients. It is diagnosed by lung biopsy. The results of treatment in patients with bone marrow failure have been poor. Phycomyocosis, cryptococcus and coccidiomycosis are other potential pathogens, which when identified must be treated in the same fashion with amphotericin. Results of treatment have also been poor.

Haemorrhage

Haemorrhage due to thrombocytopenia is a constant concern in patients with bone marrow failure. Intracerebral bleeds and fundal haemorrhages may be catastrophic. Patients with platelet counts of less than 20×10^9/l are likely to bleed. Infections and severe anaemia impose an increased risk of bleeding, particularly into the retina.

Fresh platelets may be used to stop bleeding prophylactically. One donor unit of fresh platelets will raise the platelet count by about 10×10^9/l/m² of body surface area; six units are given every other day. For severe bleeding, blood together with twelve platelet packs should be given and repeated as necessary until haemostasis is achieved.

Complications of leukaemia

In addition to the effects of leukaemia on the bone marrow, several other complications may produce medical emergencies. Some are due to electrolyte imbalance; others are the result of extremely high white cell counts.

All forms of electrolyte imbalance have been reported in leukaemia.

Hyponatraemia is thought to be due to the syndrome of inappropriate antidiuretic hormone secretion (SIADH). It occurs in patients treated with cytotoxics such as vincristine and cyclophosphamide and in some who have not received treatment. Management is with fluid restriction as for other forms of SIADH. Hypernatraemia is probably due to hypothalamic infiltration of leukaemic cells producing diabetes insipidus and is best managed by vasopressin administration.

Hypokalaemia is often seen in acute myeloid leukaemia and may be due to the renal tubular damage induced by lysozyme. Another common cause of hypokalaemia is the administration of high doses of penicillins (particularly carbenicillin). Hyperkalaemia may occur after massive cell lysis during therapy or in association with renal impairment. This diagnosis must be made with care because leucocyte breakdown after venepuncture can produce 'pseudohyperkalaemia'.

Hypocalcaemia is occasionally seen in patients with leukaemia but almost never requires correction. Hypercalcaemia is more common and must be managed as an emergency (see below under Myeloma). It presents as polyuria, nausea or vomiting and may be due to production of a parathyroid hormone-like substance by leukaemic cells, erosion of bone, or the generation of other osteolytic substances, as occurs in myeloma. The prognosis of leukaemics with hypercalcaemia is poor. Elevation and depression of serum phosphate and magnesium levels also occurs in leukaemia though rarely reaches life-threatening levels.

Hyperuricaemia is seen with rapid turnover or lysis of leukaemic cells. It may produce episodes of gout or may lead to impaired renal function. Therefore, Allopurinol prophylaxis (200 mg bd) before therapy is mandatory. Lactic acidosis has been reported in acute leukaemia and lymphoma without hepatic impairment. It responds poorly to bicarbonate therapy and carries a bad prognosis.

High white blood cell counts can produce widespread manifestations. Extreme leucocytosis has been associated with intracranial haemorrhage in the absence of thrombocytopenia. Other complications such as priapism have been reported in chronic granulocytic leukaemia. Management consists of rapid reduction of the white cell count. Leucopheresis or cytotoxic therapy may be used in these circumstances. It is dangerous to transfuse patients with a very high white cell count until the latter is reduced as the increase in blood viscosity may cause a cerebro-vascular accident.

Myeloma

Plasma cell dyscrasias are associated with a wide spectrum of complications in addition to those related to bone marrow failure. They include hypercalcaemia, hyperviscosity, renal failure and spinal cord compression.

Hypercalcaemia is a feature of myelomatosis and is thought to result from the production of osteoclast activating factor (OAF) by plasma cells. Patients suffer from thirst, polyuria, confusion and irritability. Potential adverse effects include cardiac arrhythmias and renal impairment. Management should begin with an infusion of several litres of normal saline. Frusemide may be used when adequate hydration has been established. Corticosteroids (prednisolone 60 mg/day) may reduce calcium levels but may take up to twenty-four to forty-eight hours to have any effect. When hypercalcaemia is unremitting, calcitonin (3–6 Medical Research Council units/kg/24 hours) or intravenous mithramycin (25 μg/kg/24 hours) may be used.

Hyperviscosity is seen in association with Waldenstrom's macro-globulinaemia and rarely in association with myeloma, particularly with IgA paraproteins. It is associated with cardiac failure, bleeding, confusion and focal neurological signs. The fundi show dilated retinal veins and haemorrhages. Removal of the paraprotein is the most appropriate management and is best accomplished with plasmapheresis. If this is not readily available removal of the plasma and re-infusion of the red cells from three or four units of the patient's blood will reduce the viscosity enough to relieve symptoms.

Spinal cord compression in myeloma may be due to either vertebral collapse of an extradural plasmacytoma. The symptoms of a paraperesis and bowel or bladder dysfunction should be managed as an emergency, with an urgent myelogram and decompression followed by local radiotherapy. Radiotherapy should not be carried out without previous decompression.

Renal failure in association with myeloma may be due to dehydration, hypercalcaemia, hyperuricaemia, amyloidosis, or myeloma kidney. Management should be primarily directed towards rehydration and correction of metabolic abnormalities such as hypercalcaemia. Otherwise supportive management is required.

Polycythaemia

Polycythaemia is characterized by an elevated number of red blood cells per unit volume of plasma, leading to an elevated packed cell volume (PCV). Polycythaemia vera is due to a clonal proliferation of red cells while the secondary polycythaemias may be due to high altitude, chronic lung disease, congenital heart disease, haemoglobinopathies or inappropriate secretion of erythropoietin from renal cysts, or tumours of the kidney, cerebellum, liver or uterus. 'Stress' polycythaemia and that related to dehydration are both due to reduced plasma volume and hence are relative polycythaemias.

The major risks associated with polycythaemia are thrombosis and haemorrhage. Cerebral thrombosis is a major cause of morbidity and mortality and may be arterial or may involve the venous sinuses. Coronary, mesenteric and deep vein thrombosis are also thought to be more common in polycythaemia. Bleeding from the gastro-intestinal tract is also common and may be related to the high incidence of duodenal ulcer. A more generalized bleeding tendency which may be due to abnormal platelet function also occurs. Polycythaemic patients are at high risk of both thrombosis and bleeding in the postoperative period.

Venesection is an appropriate mode of emergency therapy for patients with polycythaemia of any cause. However, this must be done with care as it may be accompanied by cardiovascular collapse and death if fluid replacement with saline is not carried out concurrently. Particularly if the initial platelet count is high, myelosuppressive agents such as busulphan or hydroxyurea should be given as the PCV is lowered by venesection, as it is usually accompanied by a further rise in the platelet count.

In the long term, patients with polycythaemia vera require venesection, ^{32}P or chemotherapy to maintain a low PCV, although concern has been expressed about the added risks of acute leukaemia in patients treated with ^{32}P or chlorambucil.

Bleeding disorders

After a blood vessel is injured, haemostasis is achieved by a three-stage mechanism. First, there is vascular contraction. This is followed by platelet aggregation with the formation of a haemostatic plug. Finally, the clotting pathway is activated. There is a fibrinolytic mechanism designed to combat this process. Normally, clotting and lysis are in a state of equilibrium.

The bleeding disorders can be classified into those which result from disorders of the vessel wall, a deficiency or abnormal function of platelets and a deficiency of one or more clotting factors (Table 30.2). The most serious disturbance of clotting and haemostatis is disseminated intravascular coagulation (DIC) which is characterized by generalized intravascular coagulation with consumption of both platelets and clotting factors.

The patterns of bleeding in these different groups of disorders are characteristic. In the case of vessel wall or platelet abnormalities the characteristic lesion is spontaneous bleeding into the skin and viscera, i.e. purpura. In the case of the clotting factor deficiencies, spontaneous bleeding is unusual unless there is a gross deficiency. The pattern of bleeding is characterized by large ecchymoses or bleeding into viscera or joints after trauma. With DIC and generalized haemostatic failure there is extensive bleeding into the skin and mucous membranes and marked and continuous bleeding from sites of trauma, such as previous venepunctures or surgery.

In the investigation of bleeding, a careful history and physical examination is carried out. This is followed by a few simple laboratory tests which

Table 30.2. Classification of bleeding disorders

1. Purpura
   a. Thrombocytopenic purpura
      Increased platelet destruction —drug allergy (heparin)
                               —ITP
                               —SLE
                               —splenomegaly
      Decreased platelet destruction—see Bone Marrow Failure
                               —alcohol
   b. Non-thrombocytopenic purpura
      Vasculitis   —Henoch–Schönlein purpura
                               —drug allergy
                               —fat embolism
                               —idiopathic
      Thrombocytopathy   —uraemia
                               —aspirin
                               —myeloproliferative disorders
                               —dysproteinaemia
                               —FDPs (liver disease)

2. Deficiency of clotting factors
   a. Congenital   —haemophilia
                               —Christmas disease
                               —Von Willebrand's disease
   b. Acquired   —liver disease, acute or chronic
                               —vitamin K deficiency (coumarin anticoagulants, surreptitious warfarin use, malabsorption)
                               —massive transfusion

are initiated to determine the particular defect in haemostasis or coagulation. These are summarized in Table 30.3.

Thrombocytopenia

Bleeding due to thrombocytopenia secondary to bone marrow failure is best managed with fresh platelets (see Bone Marrow Failure). If the thrombocytopenia is due to immune destruction of platelets several methods of treatment are available. Drug related immune thrombocytopenia, as seen after administration of quinidine, sedormid or digitoxin, responds to stopping the drug. The low platelet counts associated with SLE or lymphoreticular diseases may respond to corticosteroid or immunosuppressive therapy. Idiopathic thrombocytopenic purpura (ITP) may present either acutely or as a chronic relapsing disease. Exacerbations of the chronic form respond poorly to corticosteroids but the condition is often cured by

Table 30.3. Tests of haemostasis and coagulation

1. *Vascular or platelet defects* Blood film Platelet count Bleeding time
2. *Coagulation* Thrombin time Partial thromboplastin time Prothrombin time Specific factor assays
3. *Fibrinolysis* Fibrin degradation products Ethanol gel test Fibrinogen level

splenectomy. In its acute form, corticosteroids may be of some help in a dose of 60 mg prednisolone/day. However, there is no strong evidence that the natural history of the disease is altered by this therapy. It is important that if corticosteroids are utilized it should be for a limited time only and long-term therapy should be avoided. Failure of response after two to three weeks is an indication for splenectomy.

Vascular purpura

The vascular purpura of scurvy should be treated with ascorbic acid. Those severe vascular purpuras associated with paraproteinaemia respond to cyto-toxic therapy or plasmapheresis. There is no effective treatment for Henoch–Schönlein purpura.

Hereditary disorders of coagulation

The management of hereditary coagulation disturbances has been greatly facilitated by the development of blood components containing specific factors. The important preparations are
1. Cryoprecipitate. This contains a variable amount of factor VIII and fibrinogen and may be used in an emergency for the treatment of factor VIII deficiency.
2. Freeze-dried factor VIII concentrates. These contain defined amounts of factor VIII and are useful for treatment of haemophiliacs.
3. Factor IX prothrombin complex concentrates (IX-PCC). This contains either factors II, IX, X or factors II, VII, IX and X and is useful for

managing factor IX deficiency, coumarin overdose or haemorrhage associated with liver disease.
4. Fresh Frozen Plasma (FFP). All the clotting factors are contained in this fraction. It may be used to manage all types of bleeding diathesis where specific factor replacement is impossible or inappropriate.

The major hereditary disorders of coagulation are haemophilia and Christmas disease, due to deficiencies of factors VIII and IX, respectively. Haemorrhage tends to occur either after surgery, or following trauma resulting in a muscle haematoma or haemarthrosis, for example. Management consists of administration of factor VIII or IX concentrates. One unit of factor VIII per kg body weight will raise activity by two per cent while a similar amount of factor IX will raise activity by one per cent. Levels of 15–20 per cent are adequate to manage minor bleeding while 40 per cent may be required if a haemarthrosis is severe. The dose must be repeated every 12–24 hours. Major surgery or serious bleeding such as that following head injury requires restoration to normal factor VIII levels.

Acquired disorders or coagulation

The use of anticoagulants and thrombolytics are the commonest causes of acquired bleeding disorders. Other conditions producing a bleeding tendency are liver disease (through ineffective generation of clotting factors), malabsorption (through poor vitamin K absorption), renal failure, massive transfusion, inhibitors of coagulation factors as seen in SLE and amyloid, and disseminated intravascular coagulation.

Oral anticoagulants

Bleeding in patients receiving oral anticoagulants is best controlled by the use of fresh frozen plasma or factor-IX-prothrombin complex concentrate. Vitamin K has a delayed effect and makes later anticoagulant therapy control difficult.

Heparin

Reversal of heparin anticoagulation may be achieved with protamine. One mg of protamine will reverse 100 units of heparin; hence, a 50 mg dose of protamine is usually sufficient. An exact reversing dose can be obtained by doing a heparin titration. Excess protamine may produce a bleeding tendency so that doses of greater than 50 mg should be used with caution.

Thrombolytics (urokinase and streptokinase)

The increasing use of these agents in venous thrombosis and myocardial infarction has led to increasing problems with fibrinolytic-induced haemorrhage. The risk of this complication is greatest in the early stages of therapy (1–12 hours) when fibrinolysis occurs in the presence of high levels of fibrin degradation products (FDPs). The half life of streptokinase is 1–2 hours and hence stopping the infusion will help control haemorrhage. Fresh blood and fresh plasma are dangerous because they provide further substrate for plasminogen activator complex. Cessation of thrombolytic therapy must be accompanied by heparin administration, or rethrombosis will occur with fibrin clots deficient in plasminogen and hence resistant to subsequent fibrinolysis.

Liver disease

There are many causes of a bleeding tendency in patients with liver disease. Reduced synthesis of clotting factors, vitamin K deficiency, increased fibrinolysis and thrombocytopenia may be responsible. Vitamin K is useful prophylactically, but for patients actively bleeding without evidence of DIC, factor IX-PCC or fresh frozen plasma should be used. Platelets may also be required.

Renal disease

Some renal patients have been recognized as losing factor IX in association with the nephrotic syndrome. Corticosteroids will correct this deficiency without the use of replacement therapy. Far commoner, is an elevation of factor V, VI and VIII levels and a hypercoagulable state for which anti-coagulation may be required.

Disseminated intravascular coagulation

A variety of conditions may lead to the coincident activation of coagulation and fibrinolytic cascades, producing a depletion of normal coagulation constituents and the clinical syndrome of disseminated intravascular co-agulation (DIC). Obstetric complications, sepsis, trauma, malignancy and a diverse array of other illnesses are all associated with this disorder. The diagnosis is suggested by a tendency to bleed and ooze, often from venepuncture sites. Laboratory findings supporting the diagnosis include micro-angiopathic haemolysis accompanied by thrombocytopenia on a blood film, prolonged prothrombin and partial thromboplastin times, depressed fibrinogen titres and elevated fibrin degradation products (FDPs).

The management of patients with DIC, including the use of heparin, remains controversial. It is most important to try to correct the underlying disorder. If severe bleeding occurs, clotting factors should be replaced with fresh frozen plasma. There is no clear evidence that heparin is beneficial in established DIC but in some circumstances it may be helpful in the early stages of the syndrome, particularly in patients with obstetric complications (amniotic fluid embolism, septic abortion, abruptio placenta), in unmatched blood transfusion reactions, and possibly, in promyelocytic leukaemia. An appropriate dose is 1000 units/hour intravenously by infusion pump, adjusted after repeated assay of the haematological parameters of DIC. The use of antithrombin III in this condition remains to be substantiated. Because of its uncertain value, heparin should only be used in patients with DIC in centres where expert haematological help is available; when in doubt it is much safer to treat the underlying cause and administer either fresh blood or fresh frozen plasma together with platelets.

Blood transfusion

Administration of blood or blood products may be associated with a variety of complications necessitating emergency management. The spectrum of these problems is wide (Table 30.4), ranging from minor febrile or urticarial reactions to serious haemolytic reactions.

Non-haemolytic reactions are identified by a fever or urticarial response and are best managed by stopping the transfusion. Circulatory overload is

Table 30.4. Transfusion reactions

Non-haemolytic transfusion reactions
Febrile reactions
Allergic reactions (urticaria)
Reaction to granulocytes or platelet antigens or plasma proteins (allotypic Ig
   determinants or IgA)
Circulatory overload
Disease transmission (malaria, CMV, hepatitis B)
Pulmonary leucoagglutination reactions
Citrate toxicity
Hypothermia
Graft v. host disease (immunosuppressed patients)

Haemolytic transfusion reactions
Immediate intravascular haemolysis
Immediate extravascular haemolysis
Delayed haemolytic reaction

---

managed with diuretics such as frusemide, which should be administered prophylactically in patients with impaired myocardial function. Respiratory complications are thought to be due to leuco-agglutination and range from mild hypoxemia to the adult respiratory disease syndrome. Supportive management is the only therapy available.

Haemolytic transfusion reactions are usually due to the transfusion of incompatible blood. Clinically, the diagnosis is suggested by fever, chills, nausea and vomiting, substernal pain and tightness and urticaria. Hypotension, circulatory collapse, loin pain and a bleeding tendency indicate severe haemolysis. Oliguria, anuria and frank DIC are the major factors which lead to death in this condition.

The diagnosis may be confirmed with laboratory evidence of free haemoglobin in the plasma or urine and a positive direct antiglobulin test.

Management involves maintaining the blood pressure and an adequate urine output (> 100 ml/hour) with saline and frusemide if necessary. Prophylactic heparin infusion (1000 units/hour) may prevent the onset of DIC. Persistent oliguria indicates the onset of acute renal failure and that dialysis is required.

Massive blood transfusion

The complications of massive blood transfusion are listed in Table 30.5. The major problems are caused by the loss of factors not adequately provided by stored blood. The latter may contain no viable platelets and has very low concentrations of some clotting factors (10 per cent of normal levels of factors V and VIII and 20 per cent of factor IX) and no ionized calcium. If the patient also has a DIC, depletion of other factors may occur.

Table 30.5. Complications associated with major blood transfusion

Coagulation abnormalities
Citrate toxicity
Altered haemoglobin function (2,3 DPG)
Acid-base abnormalities
Hypothermia
Micro-embolism
Impaired bacterial defence
Hyperkalaemia

Replacement of coagulation factors is best achieved with fresh frozen plasma, administered as 400 ml every 4–6 units of blood. Ten ml of 10 per cent Ca gluconate may be given at similar intervals to counter the effect of the citrate on calcium levels. However, it is unlikely that coagulation is ever significantly altered by hypocalcaemia, as tetany would occur before any effect on the coagulation cascade.

Hypothermia is a risk with massive transfusion. It is associated with impaired citrate and lactate metabolism and cardiac arrythmias. It can be avoided by warming blood before administration.

Concern is often expressed over the acid load which accompanies a massive blood transfusion (30–40 mEq/l of citric and lactic acid) and the deficiency of 2,3 DPG in stored blood. It is doubtful if these changes are of real clinical significance.

Further reading

Hardisty R.M. and Weatherall D.J. (1982) (eds) *Blood and its Disorders*, 2nd ed. Blackwell Scientific Publications, Oxford.
Williams W.J., Beutler E., Erslev A. and Lichtman M.A. (1983) (eds) *Haematology*, 3rd ed. McGraw-Hill, New York.
Wintrobe M.M. (1982) *Clinical Haematology*, 18th ed. Lee & Febiger, Philadelphia.

31 · Self-poisoning

J. K. ARONSON

The vigour with which one treats a case of self-poisoning varies from doing little or nothing to large-scale intensive action to maintain vital body functions. Since this is a book about emergencies, I shall deal firstly with the immediate management of the acutely ill patient and shall then enlarge on the various aspects of management which may, in part or in full, be involved in self-poisoning in general. A summary of the management is given in Table 31.1.

A. Immediate management of the acutely ill patient

1. Respiratory function

It is important to maintain a clear airway at all times. If there is anoxia, lay the patient on the left side, remove all obstructions from the mouth (including dentures) and suck out any secretions or debris. Insert an oral airway or, if the patient is unconscious and not breathing spontaneously, a cuffed endotracheal tube. Begin respiration with an Ambu bag or at least by mouth to mouth breathing. If there is cyanosis give 100 per cent oxygen. Move the patient as soon as possible to facilities for mechanically assisted ventilation.

2. Cardiovascular function

Measure the heart rate and blood pressure. If the blood pressure is below 90 mm Hg raise the end of the trolley or bed. If the blood pressure remains low set up an infusion line and give plasma volume expanders (see below).

3. Convulsions

Treat with diazepam or chlormethiazole.

4. Level of consciousness

This will already have been roughly assessed while assessing respiratory and cardiovascular functions. However, it is important to assess it more rigorously at this stage, according to the scheme laid out below, so that progress can be monitored.

Table 31.1. Management of acute self-poisoning

1. Respiratory function	check cough reflex clear out oropharyngeal obstructions/debris/ secretions lay on left side with head down insert oral airway *or* intubate if cough reflex lost give oxygen assist respiration

2. Circulatory function	check heart rate and blood pressure
	if blood pressure < 90 mm Hg systolic:
	    raise end of trolley/bed
	    give volume expanders
	    if fluid overload and oliguria give dopamine
	      or dobutamine

3. Consciousness	assess conscious level in response to standard stimuli
4. Temperature	take temperature rectally if < 36°C reheat slowly ('space blanket') if < 30°C reheat more rapidly (arm in water at 40°C if elderly, whole body if young) warm all inspired air and i.v. fluids

5. Blood and urine tests	arterial gases
	plasma urea, creatinine, and electrolytes
	plasma salicylate and paracetamol for
	    treatment guidance
	plasma barbiturates for diagnosis and likely
	    duration of effects
	urine paraquat for diagnosis
	blood glucose (salicylates)
	prothrombin time (salicylates and
	    paracetamol)

6. Gastric lavage and ipecac-
induced emesis
	within 4 hours of all drugs
	within 8 hours of anticholinergics
	    (e.g. tricyclic antidepressants)
	at any time for salicylates
	ipecac-induced emesis for choice in children
	gastric lavage for choice in adults (except
	    digitalis when emesis)
	add non-specific or specific antidotes if
	    indicated

7. Specific emergency measures	cyanide—dicobalt edetate paraquat—fuller's earth paracetamol—acetyl cysteine carbon monoxide—oxygen opiates—naloxone

5. Temperature

Measure the temperature rectally and treat hypothermia or hyperthermia as discussed below.

6. Blood tests

Blood should be taken for measurement of arterial blood gases and plasma urea, creatinine and electrolyte concentrations. Ask for measurement of plasma barbiturates. Salicylates and paracetamol do not generally cause loss of consciousness but should also be measured since multiple drug ingestion is not uncommon and the history in these circumstances is likely to be unreliable.

7. Gastric lavage

This is discussed below. It is important to avoid aspiration pneumonia and lavage should not be performed in an unconscious patient without intubation. Never induce vomiting in an unconscious patient.

8. Specific measures

Some drugs require immediate specific treatment. The most important are cyanide and paraquat, discussed below. The treatment of paracetamol poisoning should be instituted as soon as possible, without waiting for the plasma concentration result, in patients seen within 10–12 hours of ingestion. Opiate poisoning should be treated as soon as possible with naloxone and carbon monoxide poisoning with oxygen.

9. Other measures

When the emergency measures have been carried out there will be time to consider other matters, such as the important features of the history and other specific measures which may be indicated. These are dealt with in the next section.

B. General management of self-poisoning

There are five components to management:

1. Diagnosis and clinical assessment.
2. Removal of the poison from the gut.
3. General supportive measures.

4. Hastening of drug elimination.
5. Measures specific to the drug.

1. Diagnosis and clinical assessment

(a) Diagnosis

The diagnosis is often straightforward. Many patients give the history them-selves or are accompanied by a friend or relative who does so. Often, the drugs used are produced. However, not infrequently the history is not straightforward. Self-poisoning should always be a differential diagnosis in the assessment of an unconscious patient, particularly in young adults and in cases where there are decreased or absent tendon reflexes, or hypothermia without an obvious cause. Even in cases where a history *is* given, one should keep in mind the possibility that the incriminated drug may not have been the drug involved and that other drugs may have been taken instead, or in addition.

History-taking should not stop at the identification of the drug. Other useful pieces of information to be elicited are:

(i) The number of tablets, capsules, etc. taken—in an attempt to assess the probable severity of the problem. In addition, it may be helpful to know if alcohol was also taken and if so how much, in order to assess to what extent impairment of consciousness is due to alcohol, rather than to the drug. However, assessment of the extent and severity of self-poisoning from the history is frequently unreliable.

(ii) The time of overdose. This serves two purposes; firstly, to help decide whether induced emesis or gastric lavage are necessary and secondly, to help in the interpretation of plasma drug concentration measurements (see below).

(iii) Whether the patient has vomited or not. In the case of a drug, such as aspirin, it is important to find out if haematemesis has occurred. If vomiting has occurred in a drowsy or unconscious patient the possibility of aspiration must be considered.

(iv) Past history. This may give a clue to drugs that might have been readily available to the patient. In patients who have been taking drugs which induce liver enzymes (e.g. phenobarbitone, phenytoin) the effects of paracetamol on the liver may be increased. A past history of renal or hepatic disease may influence one's management. For example, forced diuresis is contra-indicated in a patient with renal failure and the effects of certain drugs (e.g. the opiates) may be expected to be more prolonged or severe in the patient with liver disease.

(v) Assessment of the seriousness of the attempt. Although strictly speaking this is not part of the acute management of self-poisoning, it is important to do it early on, in order that medical and nursing staff be made aware of the seriousness of a particular case and in order that psychiatric help be sought at a relatively early stage. Nowadays, there is a growing trend to discharge patients on the same day as their presentation to the hospital, sometimes without even admitting them to the ward, and it is important that a patient who has made a serious attempt on his or her life should not be allowed to leave without having had proper assessment by a trained psychiatrist. The signs of a serious attempt are:

1. Self-poisoning in a middle-aged or elderly patient.
2. A history of depression.
3. An admission that suicide was truly contemplated.
4. A suicide note.
5. An attempt not to be discovered.

(b) Clinical assessment

(i) Level of consciousness. It is useful to grade loss of consciousness using the following standard grading system:

0: Patient fully conscious.
1: Patient drowsy but responds to commands, or asleep but easily aroused.
2: Patient unconscious, but responds to standard minimal stimuli.
3: Patient unconscious but responds to standard maximal stimuli.
4: Patient does not respond to any stimuli.

Useful 'standard' stimuli are rubbing the sternum with the knuckles or pinching the Achilles' tendon. Pressure over the supra-orbital fissure should not be used because of the risk of damage to the eye if the hand slips.

The main virtue of this system is that it may be used to provide objective evidence of a change in conscious state over a period of time. In addition any patient who is in grade 2 or worse should not have gastric lavage carried out without being intubated with an endotracheal tube first. Impairment of consciousness to any level in patients who have taken salicylates is an important sign and suggests serious poisoning.

(ii) Respiratory function. In the comatose patient this can be assessed by direct observation, by measuring the tidal volume or minute volume if appropriate equipment is available and by measuring the blood gases.

(iii) Cardiovascular and renal function. In the comatose patient it is important to assess peripheral circulatory and renal function by measuring heart rate, blood pressure and urine output. If necessary the patient should be catheterized.

(iv) Rectal temperature. Hypothermia (rectal temperature below 36°C) occurs not uncommonly in patients who are unconscious through self-poisoning. However, poisoning with salicylates and monoamine oxidase inhibitors can cause hyperthermia.

(v) Other signs. For poisoning with some drugs other signs may be of value. For example, pupillary constriction due to narcotic analgesics, the syndrome of tinnitus, hyperpyrexia, hyperventilation and sweating due to salicylates and skin blisters due to barbiturates (although this is not a specific sign and can occur in poisoning with other drugs, such as tricyclic anti-depressants and carbon monoxide). Puncture marks and perivenous ulcers in the skin of the arms should be looked for to identify the drug addict.

(vi) Blood and urine tests. The only drugs for which plasma concentration measurement should be carried out routinely as a guide to treatment are salicylates and paracetamol. These are discussed under their separate headings. Measurement of barbiturate concentrations serves principally in making the diagnosis in cases of coma of unknown cause and in identifying the type of barbiturate involved (i.e. long- intermediate- or short-acting). However, it does not reflect prognosis because of wide inter-individual variability and should not be used as a guide to treatment.

Paraquat may be identified in gastric aspirate and urine by a simple colorimetric test. This test is useful in *excluding* the diagnosis and in monitoring progress.

In the majority of cases routine plasma urea and electrolyte measurements are not necessary. Nevertheless, they should be performed in all ill patients to assess renal and hepatic function and hydration. In some cases tests should be carried out specific to the effects of the drug (e.g. blood glucose, blood gases, and prothrombin time for aspirin, liver function tests for paracetamol).

(vii) Chest X-ray. A çhest X-ray should be taken in any drowsy or comatose patient who has vomited, to rule out aspiration pneumonia. A chest X-ray is not usually necessary in a fully conscious patient even after induced emesis or gastric lavage. A chest X-ray should also be carried out in any patient who requires long-term endotracheal intubation, to check the position of the endotracheal tube.

2. Removal of poison from the gut

If the patient is seen within four hours of self-poisoning then it is worthwhile attempting to remove tablets or capsules from the stomach by induced emesis or gastric lavage. Such procedures may also be of value up to twenty-four hours or even longer after self-poisoning with aspirin, which can cause pylorospasm, and up to eight hours after drugs with anticholinergic effects, which decrease gastro-intestinal motility (e.g. tricyclic anti-depressants). The procedures are as follows:

(a) Induced emesis

This should only be carried out in a patient with a normal cough reflex. In an emergency, vomiting may be induced by pharyngeal stimulation with a finger or the back of a spoon. In hospital, syrup of ipecacuanha, or paediatric ipecacuanha emetic draught is used in a dose of 15 ml (10 ml in a child under eighteen months) with 200 ml of water or fruit juice. It should have an effect within fifteen to thirty minutes but if not, the dose should be repeated. This regimen is effective in almost all cases. However, if vomiting does not occur within thirty minutes to one hour gastric lavage must be carried out because of the cerebral toxicity of ipecacuanha, which contains emetine.

(b) Gastric lavage

Before carrying out gastric lavage check that the cough reflex is intact. If it is not, a cuffed endotracheal tube must be inserted before gastric lavage is carried out, in order to avoid aspiration. The patient should be laid on the left side, the head below the level of the rest of the body, and a wide-bore tube should be passed via the mouth into the stomach. We use a 150 cm long tube with a 7 mm internal diameter and extra perforations in the final 10 cm or so. The usual lavage fluid is warm water, but in young children saline should be used. In some cases special solutions may be indicated (e.g. desferrioxamine lavage in iron poisoning). Volumes of 300 ml are passed, via a large funnel held above the patient, down the tube into the stomach. The funnel is then lowered beneath the level of the patient and the gastric contents allowed to drain into a bucket or aspirated with a large syringe. This procedure is repeated until the fluid returning from the stomach is clear. Some of the initial return should be kept for forensic purposes, if later required.

Neither induced emesis nor gastric lavage should be carried out in patients who have taken corrosive acids (give antacids), or alkalis (give dilute acetic or citric acid), or any volatile substances (e.g. petroleum products, such as paraffin).

In children ipecacuanha-induced emesis is the procedure of choice. However, in adults gastric lavage is still to be preferred. While ipecacuanha-induced emesis is easier to carry out it carries the risk of emetine toxicity, albeit in a minority of patients, and even when successful it does not cause complete emptying of the stomach. Aspiration is a risk if the patient becomes drowsy after having taken ipecacuanha. An added advantage of gastric lavage is that antidotes may be instilled directly into the stomach, e.g. desferrioxamine in iron poisoning and milk of magnesia in bleach poisoning. Activated charcoal instilled into the stomach may adsorb and therefore reduce the absorption of salicylates, barbiturates, tricyclic antidepressants, dextropropoxyphene (e.g. in Distalgesic), digitalis and paraffin. It may also be given orally but should not be given with ipecacuanha which it also adsorbs.

3. General supportive measures

(a) Respiration

In most cases it is sufficient to ensure an open airway, in a drowsy or unconscious patient, by keeping the patient semi-prone with the neck extended, by inserting an oral airway and by regularly sucking out secretions. If there is no cough reflex an endotracheal tube should be inserted. In all such cases blood gases should be measured. If there is hypoxia, oxygen should be given in amounts depending on the blood gases according to the following guidelines:

P_{O_2} between 8 and 11 kPa (62 and 85 mm Hg), and P_{CO_2} between 5 and 7 kPa (38 and 54 mm Hg)—give 24 per cent O_2 increasing to 28 per cent after 30 minutes if the P_{CO_2} has not risen.

P_{O_2} below 8 kPa or P_{CO_2} above 7 kPa—assisted ventilation will be required.

(b) Circulatory support

If the systolic blood pressure is below 90 mm Hg and does not rise on raising the end of the bed, volume expanders should be given, e.g. plasma or colloid solutions. However, patients are often already in positive fluid balance, or at least not fluid-depleted and great care must be taken not to cause fluid overload. For this reason a central venous pressure line should be inserted. If plasma volume expanders do not cause an increase in blood pressure, or if fluid overload occurs then cautious drug therapy is indicated. Some would recommend the use of a β_1 adrenoceptor agonist such as dobutamine (2.5–10 μg/kg/min by continuous i.v. infusion) but if one's chief concern is renal blood flow then low doses of dopamine (e.g. 5–10 μg/kg/min) may be sufficient or may be combined with dobutamine. Higher doses of dopamine (10–20 μg/kg/min) also have a β_1 adrenoceptor agonist effect. There is the risk at higher doses of these drugs of α adrenoceptor agonist effects, resulting in peripheral and renal vasoconstriction. Therefore, whatever agent is used, it is wise not to raise the systolic blood pressure above 100 mm Hg. The urine output should also be carefully monitored, if necessary by catheterization.

(c) Cardiac arrhythmias

These should be treated in the same way as after an acute myocardial infarction (e.g. lignocaine for ventricular tachyarrhythmias). However, for digitalis-induced arrhythmias, phenytoin is the treatment of choice. Supraventricular arrhythmias generally do not need treatment.

(d) Hypothermia

Hypothermia (rectal temperature below 36°C) should be treated slowly by keeping the patient in a warm environment and by the use of a foil blanket ('space blanket'). In severe cases (rectal temperatures below 30°C) more rapid warming is necessary. In the middle-aged or elderly put one arm into water at 40°C. In the young immersion of the whole body in water at 40°C is safe. All inspired air and infusion solutions should be warmed before administration.

(e) Convulsions

Convulsions may be treated with either diazepam (10 mg i.v., repeated at thirty-minute intervals to a total of 30 mg) or chlormethiazole (40–100 ml of an 0.8 per cent solution given by i.v. infusion over five to ten minutes, followed if necessary by a continuous i.v. infusion at a rate depending on the patient's response). If this fails, the patient should be anaesthetized and treated with curare and assisted ventilation.

(f) Fluid and electrolyte balance

Most patients have either normal fluid and electrolyte balance or slight fluid overload. For those who are fluid depleted (e.g. because of vomiting) but conscious, oral fluids are usually sufficient. In most unconscious patients simple replacement with two 500 ml units of 5 per cent dextrose to one 500 ml unit of physiological saline is usually sufficient. Central venous pressure monitoring may be required in severely ill patients.

4. Hastening elimination of the drug

(a) Forced diuresis

For drugs which are subject to extensive passive reabsorption by the renal tubules and whose rate of renal clearance is proportional to the rate of urine flow, forced diuresis at an altered urine pH will hasten elimination of the drug. Thus the rates of salicylate and lithium renal clearance are increased by alkaline diuresis and those of amphetamine, quinine, quinidine, and tranylcypromine by acid diuresis. A useful regimen for salicylates is discussed below.

(b) Dialysis

Removal of drug by dialysis (either haemodialysis or peritoneal dialysis) is reserved for severe cases of poisoning. It is useful only for drugs which are not widely distributed to body tissues and which are not highly bound by plasma proteins. It may be of value in serious poisoning with salicylates, barbiturates, chloral hydrate and its derivatives, iron and lithium, among others. Lists of drugs which may be removed by these dialysis procedures have been published (see, for example, Matthew and Lawson 1977).

(c) Charcoal haemoperfusion

Because charcoal adsorbs many drugs it can be used to remove drug from the circulation. It is of value even when there is high plasma protein binding but wide distribution of drug to the tissues limits its usefulness. The problems of thrombocytopenia, leucopenia, febrile reactions and charcoal emboli encountered with earlier forms of charcoal columns have been diminished by more modern preparations. However, the pharmacokinetics of column clearance of drugs from the body have not yet been thoroughly worked out. If available, charcoal haemoperfusion may be of value in serious poisoning with salicylates, barbiturates, glutethimide, meprobamate, methaqualone, theophylline, and derivatives of chloral hydrate.

5. Specific measures

(a) Salicylates

The clinical features of salicylate poisoning are tinnitus, deafness, hyperventilation, hyperpyrexia with sweating and dehydration, epigastric pain and vomiting. Patients are generally fully conscious and *any* impairment of consciousness is a sign of serious poisoning. In addition, there may be hypoglycaemia and bleeding may occur because of a reduction in the prothrombin time.

Blood gases show a respiratory alkalosis due to hyperventilation and a metabolic acidosis due to the presence of salicylic acid. In adults the alkalosis usually predominates and can be compensated for by renal mechanisms. However, in children, the metabolic acidosis tends to predominate. Moreover, since respiratory compensatory mechanisms are less efficient than renal compensatory mechanisms, poisoning in children is more serious at any given plasma salicylate concentration than it is in adults.

The plasma salicylate concentration should be measured as a guide to therapy. Nevertheless, salicylate is highly protein bound and because it is the unbound salicylate in plasma which determines its therapeutic and toxic effects, the plasma salicylate concentration (measured as *total*, i.e. protein bound + unbound, salicylate) does not accurately reflect the effects of the drug. Therefore, the plasma concentration should always be considered in conjunction with the patient's clinical state.

Gastric lavage should always be carried out no matter how long after ingestion. If the plasma salicylate concentration is above 3.6 mmol/l (1.5 mmol/l in children) and the patient has obvious signs and symptoms of toxicity then forced diuresis should be carried out. The following regimen has been found to be safe:

A mixture of physiological saline (500 ml), 5 per cent dextrose (1 litre), and 1.26 per cent sodium bicarbonate (500 ml) should be infused as a 2-litre mixture over three hours and thereafter at a rate of 1 litre/hour until clinical improvement occurs. Potassium chloride should be added at a rate of 20 mmol/hour. In children the infusion rate of this solution should be 30 ml/kg/hour and plasma electrolyte measurements should be made two to four hourly. Great care must be taken to avoid fluid overload by making sure that the bladder is emptied hourly (by catheterization if need be), by keeping painstaking fluid balance records and by measuring the blood pressure every half-hour. If necessary a central venous pressure line should also be inserted. Recent work suggests that alkalinization with bicarbonate alone may be as effective as the above cocktail.

Forced diuresis should *not* be carried out in patients with circulatory failure, renal failure, or fluid overload. In such cases peritoneal dialysis or haemodialysis are the alternatives.

Hypoglycaemia is usually reversed by the dextrose in the mixed infusion. If the prothrombin time is lengthened, vitamin K_1 should be given (10 mg i.v.).

In drowsy or unconscious patients, acidosis should be corrected with i.v. sodium bicarbonate before starting other treatment. If it is available, haemodialysis is to be preferred to forced diuresis in these patients.

(b) Paracetamol

In paracetamol poisoning there is usually little in the way of acute symptoms apart from nausea and vomiting. However, in severe poisoning (more than 15g) there are several delayed effects, the most important of which is the toxic effect on the liver. Paracetamol, in the usual analgesic doses, is metabolized about 85 per cent by conjugation with glucuronide and sulphate and about 10 per cent by conjugation with glutathione. In overdose, the former pathways are saturated and proportionately more paracetamol is metabolized via the glutathione pathway. However, hepatic glutathione is rapidly depleted and an intermediate hydroxylamine metabolite accumulates. This metabolite binds to liver cell proteins and causes irreversible damage. If it can be removed before liver damage occurs then the overall damage can be prevented or reduced and full recovery will eventually occur. Glutathione itself is of no value in treatment since it does not enter liver cells after i.v. administration. Therefore, alternative compounds have been used to provide SH groups for the conjugation of the toxic hydroxylamine metabolite. The most useful of these is acetylcysteine.

Because the signs of serious toxicity occur late, the decision on whether to treat depends on the plasma paracetamol concentration and the time after dosage. A simple method of making the decision is illustrated in Figure 31.1 which is constructed on plain paper as follows: draw vertical and horizontal axes; mark on the vertical axis values of 0.3, 0.6 and 1.2 mmol/l (plasma paracetamol concentrations) at equal intervals; mark on the horizontal axis values of 4, 8 and 12 hours (time after ingestion) at equal intervals; draw a cross at the point marking 4 hours and 1.2 mmol/l and a second cross at the point marking 12 hours and 0.3 mmol/l; join the two crosses with a straight line. Plot the value of the patient's plasma concentration against the time after ingestion. If the point falls above the line, treatment is indicated. In patients in whom ingestion occurred less than four hours before sampling, the plasma concentration is unreliable because absorption is still continuing. In all cases treatment should be started straight away and the plasma paracetamol concentration result, when available, will allow one to decide whether to continue treatment or not. This is particularly important for

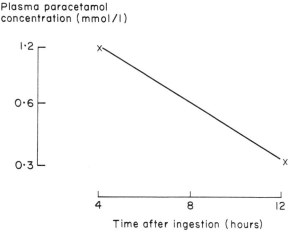

Fig. 31.1. When to treat paracetamol poisoning with acetylcysteine (see text). Adapted from Prescott *et al.* (1976).

patients who present at about ten hours after ingestion since after about ten
to twelve hours, treatment is probably of no value and may even be harmful,
if reports that liver damage is worse following treatment after ten to fifteen
hours are correct.

In patients who have been taking drugs which induce hepatic drug
metabolizing enzymes (e.g. phenobarbitone, phenytoin, rifampicin, griseo-
fulvin) the toxic effects of paracetamol may be enhanced. However, there is
no good guidance as to when treatment should be given in such cases and it is
probably wise at present to treat all such patients.

Treatment should be with intravenous acetylcysteine (Parvolex) as
follows:

150 mg/kg i.v. over 15 minutes;

50 mg/kg i.v. in 500 ml of 5 per cent dextrose over 4 hours;

100 mg/kg i.v. in 1 litre of 5 per cent dextrose over 16 hours.

Methionine is sometimes used as an alternative to i.v. acetylcysteine but
it is less reliable because it is given orally and its usefulness may be limited by
vomiting.

Liver function tests (including the prothrombin time) should be
measured on admission in all patients who require treatment. Such patients
should be kept in hospital for forty-eight hours for observation and reassessment of liver function. Abnormal liver function tests at forty-eight hours
presage severe liver damage.

In patients who take paracetamol as Distalgesic remember also to treat
dextropropoxyphene poisoning with naloxone (see below).

(c) Tricyclic antidepressants

The features of poisoning with these drugs are due to peripheral and central
anticholinergic effects and to the potentiation of sympathetic nervous
activity. The clinical results are dry mouth, dilated pupils and blurred vision,
urinary retention, tachyarrhythmias and heart block, hypotension, impairment of consciousness and of respiration, hallucinations and convulsions.

The majority (over 80 per cent) of patients require only supportive
measures but if there are life-threatening tachyarrhythmias, hypotension, or
serious cerebral effects (e.g. respiratory depression, convulsions), physostigmine should be used. It acts by inhibiting acetylcholinesterase, thereby
antagonizing the anti-cholinergic effects of tricyclic antidepressants, and
unlike other cholinesterase inhibitors such as neostigmine, it enters the
brain. It is given up to a total of 2 mg by i.v. injection at a rate of 0.2 mg/min;
the full dose need not be given if a therapeutic response occurs rapidly. The
effects of physostigmine are very variable. When it is efficacious its effects
are dramatic and occur within a few minutes. The patient wakes up and
tachyarrhythmias are abolished. However, quite often it has no effect at all.

Furthermore, its effect is short-lived and doses need to be repeated at intervals of about half-an-hour. Even if a first dose has worked, subsequent doses may sometimes have little or no effect. Physostigmine should only be used to treat life-threatening tachyarrhythmias, respiratory depression or serious cerebral effects because it has its own adverse effects, including bronchospasm, hypersalivation and an increase in bronchial secretions, vomiting, diarrhoea, gastro-intestinal spasm and convulsions.

If physostigmine is not effective tachyarrhythmias may be treated with a β-adrenoceptor antagonist, such as propranolol and convulsions with diazepam. Acidosis should be corrected with sodium bicarbonate. Brady-cardia and heart block should be treated by artificial pacing.

In passing, it may be noted that physostigmine has been reported to be of value in treating poisoning with phenothiazines, such as chlorpromazine and some antihistamines. However, its use in these circumstances has not been properly evaluated.

(d) Barbiturates

Barbiturate poisoning presents with the signs and symptoms of central nervous system depression, including any degree of impairment of con-sciousness from drowsiness to coma, restlessness, delirium, hallucinations, convulsions and respiratory depression. Other effects include hypotension, hypothermia and shock, sometimes causing renal failure. In addition, the characteristic but non-specific skin blisters may develop. They may also be seen in poisoning with, for example, tricyclic antidepressants and carbon monoxide. The effects of poisoning may persist for several days with the long-acting barbiturates, such as phenobarbitone and pentobarbitone.

Gastric lavage and supportive measures are indicated. In seriously ill patients haemodialysis or charcoal haemoperfusion may be required if deterioration occurs despite intensive support.

(e) Paraquat

This is a serious and often fatal poisoning with a herbicide used in various proprietary weed killers (e.g. Weedol, Gramoxone, Pathclear). Fatalities are much less common after ingestion of granular (domestic) forms of paraquat than after liquid (commercial) forms, which can be fatal in ingested volumes of 10 ml. Paraquat irritates skin and mucous membranes and burning sensations in the mouth and abdomen are succeeded by local ulceration, nausea and vomiting. However, the major effect takes some days to develop. They consist of pulmonary oedema due to alveolitis and bronchiolitis due to the effects of a toxic superoxide. These effects may result in fatal respiratory failure. Treatment should be started immediately and may be withdrawn if urine testing fails to reveal the presence of paraquat. The poison should be vigorously washed away from the skin and eyes and antibiotic drops applied to the eyes, if affected. Gastric lavage must be carried out as soon as possible, preferably with a 15 per cent solution of fuller's earth (i.e. 150 g/litre). In an emergency, vomiting should be induced by pharyngeal irritation. After lavage, 1 litre of a suspension of 150 g fuller's earth as an adsorbent, with 200 ml of 20 per cent mannitol as a purgative, should be left in the stomach. Bentonite 7 g may be used instead of fuller's earth but is less effective. Fuller's earth 100 g will irreversibly bind 5 g of paraquat. Thereafter, this treatment should be repeated as often as the patient can tolerate it (say half-hourly) until fuller's earth appears in the stools. During this time a nasogastric tube should be kept in position and the treatment given through the tube directly into the stomach. In addition, forced diuresis as for salicylate poisoning should be carried out, as should charcoal haemoperfusion if available. Fluid losses by purgation should be replaced intravenously.

(f) Notes on some other important poisonings

(i) Benzodiazepines. Supportive measures only.

(ii) Major tranquillizers (phenothiazines, such as chlorpromazine, and butyrophenones, such as haloperidol). Intensive supportive measures may be required. Dyskinesias should be treated with benztropine, 2 mg i.v., and convulsions with diazepam or chlormethiazole.

(iii) Monoamine oxidase inhibitors. Dopamine or dobutamine should *not* be used for treating shock. Use instead hydrocortisone, 100 mg i.v. 6-hourly. For hyperthermia use a fan and tepid sponging or chlorpromazine, 100 mg i.m. Chlorpromazine is also useful for treating the cerebral stimulatory effects of MAO inhibitors.

(iv) Lithium. Lithium excretion is hastened by forced alkaline diuresis but very careful plasma electrolyte monitoring must be carried out. Dialysis or charcoal haemoperfusion may be required.

(v) Iron. Gastric lavage should be carried out with a solution of desferrioxamine, in a concentration of 2 g/litre and 10 g of desferrioxamine in 50 ml water should be left in the stomach at the end. Desferrioxamine should also be given as soon as possible both i.m. and i.v. The doses are: i.m., 2 g (1 g in a child) repeated after 12 hours; i.v., 15 mg/kg/hour to a maximum of 80 mg/kg/day. If there is oliguria, dialysis should be started immediately.

(vi) Cyanide. Following gastric lavage, 300 ml of 25 per cent sodium thiosulphate should be left in the stomach. The traditional method of treating cyanide poisoning has been replaced by the use of dicobalt edetate (EDTA). It is given as Kelocyanor, 600 mg in 40 ml over one minute, and followed by 50 ml of 5 per cent dextrose. If recovery does not occur within a minute or two, another 300 mg of dicobalt edetate should be given. In patients who have not taken cyanide, dicobalt edetate may cause vomiting, hypotension and tachycardia; these may require treatment. The traditional alternative to dicobalt edetate is the administration of 10 ml of 3 per cent sodium nitrite, given i.v. over three minutes and followed by 25 ml of 50 per cent sodium thiosulphate, given by slow i.v. injection. Oxygen (100 per cent) should be given and acidosis should be corrected with sodium bicarbonate.

(vii) Carbon monoxide. Carbon monoxide poisoning can still occur, despite the replacement of coal gas by North Sea gas in the home, because of incomplete combustion with the formation of carbon monoxide. Of course, it may also occur in patients who poison themselves with car exhaust gases. Treatment is by removal from the source of gas and by administration of 100 per cent oxygen with assisted ventilation in patients not breathing spontaneously. In severe cases exchange transfusion may be required. Treat cerebral oedema with mannitol (500 ml of a 20 per cent solution) and cardiac arrhythmias as required.

(viii) Narcotic analgesics. Naloxone rapidly reverses the effects of opiate analgesics and other narcotic analgesics (e.g. pethidine, pentazocine, dextropropoxyphene). It is given in a dose of 0.4 mg i.v. initially, repeated every 2–3 minutes if required. A total dose of 1.2 mg is usually sufficient. In buprenorphine poisoning, only partial reversal occurs and in severe cases a respiratory stimulant, such as doxapram, may be required. Naloxone is eliminated from the body with a half-time of about an hour, i.e. faster than the narcotic analgesics. Therefore its effects may wear off.

(ix) Organophosphorus insecticides. These are very toxic and are absorbed through the skin. Rubber gloves should therefore be worn when in contact with the patient or the patient's clothes. Intensive respiratory support is required. When cyanosis has been reversed atropine should be given, 2 mg i.v. every ten minutes, until the skin is dry and there is a sinus tachycardia or other evidence of full atropinization. Since these compounds inhibit acetylcholinesterase irreversibly, a cholinesterase reactivator should be given, such as pralidoxime 30 mg/kg i.v. at a rate of no more than 500 mg/minute and repeated after thirty minutes. Convulsions should be treated with diazepam.

(x) Digitalis. In this instance, ipecacuanha-induced emesis is preferable to gastric lavage for removal of the drug from the stomach, since there is a risk of cardiac asystole during lavage. Activated charcoal may help reduce the absorption of digitalis, particularly digitoxin. In addition, an anion exchange resin, such as cholestyramine or colestipol is also effective in reducing digitoxin absorption. A temporary pacemaker should be inserted as soon as possible, even in the absence of arrhythmias or heart block. Hypokalaemia should be treated with potassium chloride, i.v. at a rate of no more than 20 mmol/hour. Hyperkalaemia may occur and is a poor prognostic sign. It should be treated with insulin, 20 units i.v. and 50 ml of 50 per cent dextrose. In severe cases dialysis may be required to treat hyperkalaemia but dialysis does not remove digitalis from the body. Tachyarrhythmias should be treated with phenytoin or propranolol and bradycardia and heart block by pacing. Atropine may be used if a pacemaker is not available.

Charcoal haemoperfusion has been advocated for digitalis poisoning but its usefulness has not been established. It may be of value for digitoxin poisoning, particularly if started very soon after ingestion.

(xi) Methanol. Give ethyl alcohol 1 ml/kg of a 50 per cent solution orally immediately, followed by 0.5 ml/kg 2-hourly. Treat acidosis with sodium bicarbonate. In severe cases haemodialysis is necessary.

Sources of information

A useful textbook describing the presentation and management of acute poisonings is that by Matthew and Lawson (1979); other useful texts are given below. For information on individual drugs one of the following poisons centres should be contacted:

Belfast	0232–40503
Cardiff	0222–33101
Dublin	Dublin 45588
Edinburgh	031–229–2477
Leeds	0532–32799
London	01–407–7600
Manchester	061–740–2254

For specific advice on paraquat poisoning one of the many paraquat treatment centres should be contacted (see the *British Medical Journal*, 1979, **ii**, p. 619).

Further reading

Gibson T.P. and Nelson H.A. (1977) Drug kinetics and artificial kidneys. *Clinical Pharmacokinetics* **2**, 403–406.

Locket S. (1978) Overdose. *British Journal of Hospital Medicine* **19**, 200–212.

Matthew H. and Lawson A.A.H. (1979) *Treatment of Common Acute Poisonings*, 4th ed. Churchill Livingstone.

Pond S., Rosenberg J., Benowitz N.L. and Takki S. (1979) Pharmacokinetics of haemoperfusion for drug overdose. *Clinical Pharmacokinetics* **4**, 329–354.

Prescott L.F., Park J., Sutherland G.R., Smith I.J. and Proudfoot A.T. (1976) Cysteamine, methionine and penicillamine in the treatment of paracetamol poisoning. *Lancet* **ii**, 109–113.

Rosenberg J., Benowitz N.L. and Pond S. (1981) Pharmacokinetics of drug over-dose. *Clinical Pharmacokinetics* **6,** 161–192.

Symposium (1977) Principles of emergency treatment for swallowed poisons. *Proceedings of the Royal Society of Medicine* **70,** 764–778.

Vale J.A. and Meredith T.J. (1981) *Poisoning: Diagnosis and Treatment*, 1st ed. Update.

Various (1984) ABC of self-poisoning. Series of articles in the *British Medical Journal*, starting July 7, Vol. 289.

32 · Acute Infections and Imported Diseases

G. PASVOL

General considerations

The appropriate management of infectious emergencies is particularly important, for delay of only a few hours in specific treatment can prove fatal. An outline of the content of this chapter is given in Table 32.1. In industrialized countries, common life-threatening infections (discussed elsewhere) include septicaemias (Chapter 9), pneumonias (Chapter 13), infectious diarrhoeas (Chapter 24) and infections of the central nervous system (Chapter 20). However, less common, but equally dangerous infectious

Table 32.1. Acute infections and imported diseases

General considerations
Outline of four important points:
(1) Diagnosis —clinical
               —acute laboratory investigations
(2) Isolation —side room
               —isolation unit
(3) Specimens
(4) Treatment—general
             —Antimicrobial
             —Immunoglobulin
Notifiable conditions.

Specific conditions (alphabetical order)
Acute tonsillitis, pharyngitis and epiglottitis
Diphtheria
Hepatitis
Leptospirosis including the Jarisch–Herxheimer reaction
Malaria
Poliomyelitis
Rabies exposure
Stevens–Johnson syndrome
Smallpox
Tetanus
Typhoid
Varicella zoster and herpes simplex infections
Viral haemorrhagic fevers

diseases, acquired both at home or abroad, continue to take their toll either because they are not recognized or because of unfamiliarity with management.

In the acute management of patients with infectious disease four important questions should be *always* asked:

(1) Diagnosis: What is the diagnosis and in particular which organs are involved and what specific agent is responsible?

(2) Isolation: Need the patient be placed in the side room of a general ward or be sent to an infectious disease unit?

(3) Specimens: Have the correct specimens been sent and are they safe for the recipient in the laboratory?

(4) Treatment: What supportive treatment and what specific chemotherapy needs to be started immediately?

(1) The diagnosis of infectious diseases is almost always made on the history; the clinical findings and laboratory tests usually only confirm the diagnosis. There are only a limited number of infectious conditions where a specific organism can, or need be sought in the emergency room. This must never be omitted when facilities are available (Table 32.2.). An exact aetiological diagnosis enables specific treatment to be started immediately.

(2) Patients with infectious diseases need not always be nursed separately from others. If the patient presents with a fever of unknown origin, an upper respiratory tract infection, diarrhoea or jaundice, it is always wise to nurse them initially in a side room. This is particularly important where immunocompromised patients are on the same ward. In such cases it is better still to remove the infected patient to an isolation unit (Table 32.3). All patients who become ill within three weeks of returning from abroad should be isolated unless they have a condition which is obviously non-infectious. All patients with tetanus, cerebral malaria or rabies must be nursed on an intensive therapy unit, especially since sudden deterioration can occur unexpectedly.

(3) In order to make an accurate and rapid diagnosis, appropriate specimens should be collected on admission and not days later as so frequently happens, resulting in a loss of valuable time. Common omissions cannot be overemphasized.

(a) The taking of blood cultures is almost always appropriate whenever infection is suspected and is especially important when the patient is to be started on antimicrobial therapy. Infections particularly in the old, very young and immunocompromised are often not accompanied by a fever especially when due to Gram-negative organisms.

(b) Where viral meningitis, encephalitis, myocarditis or pericarditis is suspected, throat swab and stool specimens are essential for diagnosis of those due to enteroviruses.

(c) Other than in bacterial infections of the urinary tract, urine samples assist in establishing the diagnosis of cytomegalovirus (CMV) infections and leptospirosis.

(d) Numerous helpful serological tests can be carried out to aid in the diagnosis of infection, e.g. anti-streptolysin O titre (ASOT), Widal in enteric fevers, etc. A sample of serum taken on admission and stored at $-20°C$ may prove invaluable in retrospect.

Table 32.2. Common infectious conditions where the specific organism can be identified immediately by laboratory tests

Condition	Specimens	Test	Organisms
Hepatitis B	Serum	Haemagglutination test and others	Hepatitis B surface antigen
Infectious mononucleosis	Serum	Test for heterophile antibody e.g. Paul–Bunnell, Monospot or equivalent	Epstein–Barr virus
Leptospirosis	Urine, blood	Dark-ground microscopy	L. species
Malaria	Blood film	Romanovsky (Leishman's or Geimsa stain)	*Plasmodia* sp.
Meningitis (pneumonia)	CSF (sputum)	Gram stain	Bacteria esp. *Meningococcus, Pneumococcus, Haemophilus, Listeria*, also *Cryptococcus*
		Countercurrent immunoelectrophoresis	*Meningococcus Pneumococcus Haemophilus*
		Latex agglutination	*Cryptococcus*
Tuberculosis	Sputum, urine, CSF, pus from abscess	Ziehl–Nielson Stain	*M. tuberculosis*
Vesicular skin lesions	Vesicle fluid	Electron microscopy	Herpesviruses esp. *herpes simplex* and *Varicella* zoster. Poxviruses (a) Variola, Vaccinia (b) Paravaccinia such as Orf

Table 32.3. Guidelines to the isolation of patients with specific infectious diseases

Infectivity and consequence if spread	Diseases	Guideline to isolation
Man to man spread common and of important consequence if transmitted	B haemolytic streptococcal throat infections Diphtheria Hepatitis A; B and Non-A or -B Poliomyelitis Salmonellae including enteric fevers Suspected smallpox or anthrax Tuberculosis Viral haemorrhagic fevers (e.g. Lassa fever, Marburg and Ebola virus infections)	Isolation unit
Man to man spread of less important consequence unless immunocompromised hosts or children are involved	Chickenpox and herpes zoster Herpes simplex Infectious mononucleosis Measles Mumps Rubella Whooping cough	Side room or isolation unit
Man to man spread almost unknown	Encephalitides Legionnaires Leptospirosis Malaria Meningitides excluding tuberculosis Rabies Tetanus	Side room where possible Intensive therapy unit where appropriate

(e) Any possible portal of entry of the infectious agent should be swabbed and transported in appropriate media. The throat, nose, vagina and skin fissures between the toes are sites commonly omitted.

(f) Unusual sites of isolation of the causative organism are sometimes of help where other sites have failed, e.g. bone marrow for enteric fevers, arterial blood for fungal infections, liver biopsy for tuberculosis.

(4) Where an exact diagnosis has been made, appropriate chemotherapy can be started immediately. However, there are commonly only three circumstances in which antimicrobial therapy should be given blindly (i.e. without identifying the causative organism). (1) In life-threatening infections. (2) In infections where the likely causative agent is obvious (e.g. streptococcal throat infections, most urinary tract infections, tetanus,

Table 32.4. Appropriate uses for human immunoglobulin in the prevention and treatment of infectious diseases. (Cunningham–Rundles et al. 1982)

Agent/condition	Target population	Preparation[a,b]	Dose[c]	Status
Hepatitis A	Family contacts Institutional outbreaks	IG	0.02 ml/kg of body weight (3.2 mg/kg of body weight)	Recommended for prevention
	Travellers exposed to unhygienic conditions	IG	0.02–0.05 ml/kg of body weight (3.2–8.0 mg/kg of body weight) every 4 months	Recommended for prevention
Hepatitis non-A, non-B	Percutaneous or mucosal exposure	IG	0.05 ml/kg of body weight (8 mg/kg of body weight)	Optional for prevention
Hepatitis B	Percutaneous or mucosal exposure	HBIG	0.05–0.07ml/kg of body weight (8–11 mg/kg of body weight) Repeat in one month	Recommended for prevention
	Newborns of mothers with HBsAg	HBIG	0.05 ml (8 mg) at birth 3, and 6 months	Recommended for prevention
	Sexual contacts of acute hepatitis B patients	HBIG	0.05 ml/kg of body weight (8 mg/kg of body weight) Repeat after one month	Optional for prevention (often too late)
Rubella	Women exposed during early pregnancy	IG	20 ml	Optional for prevention
Varicella-zoster	Immunosuppressed contacts of acute cases, or newborn contacts	VZIG[d]	15–20 units/kg of body weight minimum 125 units	Recommended for prevention

Disease	Indication	Agent	Dose	Recommendation
Measles (rubeola)	Infants less than 1 year old or immunosuppressed contacts of acute cases exposed less than 6 days previously	IG	0.25 ml/kg of body weight or 0.5 mg/kg of body weight if immunosuppressed	Recommended for prevention
Rabies	Unimmunized subjects exposed to animals	RIG	20 IU/kg of body weight	Recommended for prevention
Tetanus	Following significant exposure of unimmunized or incompletely immunized person or immediately on diagnosis of disease	TIG	250 units for prophylaxis 3000–6000 units for therapy	Recommended for prevention or treatment

[a] IG = immune globulin (human); HBIG = hepatitis B immune globulin; VZIG = varicella-zoster immune globulin; RIG = rabies immune globulin; TIG = tetanus immune globulin.

[b] Hyperimmune immunoglobulins have also been used in prophylaxis of mumps and prophylaxis and treatment of pertussis and diphtheria; there are no conclusive data available, and no recommendations can be given.

[c] Dose based on intramuscular administration of 16.5 per cent solution.

[d] Of limited availability at the present time.

meningococcal epidemics etc.). (3) Where the infection involves an inaccessible site (e.g. the chest and biliary tract). Outside these exceptions it is bad hospital practice to use antimicrobials in a blind fashion.

Human immunoglobulin is of importance in the treatment or prevention of certain infectious conditions (Table 32.4) (Cunningham-Rundles *et al.* 1982).

Notifiable conditions

The following infectious diseases are required by law in the United Kingdom (UK) to be notified by the doctor in attendance as soon as the diagnosis is made. Notifications should be made to the Medical Officer of Health of the district on forms provided by the local authority which may make additional diseases notifiable in its own area (e.g. Brucellosis). Currently these diseases include:- Anthrax, Cholera, Diphtheria, Dysentery (Amoebic or bacillary), Encephalitis, Food poisoning (including Salmonellosis), Infective jaundice, Leprosy, Leptospirosis, Malaria, Measles, Meningitis (Bacterial), Ophthalmia neonatorum, Plague, Poliomyelitis, Relapsing fever, Scarlet fever, Smallpox, Tetanus, Tuberculosis, Typhoid and Paratyphoid fevers, Typhus, Whooping cough and Yellow fever.

Specific conditions

For ease of reference these are arranged in alphabetical order.

Acute tonsillitis, pharyngitis and epiglottitis

Diagnosis

Acute tonsillitis, pharyngitis and epiglottitis present as medical emergencies when patients have difficulty in breathing, with speech or with eating. Although many micro-organisms are incriminated in upper respiratory tract infections, in adults the two most important that present as emergencies are infections with β haemolytic streptococci and the Epstein–Barr virus (infectious mononucleosis). In certain circumstances diphtheria should remain part of the differential diagnosis. When stridor is present, acute epiglottitis due to *H influenzae* must be considered as this has a high mortality and although seen mainly in children, occasionally occurs in adults (Barman *et al.* 1980; Morgenstein and Abramson 1971).

Isolation

The patient with suspected diphtheria must be sent directly to an isolation unit. The others must be kept in a side room or sent to an isolation unit.

Specimens

A full blood count and screening test for heterophile antibodies should be done urgently. Throat swabs for bacteriology and virology must be sent before therapy is started. Serum for the ASOT and serology for other upper respiratory tract pathogens should be taken.

Treatment

If a peritonsillar abscess is present particularly with associated trismus, immediate surgical drainage by an otolaryngologist should be carried out. At the same time intravenous penicillin (0.6–1.2 gms) or erythromycin (500 mg) 6-hourly should be started. It is wise to start antimicrobials even when the heterophile antibody test is positive as streptococcal infections and infectious mononucleosis often co-exist. If the initial throat swabs in infectious mononucleosis prove to be negative for streptococci, the antimicrobial can be withdrawn. The use of corticosteroids (initially hydrocortisone 100 mg 6-hourly intravenously for 24–48 hours followed by prednisolone by mouth for 5–7 days) almost always has dramatic symptomatic effects on streptococcal sore throats, infectious mononucleosis (Klein *et al.* 1969) and acute epiglottitis (Morgenstein and Abramson 1971). If acute epiglottitis is suspected, chloramphenicol (500 mg 6-hourly intravenously) is the drug of choice. The provision of an alternative airway must be considered early.

Diphtheria

Diagnosis

The index of suspicion should be high in an upper respiratory tract infection where a membrane is present, the patient is unvaccinated or has come from countries where routine vaccination against diphtheria is not the rule. It is impossible to clinically distinguish the membrane of diphtheria from that of infectious mononucleosis. Cutaneous diphtheria is common in developing countries and must be included in the differential diagnosis of skin lesions in travellers.

Isolation

All suspected cases of diphtheria must be nursed in an isolation unit.

Specimens

A swab of the affected part is essential.

Treatment

(1) After a trial dose of specific diphtheria antitoxin, 0.2 ml subcutaneously, the antitoxin should be given thirty minutes later in a dose of 10–30 thousand units intramuscularly in mild or moderate cases, or 40–100 thousand units (half given intravenously) in severe cases. Anaphylactic reactions to the horse serum require immediate treatment with sub-cutaneous or intramuscular adrenaline (1 ml of 1/1000).

(2) Erythromycin in a dose of 500 mg orally four times a day for seven days or penicillin in the same dose should be given.

(3) Carriers and unrecognized cases must be searched for by nose and throat swabbing of the family and school or work contacts.

Hepatitis

Apart from acute liver failure due to massive liver necrosis, the accidental exposure of personnel to blood with possible risk of hepatitis B is the main

Table 32.5. Guideline for action on parenteral exposure to possible hepatitis B infected blood

Blood to which exposed	HBsAg status	Action
Identifiable	Negative	Nil
	Positive	(a) HBIG* 8–11 mg/kg (usually 500 mg) intramuscularly immediately.
		(b) Collect serum from exposed to check HBsAg status.
		(c) Check HBe antigen status:- If negative no further action. If positive give second dose of HBIG (same dose) at one month.
	Unknown	Check HBsAg via screening test. Then do as outlined above.
Unidentifiable (e.g. bag of disposable medical 'sharps')	Low risk e.g. no carriers or jaundiced patients on wards.	Nil
	High risk e.g. potential carriers†, or jaundiced patients present.	HBIG 8–11 mg/kg (usually 500 mg) intramuscularly immediately and a month later.

*HBIG = hepatitis B immune globulin.
†e.g. patients from developing countries, patients with Down's syndrome, drug abusers, homosexuals.

emergency which arises as a result of hepatitis (Tedder 1980; Callender *et al.* 1982). The following steps should be undertaken as outlined on Table 32.5 (see MMWR 1981). Although hepatitis A patients should be barrier nursed, this is not necessary for hepatitis B where particular caution with blood contaminated objects should be observed.

Leptospirosis

Diagnosis

This disease has three main clinical presentations.

(1) An influenza-like illness with severe headache.

(2) An aseptic meningitis without jaundice.

(3) A severe pyrexial illness with jaundice, purpura and acute renal failure, the one most likely to present as a medical emergency.

There is usually a history of contact with sewage or water contaminated by rats urine. The onset of the illness follows on average about ten days later with fever, muscle pains and conjunctival infection. After a period of apparent improvement the patient may relapse with jaundice, meningeal involvement, haemorrhage and acute renal failure (Sitprija and Evans 1970).

Isolation

This is unnecessary as man to man transmission is unlikely.

Specimens

Urine and blood for culture and dark ground microscopy and serum for serology should be taken immediately. Dark ground microscopy particularly of urine may occasionally reveal the diagnosis immediately.

Treatment

Conflicting views remain as to the need for specific chemotherapy. However, there is evidence that if given early enough (within first week) benzyl penicillin one megaunit (0.6 g) six-hourly for seven days should be used in the more serious forms of the disease. Penicillin is said to reduce the duration of the fever, relieve symptoms, prevent relapse and possibly renal dysfunction (Mackay–Dick and Robinson 1957; Kocen 1962). Tetracyclines or amoxycillin are alternative microbials (Munnich and Lakatos 1976). Antibiotics have no effect on established liver or renal disease. Indications for dialysis are as for any case of acute renal failure. As the organism is highly sensitive to disinfectants such as hypochlorite, the risk of infection of other patients using the same haemodialysis machine is minimal. However, most renal units would reserve the use of a particular machine solely for the use of the infected patient until the course of dialysis is complete.

One complication of antimicrobial therapy in this disease, as in other spirochaetal infections such as syphilis, louse borne relapsing fever etc., is the Jarisch–Herxheimer reaction (Bryceson 1976). This usually occurs one to two hours after administration of the antimicrobial and can result in death. The reaction begins with rigors and a rise in temperature and blood pressure, and is accompanied by early hyperventilation. This is followed by a fall in temperature, severe hypotension and in some cases oliguria. Diarrhoea, vomiting, confusion and even coma may be present. It is customary to treat this with large doses of steroids e.g. hydrocortisone 1 gram per hour until recovery, although the efficacy of this treatment other than to reduce the temperature, remains unproved. More recent evidence suggests that in the Jarisch–Herxheimer reaction of relapsing fever meptazinol, and opioid antagonist, may be given 100 mg by slow intravenous injection at the time of antimicrobial treatment and a further dose of 100 mg at the time of the reaction (Teklu *et al.* 1983).

Malaria

Malaria is now the commonest imported fever seen in developed countries. The consequences of even short delays in diagnosis and treatment can be disastrous. The problem can be tackled in the emergency room by answering four questions:

(1) Has the patient got malaria?
(2) If so, is it falciparum malaria or one of 'the rest'?
(3) If it is due to *P. falciparum*, does the patient come from an area where the parasite is chloroquine resistant?
(4) Is the malaria mild, moderate or severe?

(1) *Has the patient got malaria?*

The diagnosis of malaria must be considered and excluded in every traveller who has been to a malarious area and returns with a fever. For practical purposes only Europe, North America, most of the Soviet Union, Australasia and the Southernmost portions of South Africa and of South America can be considered to be free of malaria. The longest known 'incubation' periods are one year for malaria due to *P. falciparum*, eight years for malaria due to *P. vivax* and *ovale*, and 20 years for *P. malariae*. A history of poor compliance with malarial prophylaxis and exposure to mosquito bites is highly relevant. However, it is important to emphasize that protection by prophylactic drugs can no longer be regarded as absolute due to the emergence of resistant strains of the parasite. Clinical manifestations vary from a simple pyrexial illness often with rigors, to a disease involving almost every organ in the body—brain, kidney, bone marrow, lung and liver being the most important. Malaria can present as an influenza-like illness, or with jaundice or diarrhoea, and must always be considered in these circumstances.

The cornerstone of the diagnosis is a blood film, thick or thin, air-fixed in the case of the thick film, and methanol-fixed for the thin film. Any of the Romanovsky stains may be used but the easiest is by staining the film for five minutes with a 20 per cent v/v solution of Giemsa stain in a phosphate buffer pH 7.2 (3 g of Na_2HPO_4 and 0.6 g of KH_2PO_4 per litre of distilled water). To identify a parasite, a distinct nucleus (eosinophilic) and cytoplasm (basophilic) should be seen. This will exclude common artefacts such as platelets or debris in the stain. At least 100 high power fields should be scanned before a film is regarded as negative. It is always better to repeat the fingerprick for a blood film rather than search further for parasites on the same film, as parasite numbers in the peripheral blood tend to fluctuate, especially in falciparum malaria where the mature forms sequester in the deep tissues. The presence of parasites indicates the diagnosis of malaria but their absence does not preclude it. Always treat if clinical suspicion is sufficiently strong.

(2) Is it falciparum malaria or one of 'the rest' (i.e. *vivax*, *ovale* or *malariae*)

Distinction between 'the rest' makes no difference in the management of the acute situation. However, distinction between falciparum and 'the rest' is very important. In Britain the overwhelming number of cases of falciparum malarias come from Africa, with South East Asia (East of North-East India) and South America adding a few, whereas 'the rest' (mainly *vivax*) originate from the Indian subcontinent, Middle East and North Africa. Patients with falciparum malaria are generally more ill but distinction can be reliably made on a blood film. In falciparum infections the peripheral film shows a heavy infection (up to 40 per cent of the cells infected), the ring forms are delicate, often with two chromatin dots giving the appearance of a stereo headset, multiple infected cells may be present, and the sexual forms (gametocytes) when present are crescentic-shaped. In 'the rest' the infection is light, mature forms can be present, the gametocytes are round and there is often characteristic stippling of the red cell membrane.

Treatment of 'the rest' is fairly straightforward. Patients are rarely at great risk (although rupture of the spleen can occur) and all of these parasites are chloroquine sensitive. A ten tablet course of chloroquine phosphate 250 mg. (Avochlor*) or sulphate 200 mg (Nivaquine*) (each contains 150 mg base) should be given, four immediately, two six hours later and two daily for two days. In addition, a full blood count and a further EDTA sample for the estimation of glucose-6-phosphate dehydrogenase (G6PD) should be sent, if possible. After chloroquine therapy, the patient should be put on a fourteen day regime of primaquine 7.5 mg twice daily, to eradicate exerythrocytic forms. This drug can cause haemolysis in G6PD deficient individuals. In such individuals, primaquine may be given in a 45 mg dose once a week for eight weeks, monitoring carefully for haemolysis. It is often easier to warn such a G6PD-deficient individual of the possibility of relapse and to treat such individuals only when recurrences arise. Recent evidence indicates that malaria due to *P. malariae* does not relapse, so primaquine is not necessary (Bray and Garnham 1982).

(3) If the patient has mild or moderate falciparum malaria the main question is whether he has come from a chloroquine-resistant area or not. Such areas at present (September 1984) include South America, South-East Asia and East Africa (including Kenya, Uganda, Tanzania, Madagascar, Southern Sudan, Zambia, Malawi, Zanzibar and possibly Somalia). Falciparum malaria from other areas may be treated as 'the rest' as outlined above. Primaquine is not necessary as exerythrocytic forms do not persist. Falciparum malaria from chloroquine resistant areas should be treated with quinine sulphate 10 mg/kg three times a day for seven days and can be followed by a single dose of three tablets of the combination of pyrimethamine and sulfadoxine (Fansidar*) (Hall *et al.* 1975), where the parasite is sensitive to the latter drug. In parts of Indo-China this is no longer the case.

(4) The successful management of severe falciparum malaria is a far more complex problem (Hall 1977) and requires admission to an intensive therapy unit. Antimalarials must always be given *intravenously and slowly*. As before chloroquine remains the drug of choice except in areas of chloroquine resistance where quinine is used. Twice daily blood films should be made to assess the response to treatment.

Falciparum malaria is regarded as severe when there is any evidence of major complications, namely:

(a) Cerebral malaria—any evidence in alteration of conscious level, from drowsiness to coma.
(b) Renal failure (Boonpucknavig and Sitprija 1979)
    (i) Due to massive haemolysis
    (ii) Due to heavy parasitaemia.
(c) Anaemia, especially if it is acute.
(d) Fluid and electrolyte imbalance.
(e) Pulmonary oedema leading to the adult respiratory distress syndrome (ARDS).

(f) Algid malaria with hypotension and a shock-like state.

(g) Disseminated intravascular coagulation (DIC).

The details of parenteral therapy are outlined on Table 32.6. In emergency situations where chloroquine or quinine are not available, quinidine in doses similar to quinine (White *et al.* 1981), tetracycline (Reacher *et al.* 1981) and cotrimoxazole (Hansford and Hoyland 1982) have been shown to have antimalarial activity.

Table 32.6. Treatment of severe falciparum malaria.

	Chloroquine	Quinine
Half life	±100 hours	±10 hours
Dose	10 mg/kg	10 mg/kg
Volume	500 mls	500 mls
Fluid	Normal saline	Normal saline
Infusion time	4 hours	4 hours
Frequency	every 12 hours	every 8 hours
Average no. of doses required to clear parasites	3–6	12–15

Change to oral route as soon as can be tolerated. There is no place for steroids in cerebral malaria or heparin in disseminated intravascular coagulation.

Special care must be given to fluid balance, as pulmonary oedema is very easily precipitated in these patients. Some patients on the other hand may be dehydrated. Anaemia need only be treated by transfusion if patients are haemodynamically compromised (usually when the haemoglobin drops below 5 gm/dl). The role of exchange transfusions for high parasitaemia is not as yet established but is theoretically attractive.

There is no place for corticosteroids in the treatment of cerebral malaria (Warrell *et al.* 1982), nor for heparin in the rare occurrence of DIC. Both respond to treatment with antimalarials and in the latter fresh frozen plasma can be used. In some cases of renal failure dialysis may be necessary.

Prophylaxis

An authoritive review on malaria prophylaxis is to be found in the *British Medical Journal* (1981).

Poliomyelitis

Diagnosis

This presents as a problem in the emergency room only from the point of view of isolation to prevent spread, as there is no specific therapy. Polio-myelitis must be suspected in any patient with a meningitic illness who subsequently develops a pure motor neuropathy especially when:
  (a) There is a history of incomplete vaccination.
  (b) There is a history of contact with a case or a vaccinated individual.
  (c) Recent live vaccine has been given to the patient (reported incidence paralytic disease one in 3.2 million doses distributed).
  (d) The patient has recently come from a developing country with a meningitic illness even in the absence of any motor signs.

It should be remembered that other enteroviruses (coxsackie and ECHO viruses) may present with a polio-like illness as can the Guillain-Barré syndrome from which it must be distinguished.

Isolation

All cases of suspected poliomyelitis must be sent to an isolation unit.

Specimens.

A throat swab and stool, serum and CSF specimens when obtained, will aid in diagnosis.

Suspected rabies

The emergency is usually one where a traveller has been bitten or has come into contact (e.g. licked) with a possibly rabid animal which is usually untraceable. Where possible the following information should be gathered.

  (1) Where the incident took place.
  (2) When the incident took place.
  (3) Part of the body bitten, scratched or licked with a description of the injury.
  (4) Details of the animal—description including behaviour at the time.
  (5) Name and address of its owner, whether the animal had been vac-cinated and whether alive and well.

For practical purposes Australia, the British Isles and Antarctica are the only areas of the world which can be considered to be rabies-free unless more detailed information is obtained. Unfortunately, rabies has been known to occur in huskies in Greenland and foxes in Norway.

Management (detailed in *Memorandum on Rabies*, 1977)

It is important that the wound, if recent, is debrided initially with soap and water, rinsed well and then cleaned with an iodine solution. Anti-tetanus toxoid must be given if indicated. Specific systemic treatment should be

Table 32.7. Rabies; recommendations for post-exposure treatment.

Nature of exposure	Status of biting animal irrespective of previous vaccination		Recommended treatment
	At time of exposure	During 10 days (a)	
Contact but no lesions; indirect contact; no contact	Rabid	Irrelevant	None
Licks of the skin; scratches or abrasions; minor bites (covered areas of arms, trunk or legs).	(i) Unavailable Rabid Wild animal (d)		Serum plus vaccine
	(ii) Suspected as rabid (b)	Healthy	Start vaccine. Stop if animal remains healthy for five days (a,c)
		Rabid	Start vaccine. Add serum upon positive diagnosis. Complete course of vaccine.
Licks of mucosa; major bites (multiple or on face, head, finger or neck).	Unavailable Suspected as rabid (b) Rabid domestic or wild (d) animal		Serum plus vaccine. Stop if animal remains healthy for 5 days (a,c).

(a) Observation period applies only to dogs and cats.
(b) All unprovoked bites in endemic areas should be considered suspect unless proved negative by laboratory examination (brain fluorescent antibody (FA)).
(c) Or if its brain is found negative by FA examination.
(d) Exposure to rodents and rabbits seldom if ever requires specific treatment.

carried out as detailed in Table 32.7. Most commonly, a traveller has been bitten in an area where rabies is known to occur but the animal is untraceable. Rabies immunoglobulin (RIG) plus vaccine treatment is appropriate. RIG is given in a dose of 20 iu/kg intramuscularly, half at the site of the bite and the rest in the buttock. Suturing of the wound should be delayed. Antirabies vaccine is given as a 1 ml intramuscular or a 0.1 ml intradermal dose on days 0, 3, 7 and fourteen with further booster doses at one and three months (Warrell *et al.* 1983). Treatment should be started as early as possible but where the index of suspicion is not great, overnight delay is acceptable. *No exposed person should be denied treatment whatever time interval has elapsed.* All individuals receiving treatment should be serologically tested at one month to determine the antibody response to the vaccine. Although post-exposure vaccination is now routine there is no evidence as yet that it is successful since failures have been reported.

The treatment of a suspected clinical case is quite a different matter and special precautions are necessary (*Memorandum on Rabies* 1977).

Stevens–Johnson syndrome

This condition occurs in the course of certain infectious diseases such as those due to *Mycoplasma* and herpes simplex virus or as a reaction to drugs, of which the most commonly incriminated are sulphonamides, the penicillins and phenylbutazone. The condition is characterized by maculopapular, petechial or vesicular skin lesions (erythema multiforme) with ulceration and inflammation of the oral, ocular and genital surfaces. Characteristic is the target lesion with a dark central area and surrounding ring of erythema. Apart from treatment of the underlying condition or withdrawal of the offending drug, treatment with corticosteroids initially intravenously (hydrocortisone 100 mg 4-hourly) and subsequently with a tapering dose of oral prednisolone, can be introduced and is usually indicated in severe cases.

Smallpox

Although smallpox has been officially declared eradicated globally, there are those who rightfully believe that vigilance must be maintained. Their fears are twofold. First, the smallpox virus is extremely hardy and has been known to survive thirteen years in scabs kept in an envelope! (Wolf and Croon 1968). Secondly, there still remains the possibility that monkey pox which is still endemic might adapt and infect man. Any patient presenting with a fever, backache, headache and peripheral vesicular lesions, in a single crop and under appropriate circumstances, must be regarded as suspect and redirected to an isolation unit immediately. Vaccination of all possible contacts must be considered.

Tetanus

Diagnosis: (see Edmondson 1980; Spalding and Kerr 1984)

Tetanus is caused by the neuro-exotoxin, tetanospasmin which is produced by the Gram-positive anaerobic bacillus *Clostridium tetani.* However the diagnosis is solely clinical. High risk groups are farmers, gardeners, military personnel and sportsmen. The incubation period is about one to two weeks—the shorter the incubation, the more severe the disease. Previous immunization is not a guarantee against the disease, particularly where it is incomplete.

Muscles with the shortest nerve supply are first affected. Thus stiffening of the masseter muscles (trismus, lockjaw) is an early symptom. Muscles of the neck, chest, abdomen and back are next affected with lesser involvement of the limbs. On this background of hypertonicity external stimuli provoke muscle spasms primarily involving the face (risus sardonicus), back (opisthotonus), pharynx (dysphagia), larynx, respiratory muscles and limbs. The spasms usually occur between twelve hours and five days after the onset of symptoms and may progress with alarming speed.

In severe cases there is autonomic dysfunction with tachyarrhythmias, hypertension, abnormalities of temperature and sweating. Sensation, cerebral and cerebellar function are unaffected and the patient remains fully conscious. Death results from respiratory or cardiac failure compounded by exhaustion, respiratory obstruction and infection. The spasms can sometimes result in muscle injury and even fractures. The disease usually reaches its peak in one to three weeks. Although the spasm can be easily controlled with muscle relaxants, the stiffness can remain for up to six weeks. It should be emphasized that as long as treatment maintains vital functions, full recovery is the rule.

Variations of the above clinical picture occur particularly in the partially immunized. Thus in local tetanus the stiffness and spasm are worst in the injured limb (Simons 1981). In head injuries and otitis media, cephalic tetanus can cause cranial nerve palsies, especially of the VIIth nerve, and also hydrophobic tetanus where there is spasm of the pharynx and larynx.

The diagnosis of tetanus is a clinical one as bacteriological attempts at isolation of the organism from the wound are practically always unsuccessful. Trismus can be caused by local inflammatory lesions whilst neck stiffness must be distinguished from meningitis and meningism. (The CSF is normal in tetanus). Phenothiazine intoxication can produce abnormal movements which may be confused with tetanus. Localized tenderness and spasm in the limb must be distinguished from polymyositis, polymyalgia rheumatica and other collagen vascular disorders. Differentiation of rabies from tetanus is sometimes difficult but in the former there is often restlessness, and difficulty in swallowing occurs early.

Isolation

The patient with tetanus need not be isolated. However, all personnel dealing with such a patient should have been vaccinated in the previous ten years. The patient should be nursed in a quiet dark room, initially preferably on an intensive therapy unit.

Treatment

(1) Neutralization of the exotoxin is affected by human tetanus immune-globulin (HTIG) in a dose of 3000 units i.v. This may be given slowly in normal saline as intramuscular administration of this quantity from vials of 250 units is quite impractical. Horse anti-tetanus serum (ATS) 10,000 units may be given if HTIG is not available but anaphylaxis and serum sickness are risks. Some authors do not give animal anti-tetanic serum in the belief that the risks outweigh the benefits. Since neither of these sera cross the blood–brain barrier it would be rational to give serum intrathecally. HTIG (250 i.u.) given intrathecally has been shown to be of help when given before the onset of spasms (Gupta *et al.* 1980).

(2) Antibiotics. Penicillin in a dose of 2.4 g daily in divided doses should be given for a week. Tetracycline is an alternative.

(3) Surgical debridement is a cornerstone of therapy and should be undertaken without delay.

(4) Muscle relaxants such as diazepam may need to be given in doses up to 20 mg four hourly intravenously. Failing this, muscle paralysis with curare (up to 30 mg intramuscularly half-hourly) and artificial ventilation via a tracheotomy or intubation, on an intensive therapy unit may become necessary.

(5) Careful monitoring of fluid balance and anticoagulation are necessary to prevent pulmonary embolism from venous thrombosis. Anticoagulation may be started twenty-four hours after tracheotomy.

(6) Manifestations of autonomic hyperfunction can be controlled with intravenous propranolol (starting with 40 mg eight hourly).

(7) Immunization—All patients who develop tetanus should be immunized with tetanus toxoid 0.5 ml intramuscularly immediately and then at six weeks and six months if previously not immunized. Clinical disease will not give protection.

Typhoid and paratyphoid fevers

Diagnosis

These conditions should be suspected in any patient with a history of recent (usually as little as two weeks) travel abroad, although indigenous cases continue to occur. Vaccination is not a guarantee against infection. Clinically, the symptoms are those of fever, headache, a dry cough and abdominal pain with constipation. On examination the patient is flushed, sweating, has glazed eyes, a dry cough and often confused—the 'typhoid look'. The temperature is high with a relative bradycardia and in a few cases small (1–2 mm) rose spots can be seen on the upper abdomen. It is important to emphasize that rose spots are uncommon. Splenomegaly and leucopaenia if present, are additional diagnostic pointers. Early complications are meningitis, chest infection and endocarditis. Late complications are intestinal haemorrhage, bowel perforation and osteomyelitis.

Isolation

Where the index of suspicion is high the patient should be sent without delay to an isolation unit.

Specimens

Blood cultures are essential for diagnosis and when available, stool cultures and serum for the Widal test may be of help.

Treatment

Parenteral amoxycillin has been shown to be effective in the enteric fevers (Robinson and Scragg 1980). It must be given in an intravenous dose of at least one gram four times a day, for at least a week after the temperature has returned to normal and continued for a further week by mouth at the same dosage. The stools can then be tested. Some physicians prefer intravenous chloramphenicol as the drug of first choice (one gram four times daily reducing to 500 mg per dose). Prolonged carriage of the organism when treated with chloramphenicol and the small risk of aplastic anaemia favour amoxycillin. Trimethoprim or cotrimoxazole in a dose of four tablets twice a day has also been found to be effective. In patients who are delirious, obtunded, stuporous, comatose or in shock, dexamethasone 3 mg/kg initially followed by eight doses of 1 mg/kg every six hours for up to 48 hours has been shown to reduce mortality (Hoffman et al. 1984).

Close contacts with known cases should have stools cultured to exclude carrier status. Only food handlers must be followed with care for excretion of the organism.

Varicella zoster and herpes simplex infections

Diagnosis

Varicella zoster and herpes simplex infections present as emergencies when they occur in immunosuppressed patients in which situation they have a high mortality (Juel–Jensen and MacCallum 1972). Herpes simplex encephalitis is dealt with elsewhere (Chapter 20).

Isolation

Isolation from other immunosuppressed patients is essential.

Specimens

In doubtful cases the diagnosis can be confirmed in an emergency by examination of vesicle fluid or washings from scabs under the electron microscope where herpes viruses can be identified as such but not distinguished from one another.

Table 32.8. Diagnostic pointers to some of the viral haemorrhagic fevers

Disease	Locality of known outbreaks	Clinical pointers
Dengue (Break-bone fever)	Central and Northern South America Tropical Africa Indian Subcontinent and South-East Asia	Flu-like illness Bone pain
Lassa fever	West Africa (esp. Nigeria to Sierra Leone)	Persistent fever Pharyngitis Facial oedema Proteinuria Leucopaenia
Marburg and Ebola virus disease	East, Central and Southern Africa	Maculopapular rash Conjunctivitis Bleeding
Yellow fever	Africa, South of the Sahara to Northern Zambia South America	Jaundice Bleeding No vaccine > 10 years Exposure to mosquitoes

Specific treatment

Acyclovir in a dose of 5 mg/kg given intravenously over one hour every eight hours for five days can be given for herpes simplex infections and double the dose (10 mg/kg) for varicella zoster infections. An alternative for varicella zoster infections is vidarabine 10–15 mg/kg daily, given intravenously in a single dose for five days. An alternative for herpes simplex is cytarabine 3–5 mg/kg intravenously daily also for five days. Since, these latter two drugs have more side effects on the bone marrow and central nervous system than acyclovir the advantages of these drugs must be weighed against these risks. When the eye is involved, topical idoxuridine or acyclovir should be used in addition to systemic therapy. Varicella zoster immune-globulin (VZIG) may modify the attack of chickenpox in the immunosuppressed (see Table 32.4).

Viral haemorrhagic fevers (see MMWR 1983)

Whenever Lassa fever (Memorandum on Lassa Fever 1976), Marburg or Ebola virus diseases, Yellow fever, Dengue fever or other viral haemor-rhagic fever are suspected in travellers from abroad with fever, relative bradycardia, headache, an influenza-like illness and severe systemic illness, they should be redirected to an isolation unit. The areas of known outbreaks of the various diseases are shown on Table 32.8. In all cases malaria should first be excluded by blood films. Sufficient serum should always be saved for later serological testing. Immune sera from convalescent patients has been found to be of therapeutic help in some cases.

Further reading

Barman S.N., Bell H. and Chazan B.I. (1980) Acute epiglottitis in an adult. *Post-graduate Medical Journal* **56**, 504–506.
Boonpucknavig V. and Sitprija V. (1979) Renal disease in acute *Plasmodium falci-parum* infection in man. *Kidney International* **16**, 44–52.
Bray R.S. and Garnham P.C.C. (1982) The life-cycle of primate malaria parasites. *British Medical Bulletin* **38**, 117–122.
British Medical Journal, Report of meetings convened by the Ross Institute (1981) Malaria prevention in travellers from the United Kingdom. *British Medical Journal* **283**, 214–218.
Bryceson A.D.M. (1976) Clinical pathology of the Jarisch-Herxheimer reaction. *Journal of Infectious Diseases* **133**, 696–704.
Callender M.E., White Y.S. and Williams, R. (1982) Hepatitis B virus infection in medical and health care personnel. *British Medical Journal* **284**, 324–326.
Cunningham-Rundles C., Hanson L.A., Hitzig W.H., Knapp W., Lambert P.-H., Nydegger U.E., Prince A.M., Rosen F.S., Seligmann M., Soothill J.F.,

Thompson R.A., Torrigiani G. and Wedgwood R.J. (1982) Appropriate uses of human immunoglobulin in clinical practice: Memorandum from an IUIS/WHO Meeting. *Bulletin of the World Health Organization* **60**, 43–47.

Edmondson R.S. (1980) Tetanus. *British Journal of Hospital Medicine* **23**, 596–602.

Gupta P.S., Kapoor R., Goyal S., Batra V.K. and Jain B.K. (1980) Intrathecal human tetanus immunoglobulin in early tetanus. *Lancet* ii, 439–440.

Hall A.P. (1977) The treatment of severe falciparum malaria. *Transactions of the Royal Society of Tropical Medicine and Hygiene* **71**, 367–379.

Hall A.P., Doberstyn E.B., Mettaprakong V. and Sonkom P. (1975) Falciparum malaria cured by Quinine followed by Sulfadoxine-Pyrimethamine. *British Medical Journal* **2**, 15–17.

Hansford C.F. and Hoyland J. (1982) An evaluation of co-trimoxazole in the treatment of *Plasmodium falciparum* malaria. *South African Medical Journal* **61**, 512–514.

Hoffman S.L., Punjabi N.H., Kumala S., Moechtar M.A., Pulungsih S.P., Rivai A.R., Rockhill R.C., Woodward T.E. and Loedin A.A. (1984) Reduction of mortality in chloramphenicol-heated severe typhoid fever by high-dose dexamethasone. *New England Journal of Medicine* **310**, 82–88.

Juel-Jensen B.E. and MacCallum F.O. (1972) *Herpes simplex varicella and zoster; clinical manifestations and treatment.* William Heinemann, London.

Klein E.M., Cochran J.F. and Buck R.L. (1969) The effects of short-term corticosteroid therapy on the symptoms of infectious mononucleosis pharyngotonsillitis—a double-blind study. *Journal of the American College of Health Associations* **17**, 446–452.

Kocen R.S. (1962) Leptospirosis. A comparison of symptomatic and penicillin therapy. *British Medical Journal* **1**, 1181–1183.

Mackay-Dick J. and Robinson J.F. (1957) Penicillin in the treatment of 84 cases of leptospirosis in Malaya. *Journal of the Royal Army Corps* **103**, 186–197.

Memorandum on Lassa Fever (1976) Department of Health and Social Security and the Welsh Office. Her Majesty's Stationery Office, London.

Memorandum on Rabies (1977) Department of Health and Social Security and the Welsh Office. Her Majesty's Stationery Office, London.

MMWR (1981) CDC. Immune globulins for protection against viral hepatitis. *Morbidity and Mortality Weekly Reports*, Communicable Disease Centre, Georgia, Atlanta **30**, 423–435.

MMWR (1983) CDC. Viral hemorrhagic fever: Initial management of suspected and confirmed cases. *Morbidity and Mortality Weekly Reports*, Supplement No. 25, Communicable Disease Centre, Georgia, Atlanta **32**, 27–39.

Morgenstein K.M. and Abramson A.L. (1971) Acute epiglottitis in adults. *Laryngoscope* **81**, 1066–1073.

Munnich D. and Lakatos M. (1976) Treatment of human leptospira infections with ampicillin or·with amoxycillin. *Chemotherapy* **22**, 372–380.

Reacher M., Campbell C.C., Freeman J., Doberstyn E.B. and Brandling-Bennett A.D. (1981) Drug therapy for *Plasmodium falciparum* malaria resistant to Pyrimethamine-Sulfadoxine (Fansidar): A study of alternate regimens in Eastern Thailand. *Lancet* ii, 1066–1069.

Robinson O.P.W. and Scragg J.N. (1980) Parenteral amoxycillin therapy in typhoid fever in Nelson J.I. and Grassi C. (eds) *Current Chemotherapy and Infectious Disease* Vol. II, pp. 929–930. American Society of Microbiology, Washington D.C.

Simons E.R. (ed.) (1981) Local tetanus. *Johns Hopkins Medical Journal* **149**, 84–88.

Sitprija V. and Evans H. (1970) The kidney in human leptospirosis. *American Journal of Medicine* **49**, 780–788.

Spalding J.M.K. and Kerr J.H. (1984) Tetanus (Chapter 86) in Warren, K.S. and Mahmoud, A.A.F. (eds) *Tropical and Geographical Medicine.* pp. 821–825. McGraw Hill Book Co., New York.

Tedder R.S. (1980) Hepatitis B in hospitals. *British Journal of Hospital Medicine* **23**, 66–70.

Teklu B., Habte-Michael A., Warrell D.A., White N.J. and Wright D.J.M. (1983) Meptazinol diminishes the Jarisch–Hercheimer reaction of relapsing-fever. *Lancet* **i**, 835–839.

Warrell D.A., Looareesuwan S., Warrell M.J., Kasemsarn P., Intaraprasert R., Bunnag D. and Harinasuta T. (1982) Dexamethasone proves deleterious in cerebral malaria. A double-blind trial in 100 comatose patients. *New England Journal of Medicine* **306**, 313–319.

Warrell M.J. *et al.* (1983) An economical regimen of human diploid cell strain anti-rabies vaccine for post-exposure prophylaxis. *Lancet* **ii**, 301–304.

White N.J., Looareesuwan S., Warrell D.A., Chongsuphajaisiddhi T., Bunnag D. and Harinasuta T. (1981) Quinidine in falciparum malaria. *Lancet* **ii**, 1069–1071.

Wolff H.F. and Croon J.J.A.B. (1968) The survival of smallpox virus (variola minor) in natural circumstances. *Bulletin of the World Health Organization* **38**, 492–493.

33 · Medical Emergencies in Elderly Patients

G. K. WILCOCK

It is impossible to cover all geriatric emergencies in a single chapter and many acute emergencies in the elderly fall within the province of the other chapters. The following sections are chosen on a somewhat arbitrary basis but include important problems which are not covered elsewhere.

Accidental hypothermia

Accidental hypothermia is diagnosed when the body core temperature falls below 35°C (95°F) as measured from the rectal temperature or that of a freshly passed specimen of urine. A Royal College of Physicians Report (1966) showed that in a survey of ten hospitals in England and Scotland during the three months of the Winter in 1965, the incidence of admission with hypothermia was 0.7 per cent (126 cases) of all admissions. Just over 40 per cent of these were sixty-five years or over with an incidence of 1.2 per cent. Applied to the country as a whole this would have meant that in the region of 3800 elderly people would have been admitted to hospital with hypothermia during that period. The follow-up study some ten years later reported a higher incidence—3.6 per cent of all elderly patients were found to be hypothermic upon admission to hospital. A community study of people aged sixty-five years or over conducted by Fox and his colleagues (1973) found the incidence of hypothermia, based on urine temperature, to be in the region of 0.5 per cent, while a further 10 per cent of those surveyed were judged to be 'at risk' since they had core temperatures of between 35 and 35.5°C.

Aetiology

(1) Exposure to cold

Fox *et al.* (1973) found 75 per cent of those studied had living-rooms where the morning temperature was less than 18.3°C—the minimum recommended by the Parker-Morris Report for council housing (1977). In 10 per cent of cases the environmental temperature was extremely low.

(2) Impaired thermo-regulation

It is now well established that many elderly patients suffer some impairment of the ability to shiver (Fox *et al.* 1973) and similarly that a significant proportion exhibit impaired autonomic responses as they age, including a reduced ability to vasoconstrict and also to perceive a fall in temperature (Collins *et al.* 1977).

(3) Brown adipose tissue

The role of brown adipose tissue is controversial and the reader is referred to Johnstone *et al.* (1963) who reported that shivering is the only means of increasing metabolism in response to cold in adults, while others (Aherne and Hull 1965; Heaton 1973) believe that brown adipose tissue may also be relevant.

(4) Pathological conditions

These may either predispose to the effects of a low environmental temperature, or contribute to the hypothermia itself, or both, e.g.
(a) Loss of metabolic heat production—hypothyroidism, hypopituitarism, loss of muscle activity, immobility due to stroke, arthritis, Parkinson's disease etc.
(b) Autonomic dysfunction—as in diabetes mellitus, Parkinson's disease etc.
(c) Tendency to fall with loss of muscle heat—stroke, arthritis, postural hypotension (often itself due to autonomic abnormality) etc.
(d) Failure to perceive a fall in environmental temperature, e.g. acute confusional states and dementia.
(e) Iatrogenic, especially drugs—phenothiazines, antidepressants, hypnotics (alcohol may also be a contributory factor) etc.
(f) Severe illness.

Clinical features and diagnosis

A high index of suspicion is needed not only in the coldest of the winter months but also in the spring and autumn, since some patients with a moderately low resting temperature later develop hypothermia, even in a warm environment (Johnstone and Park 1973). The rectal temperature, taken with a low reading rectal thermometer, should be measured whenever hypothermia is suspected.

    The clinical features include a feeling of coldness on the trunk and a patient who is pale and often confused or unconscious. Cardiovascular signs include a sinus bradycardia or slow atrial fibrillation, pulmonary oedema, a J-wave and some degree of AV-block or intraventricular conduction delay on an ECG, and a low blood pressure which is associated with a poor prognosis. In the central nervous system the reflexes and pupillary reactions are usually sluggish, the plantars may become extensor and muscular rigidity is common, sometimes mistakenly taken as indicating intra-abdominal pathology or meningism. A reduced respiratory rate may result in carbon dioxide retention with severe acidosis, but the P_{CO_2} may be low because of reduced metabolism. Undetectable bronchopneumonia is common. Gastric dilatation occurs not infrequently and pancreatitis is present in many cases, although a high amylase does not necessarily confirm this diagnosis, neither does an increased transaminase level always indicate hepatic damage (MacLean *et al.* 1968). The latter, together with a raised creatine-kinase, may rather indicate muscle damage. Oliguria is usually present because of a reduced filtration rate, or sometimes acute tubular necrosis.

Management

The patient should be managed along the following lines:

(1) Re-warming

Slow re-warming is the treatment of choice, using blankets in a warm room (approximately 25°C) to raise the body temperature by approximately 0.5°C per hour. The rectal temperature and blood pressure should be monitored continuously and should the latter fall, the patient must be cooled by lowering the room temperature, re-starting warming as the blood pressure stabilizes.

(2) Cardiac monitoring

Cardiac monitoring is essential and dysrhythmias are treated in the usual way, although tachyarrhythmias can be especially difficult to control.

(3) Central venous pressure monitoring

A CVP line is essential in the majority of patients to reduce the risk of pulmonary oedema, even if only a small volume of fluid is being administered. All fluids administered intravenously should be warmed to body temperature before infusion and unless there is evidence of dehydration, only the minimum necessary should be given.

(4) Bicarbonate infusion

In the presence of a severe metabolic acidosis it may be necessary to give bicarbonate but in many instances the pH will correct itself with supportive treatment alone.

(5) Blood glucose levels

As the patient warms up and the temperature rises there is a danger of hypoglycaemia and hypokalaemia developing, as insulin is inactive at low temperatures and builds up in the circulation. An elevated plasma glucose in the early stages of re-warming should not be treated with insulin and will usually fall as the temperature rises.

(6) Urea and electrolytes

The danger of hypokalaemia has already been mentioned but hyper-kalaemia may also occur. Therefore, frequent estimation of the urea and electrolytes is necessary until the patient is stable. Arterial blood should be used for all investigations if possible, since there is usually significant venous stagnation in peripheral vessels.

(7) Oxygen

Oxygen should be given to all hypothermic patients. If they are very hypo-thermic, e.g. with a core temperature below 32°C, intermittent positive pressure ventilation may also be needed, since some hypothermic patients rely upon the hypoxia to drive their respiratory centre (Ledingham and Mone 1972).

(8) Steroids

The widespread practice of administering intravenous steroids to hypo-thermic patients is probably misconceived. Plasma cortisol levels are elevated and there is evidence that cortisol utilization is decreased (MacLean and Emslie-Smith 1972).

(9) Antibiotics

A wide spectrum antibiotic should be administered to all patients until they have recovered sufficiently to be certain that clinically undetectable bronchopneumonia or other infection is not present.

Finally, there is no place for tri-iodothyronine, even in the presence of myxoedema, until the patient has regained a more normal temperature. Even then, observe the usual caution with regards to the size of the dose.

Prevention

In addition to protecting those at risk from exposure by encouraging adequate heating and clothing, it is important to remember to avoid potentially hazardous drugs and to screen patients with hypothermia for any underlying physical disorder that might be implicated in its aetiology.

Chronic subdural haematoma

Like so many conditions in the elderly, this is easily missed if a high index of suspicion is not maintained, especially in patients taking anticoagulants (Wiener and Nathanson 1962). Small veins crossing the subdural space to the dural sinuses are easily ruptured, particularly if there has been some loss of brain substance, which may also allow a haematoma to become quite large before it is apparent.

Previous trauma, which may be slight or forgotten, probably occurs in between half and three-quarters of cases (Fogelholm *et al.* 1975). The clot, which is usually frontal or parietal, liquefies and its osmotic pressure may rise because of the presence of red cell breakdown products, attracting CSF and enlarging. After two to three weeks it is usually walled off and surrounded by a vascular membrane.

Clinical features and diagnosis

The classical picture of a fluctuating level of consciousness is less common than usually supposed, although impairment of the level of consciousness is very frequent. The Nottingham study indicated that a hemiplegia was also a frequent presenting feature, although relatively speaking, the signs were often less marked than one would expect from the level of consciousness (Dronfield *et al.* 1977). Corticospinal tract signs may be bilateral. A variety of other neurological symptoms and signs can occur, including headaches, memory impairment, coma, papilloedema, dilatation of the pupil and it must be remembered that a large clot may produce bilateral or brain stem signs.

Shift of mid-line structures, e.g. a calcified pineal, may be visualized on a skull X-ray, C.T. scan or echo-encephalogram but bilateral haematomas may prevent this being recognized. Angiography is the most reliable means of diagnosis in difficult cases but exploratory burr holes may be preferable in an older patient.

Management

Evacuation is the only reliable means of treatment and should rarely, if ever, be withheld simply on the basis of a patient's age even though the outcome is sometimes disappointing (Cameron 1978).

Acute confusional states

Acute confusional states are frequently encountered, presenting with clouding of consciousness (but not true coma), disorientation in time and space, disturbance of thought processes and of perception leading to inappropriate illusions, delusions and hallucinations. Many patients are agitated, apparently picking distraughtly at their bed-clothes, or attempting to wander up and down, whereas others are withdrawn and apathetic.

Diagnosis

The patient's state of mind is usually obvious and it is the underlying cause that needs to be sought and diagnosed. As usual, it is important to obtain a history from a reliable third party and also to consult previous medical notes, whether hospital or general practice. Physical examination is often extremely helpful but equally often hampered by an uncooperative and difficult patient. The two commonest causes in the elderly are probably infection and drugs. Respiratory tract and urinary tract infections spring to mind immediately but other more cryptic infections can be involved, including subacute bacterial endocarditis, tuberculosis, paracolic abscess, empyema of the gall-bladder, pyogenic arthritis and meningitis. In the elderly, the usual signs of infection may be absent and they may have a normal temperature and white cell count. Blood cultures may yield useful and helpful information.

Almost any drug can cause confusion but the most common offenders include anti-depressants, anti-epileptic preparations, anti-parkinsonian drugs and hypnotics and sedatives.

Withdrawal of tranquillizing drugs, as well as alcohol, can be responsible too (Victor & Adams 1953). Digoxin, particularly in the presence of impaired renal function or hypokalaemia, may reach toxic levels and produce confusion. In addition, diuretics can induce electrolyte deficiencies and dehydration, which may also cause confusion.

Both hyper- and hypoglycaemia may be responsible and the latter should be considered in any patient treated for diabetes mellitus, especially if taking some of the longer-acting, renally cleared, sulphonylureas, e.g. chlorpropramide.

A dementing illness of whatever cause may appear to have a sudden onset if it is abruptly unmasked, e.g. with the death of a spouse who had previously been accommodating for the altered behaviour.

Amongst the intracranial conditions which may lead to confusion, the commoner include cerebrovascular accident, subdural haematoma and the effects of intracerebral space occupying lesions (tumours and cerebral abscesses in particular). Meningitis is occasionally the cause.

Nutritional deficiencies, anaemia, myocardial infarction, congestive cardiac failure, anoxia and even non-metastatic sequelae of extracerebral tumours are amongst the many other conditions that have been implicated as a cause of acute confusion.

Management

This falls most readily under two headings. The first is detection and treatment of the underlying cause. As usual the history and examination backed up by routine laboratory investigations, i.e. electrolytes and biochemical screen, full blood count, chest X-ray, ECG, MSU, and any others particularly indicated by the clinical findings. In some patients a skull X-ray, lumbar puncture or C.T. scan are helpful, but are probably best undertaken only if there is a specific indication or a complete blank has been drawn in the diagnosis.

Secondly, and of equal importance, is the approach to management of the patient while awaiting return to a more normal intellectual state. Fear and anxiety are frequently obvious even to the untrained observer and these can communicate themselves to the patient's attendants or relatives, so that they in turn may feel distressed, worried and unsure how best to react. It is important to repeatedly identify oneself to the patient if necessary and explain firmly but kindly what one is doing and why. Failure to do this may easily aggravate the patient's state of mind by fuelling the disturbances of thought process and perception. In many patients it is difficult to believe that this is helpful but it is nevertheless important to adopt such an approach. Pain and discomfort, including bladder and bowel function, should be relieved promptly. If possible, the patient should be put in a well-lit environment to avoid misleading impressions from shadows and unfamiliar shapes. A familiar object or two in their immediate surroundings may also aid a return to reality.

It is important to avoid prescribing drugs if at all possible and particularly chlorpromazine. If therapeutic intervention is necessary, the prescription of hypnotics and sedatives which merely reduce the patient to a state of drowsiness or stupor should be avoided. Instead, those drugs which help to modify behaviour and make the patient more accessible to suggestion and less likely to suffer from delusions and hallucinations, should be employed. These include some phenothiazines, e.g. thioridazine and promazine, and butyrophenones, e.g. haloperidol. The latter is probably preferable but it must be remembered that it has a long half-life. It is important to watch carefully for side-effects, especially extra-pyramidal rigidity and postural hypotension. The appropriate dose is arrived at by trial and error. However, in the elderly one starts with the minimum dose, working up through the therapeutic range, as appropriate.

Giant cell arteritis

This has to be considered along with polymyalgia rheumatica with which it probably exists as a continuous spectrum, occurring particularly in elderly women. However, for the purposes of this account the temporal arteritis end of the spectrum will be concentrated upon but many aspects of the management and complications should also be considered in patients with polymyalgia rheumatica.

It is particularly important to remember that the temporal arteries may not be involved and even if they are, the presence of 'skip lesions' may lead to a negative result from arterial biopsy.

Clinical features and diagnosis

It may present with general constitutional symptoms, such as malaise, weakness, weight loss and low grade pyrexia. However, there are often more specific local symptoms, such as headache; thick tender non-pulsatile temporal or occipital arteries which produce scalp tenderness; sudden blindness due to occlusion of a central retinal artery (which may occur in up to 20 per cent of untreated patients); or less commonly a cerebrovascular accident. Eye problems are reported to be present in 50 per cent of people with the temporal arteritis end of the spectrum. Other neurological deficits can occur and it may of course also present as polymyalgia rheumatica with painful, tender and stiff shoulder and pelvic girdle muscles and the constitutional changes described above.

This spectrum of disease should always be considered in any patient in whom there is an unexplained general constitutional illness, occular problem, or cerebrovascular accident.

Most patients will have a mild degree of normochromic normocytic anaemia, an ESR that is eighty or above and often a slight leucocytosis. Biopsy of an appropriate artery may help but a negative result does not exclude the diagnosis. Arteriography is practiced in some centres. Auto-antibodies are not usually detected but peripheral blood lymphocytes from patients, with the polymyalgia rheumatica end of the spectrum, have been shown to be stimulated *in vitro* by an arterial homogenate, suggesting the possibility of an auto-immune basis (Hazleman *et al.* 1975).

A therapeutic trial of high dose steroids is often diagnostic in itself, since there is usually a dramatic relief of the systemic symptoms.

Management

If the diagnosis has been made, or even if there is only a high index of suspicion, steroid treatment is indicated (40–60 mg of prednisolone daily in divided doses). This should be continued for ten days, unless the diagnosis has been disproved and then the steroids slowly tailed off until either a dose of 5–10 mg daily is reached, the symptoms recur, or the ESR increases. It is imperative not to await the outcome of temporal artery biopsy before starting the patient on treatment because of the risk of complications, especially blindness. Even if the patient is taking high dose steroids, a delay of 24–48 hours before undertaking the biopsy does not always appear to alter the pathological findings. Steroids may eventually be withdrawn although this can take up to two years, or even longer.

It is important, especially in elderly people, to remember all the problems of high dose and maintenance steroid treatment. These include fluid retention, electrolyte imbalance, especially hypokalaemia and an increase incidence of fractures caused by osteoporosis.

Social admissions—their prevention and early discharge

Whenever admission is requested for a patient, especially over the age of seventy years, it is important to establish why this is necessary at the time of the request. If the patient has an acute illness which requires the facilities of a district general hospital, or is otherwise ill and has no-one to look after him and an alternative bed is not available (e.g. in the geriatric unit or a community hospital) then clearly admission is essential. However, very often the request for admission will reflect more the build up of tension within those caring for him or her. Sometimes this is apparently precipitated by an intervening 'acute problem', commonly a respiratory tract infection, which legitimizes the admission and makes it respectable, at least superficially, when in reality the extra demands in terms of nursing care may be minimal. Under these circumstances admission to an acute general hospital bed is often inappropriate both for the patient and for the hospital. Carers will frequently be happy and willing to carry on coping if they know that something is going to be done, that they will be supported as much as is possible and that they can be made to feel that they are no longer alone. It is in this situation that a domiciliary visit by a geriatrician, especially if it can be arranged within twenty-four hours, will prevent many admissions to an acute bed, at the same time enabling the medical approach to be tailored more effectively to the patient's particular need. This can vary from the use of the Day Hospital to rehabilitate the patient suffering a mild stroke (with the provision of a rehabilitation bed in due course if necessary), to arranging care in an old people's home or mobilizing enough social services support to enable carers to manage, either in the long or the short term.

In summary, the answer to the question 'why is admission needed now rather than yesterday or tomorrow?' will often indicate whether it is worth considering recommending a domiciliary visit to investigate possible alternatives. One also has to remember that general practitioners requesting admissions that do not necessarily seem appropriate for an acute medical unit are themselves under pressure, as well as being uncertain how they may otherwise best tackle the problem. It is important always to be tactful in these circumstances, and to remember that the general practitioner's special knowledge of the family's circumstances may lead him to insist upon admission even when alternatives are offered.

Resettlement

The basis of resettlement lies in matching a patient's level of independence before admission, assuming this was adequate, to that which he is capable of at the projected point of discharge. It is impossible to give strict rules that will lead to satisfactory discharge in all cases and each person's resettlement is an individual matter. However, a few basic guide-lines are given below. It is important to remember that it is one's duty to attempt to allow a patient to resettle into which ever environment he or she wishes, rather than to try and make them conform to one's own picture of their future.

If it is apparent that the patient is not going to be as independent as before admission, one then has to decide whether it is possible to plug the gap with the resources that are available, e.g. including an attendance at a day hospital (which implies a therapeutic need) or at a day centre or day care in an old people's home (usually as a social outlet or 'granny sitting service'), meals-on-wheels, district nurse to help with bathing, dressing etc. and home-help. If there is any doubt at all about the practicality of discharge or a considerable difference in level of functioning at the time of the projected discharge, a home visit by the occupational therapist, physiotherapist and medical social worker together with an involved local person, as well as the patient, will help iron out many snags and allow an assessment of its feasibility. In many cases it would be essential to involve the community nurse, health visitor or general practitioner, as well as members of the hospital team.

If discharge to the patient's own home is inappropriate or impossible one has to assist the patient to come to terms with this situation. It is here that the medical social worker can be very helpful, as well as in suggesting suitable alternative accommodation.

The unrealistic patient

Occasionally one comes across an elderly patient who insists on returning home, even though it is clear to those caring for the patient that he or she will not be able to manage. It is often best to tackle this situation along the following lines: a home visit with the patient left on their own for an hour or two may lead to a realization that he or she really cannot cope. If this fails to work, one is often left with no option but to allow the patient to return home with as much social support as possible. It is necessary to make sure that the relatives, neighbours, GP, health visitor and district nurse etc. realize that the patient is not being heartlessly discharged home and that one is almost expecting the discharge to fail. This often removes much of the anxiety surrounding the discharge, particularly in the community. In addition, it helps considerably if it is known that the bed will be kept for two or three days or alternative measures taken to ensure immediate re-admission if necessary. It is surprising how often the patient manages.

Further reading

Aherne W. and Hull D. (1965) Brown adipose tissue. *Lancet* **i**, 765.

Cameron M.M. (1978) Chronic subdural haematoma: a review of 114 cases. *Journal of Neurology, Neurosurgery and Psychiatry* **41**, 834–839.

Collins K.J., Dore C., Exton-Smith A.N., Fox R.H., McDonald I.C. and Woodward P.M. (1977) Accidental hypothermia and impaired temperature homeostasis in the elderly. *British Medical Journal* **1**, 353–356.

Department of the Environment (1977) *Homes for Today and Tomorrow*. 10th Imp. (HMSO London).

Dronfield M.W., Mead G.M. and Langman M.J.S. (1977) Survival and death from subdural haematoma on medical wards. *Postgraduate Medical Journal* **53**, 57–60.

Fogelhom R., Heiskaneno O. and Waltimo O. (1975) Chronic subdural haematoma in adults. Influence of patient's age on symptoms, signs and thickness of haematoma. *Journal of Neurosurgery* **42**, 43–46.

Fox R.H., Woodward P.M., Exton-Smith A.N., Green M.F., Donnison D.V. and Wicks M.H. (1973) Body temperatures in the elderly: a national study of physiological, social and environmental conditions. *British Medical Journal* **1**, 200–206.

Hazleman B.L., McLennan I.C.M. and Esiri M.M. (1975) Lymphocyte proliferation to artery antigen as a positive diagnostic test in polymyalgia rheumatica. *Annals of Rheumatic Disease* **34**, 122–127.

Heaton J.M. (1973) A study of brown adipose tissue in hypothermia. *Journal of Pathology* **110**, 105–108.

Johnstone R.H., Smith A.C. and Spalding J.M.K. (1963) Oxygen consumption of paralysed men exposed to cold. *Journal of Physiology* London **169**, 584–591.

Johnstone R.H. and Park D.M. (1973) Intermittent hypothermia. Independence of central and reflex thermo-regulatory mechanisms. *Journal of Neurology, Neurosurgery and Psychiatry* **36**, 411–416.

Ledingham I. McA. and Mone J.G. (1972) Treatment after exposure to cold. *Lancet* **i,** 534–535.

MacLean D., Griffiths P.D. and Emslie-Smith D. (1968) Serum enzymes in relation to electrocardiographic changes in accidental hypothermia. *Lancet* **ii,** 266–271.

MacLean D. and Emslie-Smith D. (1972) *Accidental Hypothermia.* Blackwell Scientific Publications, Oxford.

Royal College of Physicians, London (1966) *Report of the Committee on Accidental Hypothermia.*

Victor M. and Adams R.D. (1953) *The Effect of Alcohol on the Nervous System in Metabolic and Toxic Diseases of the Nervous System.* Williams and Wilkins, Baltimore.

Wiener L.M. and Nathanson M. (1962) The relationship of subdural haematoma and anticoagulant therapy. *Archives of Neurology and Psychiatry Chicago* **6,** 282–286.

34 · Psychiatric Emergencies: Principles of Assessment and Management

E. B. O. SMITH

In the minds of a majority of physicians the psychiatric emergency stands apart from others encountered in medical practice. It is often perceived as a time-consuming affair involving intensely emotional, sometimes violent, and occasionally unattractive people. The behaviour and attitudes of many patients may seem socially inappropriate, unreasonable and occasionally bizarre and they frequently defy understanding based only on common sense and the application of general medical knowledge. The nagging fear of missing physical or mental illness requiring urgent treatment, the competing demands of other overtly sick or injured people and anxiety about the safety of other patients, staff and themselves may combine to produce a stressful and demanding situation. By their very nature psychiatric emergencies require rapid judgements to be made on psychological, social and medical issues based on incomplete, but not necessarily inadequate, information. Confronted with such tasks in vexatious, manipulative or unpredictable patients it is hardly surprising that many inexperienced doctors find this a daunting situation, particularly if their basic psychiatric training and knowledge has been neglected or unsound. It is the aim of the present chapter to suggest that with a modest knowledge of certain principles and techniques, basic interviewing and assessment skills, and access to effective psychiatric and social services, most psychiatric emergencies can be competently dealt with by most doctors.

It is an exceedingly difficult task to define psychiatric emergencies except in the most general terms since every type of emotional, cognitive and behavioural disorder may be encountered in such situations. As Berrios (1982) has pointed out, other than for purposes of epidemiological or operational research, there is no advantage in precise definitions in clinical practice. The genesis of a psychiatric emergency is a complex matter involving the interaction of individual psychological, socio-economic, interpersonal, and physical factors of the moment. Most, but by no means all, patients may be regarded as being in some form of emotional crisis. Interesting and sometimes ingenious attempts have been made by theorists to establish general explanations for human crises and guidelines for successful interventions but such activity appears to have had only a marginal effect on the management of emergency situations. Nevertheless, as many experienced general practitioners and psychiatrists know, crises, despite their complexity, offer opportunities for furthering the understanding of individuals and their problems and can be occasions for advantageous change. However, crises are short-lived and successful intervention calls for commitment and a willingness to work intensely with the patient and other people who are closely involved in a brief period of time.

The frequency with which an individual clinician will encounter a psychiatric emergency in the general hospital or community will depend largely on the extent of social and psychiatric morbidity locally and on the provision of effective social, psychiatric and other helping agencies. The presence in the local community of the Samaritans, other telephone counselling services, night refuges, hostels and self-help groups will not only provide alternative sources of help lessening further the demands on medical services but will also act as valuable resources in resolving emergencies.

Preparation

Adequate planning and appropriate training and supervision for staff likely to be involved in coping with psychiatric emergencies must be the basis for an effective service. A multi-disciplinary approach is needed since no individual possesses the skills and knowledge required to respond to all the problems presented by such a heterogeneous group of patients. Local policies for managing those who have deliberately harmed themselves, who have abused drugs or alcohol, or who are psychotic, severely mentally handicapped or violent should be defined and reviewed from time to time.

In order to support their colleagues in the community and general hospital and to ensure appropriate use of psychiatric facilities, those responsible for planning psychiatric services should give high priority to resources for emergency assessment and care. Johnson (1969) found that 53 per cent, and Waters and Northover (1972) 42 per cent, of all psychiatric admissions arose from emergency consultations. In general hospitals in the United States the psychiatric emergency room has provided the major resources for coping with these demands (Gerson and Bassuk 1980). In the United Kingdom, where psychiatric teams collaborate closely with primary medical and social work services, only a few districts have found the need to provide special facilities, such as an emergency clinic or a community-based crisis intervention team (Brothwood 1965). The emergence of liaison psychiatry as a relatively new feature in British psychiatric services may lead to improvement in the quality of emergency care within the general hospital. In Oxford over the past eight years a multi-disciplinary psychiatric emergency team, located within the John Radcliffe Hospital has provided a 24-hour service to the wards and the Accident and Emergency Department and carries the responsibility for the assessment and management of all cases of deliberate self-harm (Hawton et al. 1979).

Staff in casualty departments and in wards where psychiatric emergencies are frequent need careful selection, training and supportive supervision. There should be planning and training for the management of aggressive and violent patients and everyone concerned should be aware of carefully selected and equipped areas and interview rooms designated for the management of disturbed people. Good communications are essential in crises. The telephone numbers of psychiatrists, approved social workers and general practitioners on call should be instantly available, as well as those of every other potentially valuable community facility for drug- or alcohol-dependent, homeless, bereaved, abused or severely handicapped individuals. Ready access to previous case notes outside normal working hours will pay dividends in saving time and inappropriate responses. As Waldron (1982) has emphasized, neglect of such simple preparations may easily complicate and perpetuate emergency situations, create professional misunderstandings and lead to unsatisfactory outcomes.

Most cities and large towns in the United Kingdom have multi-racial societies with ethnic minorities containing some people who have linguistic and cultural difficulties when seeking help, especially in an emergency. In psychiatric crises there may be disadvantages in relying on relatives or friends to act as translators. Therefore, it is important for all major hospitals to maintain lists of competent interpreters who are willing to be called in to assist even at unsociable hours. The good interpreter should understand both languages and cultures well, be able to establish an easy rapport with both patient and staff, and be capable of making linguistic and cultural interpretations (Cox 1976).

The individual doctor needs to ensure that interviewing skills are sound when time is limited, that he or she is competent in examining the mental state, is familiar with a few psychotropic drugs, and is acquainted with procedures under the new Mental Health Act 1983. An awareness of the common problems and presenting syndromes is needed but an extensive knowledge of psychiatry is not required. The management of emotional and behavioural disorder in mental illnesses of widely differing aetiology will often be the same.

Approach to the patient

Traditionally, in the medical or surgical emergency, the doctor takes immediate responsibility for the diagnosis and treatment of the illness. He is used to making decisions for the patient while encouraging him to accept the sick role with its privileges and obligations. There is an expectation that information will be given as and when required, that the patient will be as co-operative as possible and that any treatment offered will be accepted gratefully. There is usually an unspoken assumption that the patient is not responsible for their misfortune and, therefore, is deserving of sympathy, although the expression of emotion to any extent is discouraged as being unhelpful. In marked contrast such an approach to the psychiatric emergency is inappropriate and likely to have an adverse effect on the patient and the outcome. Unless and until it is necessary to transfer responsibility away from the patient by the emergence of evidence of overwhelming emotional disorder, psychosis, severe mental handicap or serious disturbance of cognitive functioning, the clinician and the other professionals involved should avoid unilateral decision-taking. It should be explicit that those involved are working with the patients and their families on the problems and not on their behalf. Such a policy encourages mature attitudes and behaviour, discourages collusion in manipulative manoeuvres and the reinforcement of maladaptive coping strategies, and ensures that the patient shares responsibility for the outcome of the situation. To neglect it not only leads to ethical dilemmas and pitfalls, but will leave many patients feeling incensed, resentful and devalued by being treated like children in the sick role.

Since none may claim absolute immunity from conditions which lead to a psychological crisis it follows that every type of personality and a wide range of emotional and behavioural disorder may be encountered. Although studies of services have shown that a substantial proportion of patients presenting as emergencies have had previous contact with psychiatric services only a minority show formal psychiatric illness. Many appear strange and threatening, ill-kempt and self-neglected, or excessively demanding of attention and sympathy. Others may be brought to hospital or surgery against their wishes, resent medical attention and respond in a suspicious or aggressive way. The task of relating to such people is never an easy one and it is hardly surprising that they provide a breeding ground for prejudice, misunderstanding and neglect. Nevertheless, the experienced and effective clinician is mindful of the way that even the most socially and psychologically deviant may be victims of pathological parenting, damaging life experiences, illness or circumstances and will concentrate on the tasks of identifying the present problems, assessing the mental and physical states, understanding the crisis despite its complexity and offering relevant help.

The most successful interventions will occur when the doctor is able to communicate genuine interest and accurate empathy in a calm, apparently unhurried and attentive way. People in emotional crises even in the extremes of high or low arousal remain sensitive and are quick to detect insincerity and lack of interest. Temptations to deceive the patient or to create false expectations to achieve a temporary resolution of the crisis should be resisted. There is also a need to actively avoid damaging inadvertently any pre-existing relationships in the patient's life or to prejudice future ones. The legitimacy of feelings should be accepted but when seemingly spurious emotions are encountered the problems they create should be discussed openly. Many patients have acted impulsively and out of character and need help as they struggle to regain their dignity and self-esteem. With those who seek to manipulate it is essential to be firm and frank, retaining a helpful optimistic attitude to their problems while setting limits, yet avoiding confrontations which may be perceived as threatening.

Assessment

The interviewing situation is seldom ideal in an emergency, particularly in the general hospital. Dehumanizing arrangements should be avoided as much as possible and confidentiality protected. In the casualty department a safe area should be designated, free of potential weapons and equipped with an alarm bell. It is unwise to see an unpredictable and potentially aggressive patient in a secluded setting and it is sensible to have other people visibly available in the background. Unless there is a medical or surgical indication for it, the patient should not be interviewed in a bed or on a trolley, but seated in a chair. With restless, agitated people it is normally preferable to accompany them on their perambulations. Patients, relatives and other informants should be interviewed individually.

Before meeting the patient, the assessing clinician should learn as much as possible from those who have brought him to attention. Ambulance drivers, police officers and others who may be a source of clarification after the initial assessment should be invited to wait if possible. Previous case notes should be requested and nursing staff already in contact with the patient should be questioned about behaviour with them.

On meeting the patient the doctor should introduce himself, offer to shake hands and proceed to interview in a style which, as much as possible, is conversational rather than inquisitorial. Intense listening and constant observation are needed throughout and note writing should be avoided as much as possible. History-taking which is problem-orientated, with attention to events and experiences leading up to the crisis and the identification of other significant individuals, should be followed by enquiries about previous crises, illnesses and contact with medical, social work and other agencies. The present social circumstances, existing sources of support and the quality of relationships with the general practitioner and other professionals need evaluation. In every case it is essential to enquire about the use and abuse of alcohol and drugs which may have been introduced or withdrawn recently. When physical illness is present or suspected the patient's psychological reactions to it (Lloyd 1977) and their own perceptions of its nature, treatment and prognosis demand exploration. Attitudes to psychiatric treatment and to other forms of help and the patient's expectations are highly relevant to understanding and managing the crisis.

Throughout the consultation the recent and present mental states are carefully evaluated. The patient's appearance and demeanour, clarity or otherwise of consciousness, cognitive functioning, mood state, form and content of talk and perceptual experiences are examined. Direct enquiries about thoughts or fears of harming themselves or others should be made. The level of self-esteem and any recent fall in it should be gauged. When abnormalities of mood, thought or perception are encountered, their duration, nature and, where applicable, content must be studied. The patient's capacity to relate to the interviewer, subtle changes in rapport, and any inconsistencies in the mental state may be extremely valuable in understanding the crisis. Some idea of the patient's normal level of intellectual functioning can usually be formed. While it is not a time for making comprehensive assessments of personalities, underlying and enduring emotional problems may become visible in the emergency situation.

An essential part of the assessment is a consideration of the patient's physical health and a physical examination should not be neglected. In a study of a hundred consecutive new patients referred to an emergency clinic in a psychiatric hospital, Eastwood and his colleagues (1970) found that 24 per cent were suffering physical disorders known to their general practitioners while 16 per cent had previously unrecognized abnormalities.

Towards the end of the interview and examination, if the mental state of the patient permits, it is good practice to invite the patient to review the list of problems exposed (including those that belong to the clinician), and to discuss ways of dealing with them. Permission to talk to relatives and other people who might help should then be sought. In every case an attempt should be made to talk to the patient's general practitioner. Relatives, other significant people in the patient's life, other hospitals and social work agencies may provide further information to complete the assessment.

Evaluating the crisis

In order to respond appropriately and effectively it is necessary to understand the often complex genesis of a psychiatric emergency. Even when information gathering has been comprehensive and the assessment interview sound, there may be emotions or behaviour which are puzzling or incomprehensible. Misinterpretation in some cases may lead to unnecessary and inappropriate admission, failure to diagnose what may be a life-threatening condition, or the reinforcement of maladaptive coping behaviour. However, such outcomes will be avoided if the total situation is studied as well as the patient, if a number of pitfalls are kept in mind and if advice is sought from relevant sources.

For the physician the most obvious and comfortable task is to confirm or exclude the possibility of physical illness. This should never be a prolonged process which postpones or neglects the evaluation of psychological or social issues. Deciding whether or not physical symptoms have a psychological basis is not always easy. Cohen (1982) has suggested three criteria which may be applied. First, the nature of the symptoms themselves; secondly, the presence of features which one would not expect to find if the symptoms had an exclusively organic basis; and thirdly, whether the symptoms fit into the pattern of the patient's life history.

When evidence of formal psychiatric illness is found it should not be assumed that this explains all the patient's behaviour. Many patients handicapped by neurotic or psychotic disorder are particularly vulnerable to stress or the consequences of disturbed human relationships, and they can easily become a scapegoat in situations or be subtly manipulated by other people in their lives. In immigrants the evaluation of disturbed behaviour and sometimes dramatic emotional disorder calls for caution and an awareness that there are considerable cultural variations in reacting to stress, in signalling distress and in the manifestation of the functional psychoses (Rack 1983).

Occasionally, aspects of a crisis seem to defy all attempts at understanding. Sometimes an analysis of the various roles which the patient occupies simultaneously may throw light on the problem. For example, an apparently mentally-intact and otherwise sensible man accepted that he needed, but nevertheless refused, treatment for alcoholism. Analysis revealed that he would be admitting the validity of his wife's long-standing claim that treatment was necessary thus altering the precarious balance in their relationship. Other explanations for apparently incomprehensible crisis behaviour may lie in what it might stop happening, in the manipulation of other people, or in underlying and disguised psychotic processes.

Not all patients are in crisis and of those that are, a minority will be re-enacting behaviour shown in previous crises. Such patients require very careful management if reinforcement of maladaptive coping strategies and tactics is to be avoided. This may be an exceedingly difficult task when repetitive and sometimes quite serious self-injury is a means of gaining psychiatric admission.

Principles of treatment

The therapeutic value of the assessment interview should not be underestimated and many anxious and distressed patients benefit from relatively brief relationships with the doctor and other members of the staff. The opportunity to ventilate emotions, to verbalize problems, to share loss and grief, and to receive reassurances often leads to a dramatic change especially in acute anxiety states. Furthermore, with the passage of time, spontaneous changes may occur in the mental state as, for example, when acute alcohol intoxication is responsible for the situation. In many cases if the needs of the patient are accurately identified and satisfied there may be a dramatic resolution of the crisis although this may also follow a successful but undesirable manipulation of others by the patient.

However, in many other cases some form of psychiatric or social work involvement is indicated. When this appears likely, contact with those on call should be established as early as possible so that suitable arrangements can be planned. When communicating with the psychiatrist the physician should give a clear account of all he has learned, emphasizing the problems in management and should not be afraid to reveal his own diagnostic difficulties, anxieties and other reactions to the situation.

Only a minority of people presenting with psychiatric emergencies will require admission to a psychiatric or medical bed and of those that do, most will be co-operative and accept it sensibly if reluctantly. In areas where psychiatric services are comprehensive and particularly when there are psychiatric beds in the general hospital, it may be possible to give high quality physical and psychiatric nursing care in the same unit. Reasons for admission should be clear, carefully considered and never based on ex-pediency to shelve or pass on difficult problems. Removal to a medical or psychiatric bed from the community merely for the convenience of relatives, hospital staff, or anyone else must be prevented. Whereas admission to a medical ward for purely social or psychiatric reasons is in the interests of neither patient nor hospital, beds designated for brief periods of observation are invaluable to both physician and psychiatrist. In Oxford all patients admitted following deliberate self-harm are nursed in a short-stay ward, usually for twenty-four hours or less, enabling both physical resuscitation and psychiatric assessment to be accomplished and an appropriate inter-vention planned.

Ideally, every patient being accepted for admission to a psychiatric bed should be seen prior to admission by a psychiatrist and preferably one who will continue to treat the patient in hospital. Apart from adhering to the fundamental principle of continuity of a therapeutic relationship, such a policy is remarkably effective in ensuring that the admission is appropriate and in the long-term interests of the patient. Where this is not feasible the admission must be fully discussed and planned by telephone with the psychiatrist receiving the patient. No psychiatric hospital is obliged in law to accept any patient even when the admission is under a compulsory order. Prior to transfer it must be made clear to the patient where they are going and deception to achieve an uneventful journey should be avoided. Trans-port should be by ambulance with a competent escort carrying all relevant documents and clinical notes or a letter giving full details including drugs administered.

The emergency situation is not an occasion for initiating the longer-term treatment of mental illness. Management is directed to the relief of distress, the protection of the patient and others who may be threatened, the provision of sanctuary and when necessary an environment offering opportunities for more prolonged observation. To achieve these objectives it may be necessary occasionally to restrain or tranquillize the patient or to compel admission to a psychiatric unit.

Restraint

The aim of restraint must only be to protect and calm the patient. It is used only when absolutely necessary and when other verbal measures have failed. Doctors and nurses acting in good faith in life-threatening situations by imposing restraint and if necessary medication are protected by common law. Such restraint should be offered in a firm but not threatening way, should be the minimum necessary and should always be preceded and accompanied by explanation to the patient. It should not be prolonged and there should be frequent trials of cautious withdrawal. An adequate number of staff is essential. Holding the patient by the limbs and main joints is usually the most effective and safest way of handling. It is always preferable to leave such measures to trained staff acting under an experienced leader.

Medication

In modern psychiatric practice there are three groups of drugs which are invaluable in the emergency situation, namely butyrophenones, phenothiazine derivatives and benzodiazepines. Every doctor should be familiar with at least one in each group. Barbiturates should not be used since they increase irritability, lead to disinhibition and loss of control and cause heavy sedation rather than tranquillization. Paraldehyde—which can be valuable in the treatment of status epilepticus, while having a reputation for safety and effectiveness, requires large and painful injections, is unpleasant to use, can only be given very quickly from plastic syringes and may produce abscesses—is now obsolete in psychiatric practice. Treatment with antidepressants, lithium and long-acting depot antipsychotic preparations should never be initiated in an emergency situation.

Before the drug is administered the patient should be told that the objective is to make him tranquil and comfortable and not to induce unconsciousness. When repeated doses of some major tranquillizers are necessary to gain control there is a possibility of inducing continuous narcosis which demands intensive nursing and medical care, neglect of which may lead to fluid and electrolyte imbalance and circulatory collapse.

The choice of dosage in acute psychiatric disorder is often difficult especially with physically ill or frail patients in states of high arousal. There is a tendency for inexperienced clinicians to give an inadequate dosage which has little effect on the mental state and also to give either repeated inadequate doses which eventually accumulate and then oversedate the patient, or to switch inappropriately to another drug. When choosing a reasonable dosage, age, body weight, physical status, level of arousal and degree of behavioural disturbance need to be taken into consideration.

Chlorpromazine has a time-honoured and established place in acute psychiatric conditions. When given in higher doses, especially systemically it has a marked sedative effect which can be a disadvantage especially in acute organic reactions. It may cause serious hypotension and cannot be given intravenously with safety. The dose range is 50–100 mg intramuscularly, with repetition permissible in 30–60 minutes if the response is inadequate. Some psychiatrists prefer thioridazine in a similar dose range particularly in the elderly. Anticholinergic and extrapyramidal symptoms may soon appear with phenothiazine derivatives and add to the patient's distress.

Haloperidol is probably now the most widely used drug in the management of acute behavioural disturbances. With a powerful anti-psychotic effect it is much less sedating than the phenothiazine derivatives, is less likely to cause hypotension and can be given by *slow* intravenous injection. Intramuscularly the dose range is 10–30 mg and up to 20 mg can be given intravenously. While anti-cholinergic symptoms are less of a problem compared with the phenothiazine derivatives, dystonic reactions and other extrapyramidal side-effects are more frequent and severe. For this reason many clinicians follow intravenous or intramuscular injections with procyclidine 5 mg by the same route. Once good control of symptoms and behaviour has been obtained, twice daily administration of haloperidol is usually sufficient since the drug has a long half-life. High doses of haloperidol should be used with caution in patients who are established on lithium therapy.

Benzodiazepines also have a place in emergencies. Diazepam 5–10 mg intramuscularly or intravenously may be necessary when other measures have failed to control acute anxiety states and panic attacks and to facilitate medical procedures in apprehensive patients. Caution is required in the elderly, frail and in anyone when there is a risk of respiratory failure. Chlomethiazole is often used in the management of alcohol withdrawal.

Compulsory hospitalization

To deprive anyone of their liberty by compulsory admission as a psychiatric patient even for a brief period of assessment is a serious step. It should only be considered when it is warranted either by the nature or degree of mental disorder present, or is in the interests of the patient's health or safety, or is with a view to protect other persons and when informal admission has proved to be impossible. Compared with its predecessor of 1959, the Mental Health Act 1983 imposes stricter criteria and safeguards for the admission and treatment of patients and increases the involvement of social workers in the processes of detention. To appreciate and understand the complexities of the new Act the reader is advised to consult Blueglass (1983) who gives an admirably lucid account of its provisions. For present purposes it is necessary to consider the procedures to admit for assessment, to retain a patient who is already in hospital and to protect the mentally disordered in public places. Before doing so it is important to define key roles occupied by the patient, relative, social worker and doctor.

A Patient under the Act means a person who is suffering or appearing to be suffering from mental disorder; it cannot be invoked to impose the treatment of physical illness alone. The 'Nearest Relative' has a crucial role and is determined by position in a hierarchical list which involves individuals who have been living in a close relationship with the patient but are not blood relatives. An Approved Social Worker is an officer of a local social services authority with special training and responsibilities and who is empowered to apply for the patient's admission under the Act having ensured that this is the most appropriate way of dealing with the case. Medical recommendations may only be made by registered medical practitioners who have examined the patient personally. Where two doctors are required one must be an Approved Doctor under Section 12, recognized as having special experience in the diagnosis and treatment of mental disorder. Only one of the doctors may be on the staff of the hospital to which the patient is to be admitted unless this would involve a delay of more than forty-eight hours from the completion of the first recommendation and the admission is in the best interests of the patient. Even then, one of the doctors must not be working under the direction of the other at that hospital, one of them must work at the hospital for less than half the time under his contract with the Health Service and it must not be a private hospital or nursing home. Neither may act as the applicant for the patient's admission, be a partner or assistant of either the applicant or the other doctor giving the recommendation, or receive payments for the maintenance of the patient. One of the two doctors should have had previous acquaintance with the patient either as the family doctor or from treating him as a consultant in the past, although there may be occasions when it is impossible to apply this principle.

Admission for Assessment may be made under Section 2 of the Act on the application of the nearest relative or a social worker either of whom must have seen the patient in the previous fourteen days. Unless it would involve undue delay, the social worker must consult the nearest relative who has the right to disallow admission. Two medical recommendations are required, one being by an Approved Doctor, and both must state that (a) the patient is suffering from a mental disorder of a nature or degree which warrants detention in a hospital for assessment (or for assessment followed by medical treatment) for at least a limited period; and (b) that he or she ought to be so detained in the interests of his or her own health or safety, or with a view to the protection of other persons. If the doctors examine the patient individually not more than five clear days must elapse between the examinations. The patient may be detained for twenty-eight days beginning with the day of admission and has the right of appeal to a Mental Health Review Tribunal within the first fourteen days of admission.

Admission for Assessment in an Emergency under Section 4 is appropriate only in genuine emergency situations where there is insufficient time to arrange a second medical recommendation. Application is made by the nearest relative or an Approved Social Worker, either of whom must have seen the patient in the previous twenty-four hours. The application may be supported by one medical recommendation but given preferably by a doctor who is already acquainted with the patient. The patient must be admitted within twenty-four hours of the time of the examination or the application if that is made earlier. The patient may be detained for only seventy-two hours unless a second medical recommendation is received thereby allowing Section 2 of the Act to be applied. An Emergency Application only allows assessment and does not permit treatment within the meaning of the Act. Urgent treatment to relieve serious suffering or to save life may be necessary and is covered by the authority of common law. The grounds for admission are identical with those applying under Section 2 with the additional requirement that admission is of urgent necessity and compliance with the requirements of Section 2 would involve undesirable delay.

Patients already in any hospital receiving any form of in-patient treatment on an informal basis may be detained under Section 5 of the Act. It provides a mechanism to protect the patient or endangered others when the patient is intending to leave hospital and there appear to be grounds for an application for compulsory admission to hospital under Sections 2 or 3. Only the doctor in charge of the patient's treatment or his nominated deputy may make a report in writing to the managers of the hospital stating that the patient is presenting a danger to himself or others and that an application for compulsory admission appears necessary. Only a single and suitably qualified deputy may be nominated and that person must apply an independent clinical judgement. The detention may last for only seventy-two hours from the moment the report to the managers is signed. Since there may be delay before the doctor in charge or his deputy can examine the patient, particularly in certain psychiatric hospitals under Section 5(4) of the Act, psychiatric nurses of a prescribed class may detain a patient *already receiving treatment for mental disorder* for up to six hours while the appropriate doctor is found.

When a mentally disordered person is found in a public place and appears to be in immediate need of care and control, a police constable is authorized under Section 136 to remove him to a 'place of safety' if it appears necessary to do so in the interests of that person or to protect other people. Places of safety include a hospital, a police station, a residential home for mentally disordered persons or any suitable place whose occupier is willing temporarily to receive the patient. Detention under this Section must not exceed seventy-two hours, which is ample time for the assessment of the person and the arrangement of further compulsory care if necessary.

After the crisis

Immediately the emergency is over attention should be directed to ensuring that good communications are completed, the on-going care of the patient and others disturbed by it are not neglected, and that opportunities for learning from it are not lost. Clinical notes should be concise and factual with precise descriptions of the problems exposed, the mental state found, actions taken and future ones planned. Pejorative labelling of personalities and indulgence in theorizing about the genesis of the mental disorder are unhelpful.

Pre-existing harmonious relationships are easily damaged by some psychiatric emergencies and inexperienced staff members and even other patients may be left feeling inappropriately responsible, guilty or anxious. Where professionals from different services only meet in emergency situations, opportunities to meet and share problems are of great benefit. At the John Radcliffe Hospital for some years members of the psychiatric emergency team have held regular, informal meetings with colleagues in the Accident and Emergency Department and the Short-Stay Wards.

Wherever possible the continuing psychological care of the patient should remain with whoever provides the major psycho-social assessment and counselling contribution in the crisis, unless there are advantages in transferring care to other medical or social agencies. Every opportunity to help the patient to cope more appropriately with any future crisis must be grasped. Since its inception in 1975 the Radcliffe Psychiatric Consultation Service has operated an Open Access facility giving patients a card with a special telephone number by which they can receive prompt help in future crises.

References further reading

Berrios G.E. (1982) Psychiatric emergencies. *Hospital Update* **8**, 303–314.
Bluglass R. (1983) *A Guide to the Mental Health Act, 1983.* Churchill Livingstone Edinburgh.
Brothwood J. (1965) The work of a psychiatric emergency clinic. *British Journal of Psychiatry* **iii**, 631–634.

Cohen S.I. (1982) The evaluation of patients with somatic symptoms—the 'difficult' diagnostic problem. In Creed F. and Pfeffer J.M. eds. *Medicine and Psychiatry: A Practical Approach*. Pitman Books, London.

Cox J.L. (1976) Psychiatric assessment and the immigrant patient. *British Journal of Hospital Medicine* **16**, 38–40.

Eastwood M.R., Mindham, R.H.S. and Tennent T.G. (1970). The physical status of psychiatric emergencies. *British Journal of Psychiatry* **116**, 545–550.

Gerson S. and Bassuk E. (1980) Psychiatric emergencies: an overview. *American Journal of Psychiatry* **137**, 1–12.

Hawton K., Gath D. and Smith E. (1979) Management of attempted suicide in Oxford. *British Medical Journal* **2**, 1040–1042.

Johnson J. (1969) Psychiatric emergencies in the community. *Comprehensive Psychiatry* **10**, 275–283.

Lloyd G.G. (1977) Psychological reactions to physical illness. *British Journal of Hospital Medicine* **18**, 352–358.

Rack P.H. (1983) Psychiatric disorders in immigrants. *Medicine International* **34**, U134–137.

Waldron G. (1982) Psychiatric emergencies. In Creed F. and Pfeffer J.M., eds. *Medicine and Psychiatry: A Practical Approach*. Pitman Books, London.

Waters M.A. and Northover J. (1972) Patterns of emergency care: an operational study. *Social Psychiatry* **7**, 127–138.

35 · Psychiatric Emergencies: Common Clinical Situations

E. B. O. SMITH

While it is impossible to cover comprehensively the range of emergency situations, some consideration needs to be given to specific aspects of assessment and management in some of those met in general medical practice.

The commonest emotional crises stem from bereavement, separation, loss of health, self-esteem or resources, interpersonal problems, unexpected life-events or the threat of these in the future (Bancroft 1979). The majority of individuals facing such stresses succeed in coping with their feelings, particularly if they are able to express their emotions and when they find solutions to their problems. Inadequate personal resources, the adoption of maladaptive coping behaviours and psychological defences, or an inaccurate perception of appropriate help may lead an individual to seek medical treatment. Acute anxiety states, depressive reactions, dissociative hysterical conditions, inappropriate adoption of the role of the physically ill, deliberate self-harm and a behavioural repertoire which includes anxiety-arousing and manipulative behaviours, may then be found. Most will respond to the measures already outlined offered by a genuinely concerned counsellor who helps the patient to find and express the underlying feelings, to define the problems, and to choose more effective ways of coping with their distress. Only rarely should it be necessary to prescribe psychotropic medication, offer the sanctuary of admission to a psychiatric bed, or take other steps to solve problems on the patient's behalf. In evaluating the crisis it is important to accurately detect who is being reproached for failing to offer sufficient affection, expected to behave in a particular way, or being influenced to appreciate a disguised emotion or attitude. Recognition of such dynamic factors is crucial to understanding and responding to the situation.

Alcohol-related emergencies

Alcohol frequently plays a major role in generating psychiatric emergencies either from abuse by the patient or by another significant person. It may cause psychiatric and neurological disorders arising directly from central and peripheral neuronal damage and liver disease. It is also responsible for syndromes associated with withdrawal. Its chronic abuse causes major social and marital pathology and often leads to individual self-neglect, malnutrition, poverty and homelessness. Depressive states, paranoid conditions, morbid jealousy, self-destructive behaviour and suicide, child abuse, criminal behaviour and homicide are frequently linked with it. Its very ubiquity combined with the difficulty of successfully treating the victim ensures that alcoholism is a constant cause of misunderstanding, neglect and antipathy in individual cases. Acute alcohol intoxication in itself does not constitute a psychiatric emergency although the behaviour it releases may do so. A common problem is the chronic abuser who, while still intoxicated, seeks immediate admission and in a remorseful state of mind declares that he wishes to be cured. Clinicians in charge of detoxication centres are very conscious that many such patients reject help the next day. Nevertheless, at times of crisis it is sometimes possible to influence a patient's attitude to his problems and to facilitate new help-seeking behaviour. The nature and extent of the physician's response will be largely governed by the policies and facilities offered by his psychiatric colleagues. Testing of the patient's motivation by suggesting that he or she should, on their own initiative, seek treatment at the appropriate agency, perhaps after an interval, has the merit of selecting those most likely to benefit from often scarce facilities. Unfortunately this tactic leaves the majority beyond effective help.

Threat of suicide

One of the commonest problems is the patient who discloses, spontaneously or in response to questioning, the intention or fear of deliberate self-harm. The assessment of all distressed, depressed or mentally disturbed patients should include direct enquiries about such ideas and feelings. It is fallacious to believe that such open discussion increases the risk of suicidal behaviour; the majority of patients appreciate the opportunity of sharing the burden of entertaining suicidal ideas with a concerned and sympathetic counsellor. When a spontaneous declaration of suicidal intent or risk is made, it must always be taken seriously. Over two-thirds of those who die by suicide have been shown to have given a warning of the possibility. Even in the small minority of people who consciously use such threats as a manipulative device, the motive is usually to emphasize the seriousness of their distress.

The assessment of the individual patient to determine the risk of self-destruction is not always an easy one. Surveys of suicide in the general population have disclosed general factors. The risk increases with age, is higher in males than females and in those who live alone or are rejected, including the unmarried, widowed and divorced. Unemployment as a general factor becomes weaker during periods of economic recession. However, in some individuals the loss of the working role through redundancy or premature retirement increases vulnerability to depressive states. Alcoholism, drug dependence and chronically painful or disabling illness are other general factors. Severe depressive states and hypomania carry a particularly high risk, while in schizophrenia the risk is much lower, although the event is not easy to predict.

In the individual patient, while taking account of these general factors, it is necessary to explore and understand the patient's recent life experiences, the development of the present mental state and to be alert for more specific indicators of increased risk. A recent and marked fall in the level of self-esteem is a particularly strong one, especially in obsessional personalities. A family history of suicide and previous attempts on the part of the patient increase the chances of a further serious attempt. Depressive states carry the highest risk of suicide, especially when low mood is accompanied by the following: guilt and self-depreciatory attitudes, hypochondriacal or delusional preoccupations, or severe insomnia with restlessness and early morning waking. Depressed patients who have previously been indecisive and retarded may become actively suicidal after treatment has been initiated. In every patient any factors which might increase impulsiveness should be sought such as alcohol or drug-abuse and the availability of particular means of self-injury. The effect of the patient's mental state on relatives and other significant people must be judged and the possibility of harm to them considered.

As in the management of all psychiatric emergencies the clinician should adopt a firmly optimistic approach, taking seriously all the problems that have been revealed and, with the patient, formulating a plan of action to solve them. In many cases the prospect of help, the clarification of problems and the therapeutic nature of the consultation may have a favourable effect on the mental state. If at the end of the assessment the risk of suicide remains high and especially when serious psychiatric disorder has been found, the patient should be referred for immediate assessment by a psychiatrist. In the meantime he or she should be nursed with discrete observation and sensible precautions away from any potential instruments of self-harm.

If it is suspected that the patient is being disingenuous or manipulative, it will be necessary to insist on a clarification and declaration of the response they are expecting. When this is unrealistic or inappropriate, limits must be set and refusal to collude must be explicit while at the same time alternative offers of help maintained.

Deliberate self-poisoning

Over 90 per cent of patients admitted to hospitals following deliberate self-harm have taken an overdose of a drug or ingested a potentially injurious substance. During the past two decades it has become a fashionable behaviour in crisis in the Western world and is responsible for over 100,000 admissions to general hospitals in the United Kingdom every year. In a high proportion of patients the act is impulsive, emotionally determined and considered only in the previous hour or so. Motivation is usually complex and in only a minority does there appear to be an unequivocal desire to die. After the event, with the exception of this minority, patients select as the major motives the need to escape from an intolerable situation which no other action could give, loss of control, and the necessity to communicate their feelings to others. However, psychiatrists interpret the same acts as manipulating the emotions and behaviour of others, communicating hostility and help-seeking (Bancroft et al. 1979). While the majority of patients describe psychological symptoms, less than 8 per cent show formal psychiatric illness. Deliberate self-harm is rare in childhood, more common in girls than in boys in the adolescent years and commonest under the age of 35 years. Twice as many women as men show the behaviour although in recent years this sexual difference has shown signs of lessening. Psychotropic drugs and non-opiate analgesics are now the commonest substances taken. Alcohol has frequently been taken a few hours before, or at the time of, the overdose.

Once resuscitation and other medical treatments have been completed, assessment should follow the principles outlined in the last chapter. A detailed account of events leading up to and the circumstances of the act should be obtained. The degree of suicidal intent can be judged from the degree of premeditation, the nature of the planning and precautions against discovery, verbal and written communications before the attempt, the timing and isolation of the act, and actions to summon help after it. Relevant aspects of the family and personal history including previous episodes of deliberate self-harm and other crises should be elicited and an assessment made of the patient's coping resources including potentially supportive relationships. A review of all recent and current problems will usually reveal crises in relationships with sexual partners, spouses, other family members or key figures. Alcoholism, drug-abuse, physical ill-health, sexual difficulties, unemployment, financial embarrassment and involvement with the processes of the law as an offender are other common problems. During the interview the mental state must be carefully assessed and any degree of continuing suicidal risk determined. By the end of the interview the assessor should feel able to understand why the act occurred; if this is not the case, the possibility that information is being witheld or that the patient is suffering from a covert psychotic state should be considered.

With the patient's permission, other significant people in the crisis should be interviewed and the family practitioner contacted by telephone. Where necessary, advice and opinions should be obtained from psychiatrists, social workers or other professionals. The clinician and patient should then review the situation, re-defining problems where necessary, establish realistic goals and, if appropriate, establish a therapeutic contract. Only a minority, less than ten per cent where adequate resources for crisis intervention exist, require admission to a psychiatric bed. Future management should be flexible, problem-orientated and wherever possible involve other significant people in the patient's life. Psychotropic medication, if prescribed at all, should be limited and used only briefly. An essential part of the intervention is to assess the risk of repetition of self-harm and the possibility of eventual suicide. It is also important to endeavour to provide alternative and more appropriate help in future crises. Prediction of repetition, the problem of chronic repeaters, the provision of special services for this group of patients and techniques of management are beyond the scope of this chapter and should be sought elsewhere (Hawton and Catalan 1982; Gelder *et al.* 1983).

Deliberate self-injury

Forms of self-injury other than by self-poisoning occurred in 13 per cent of all cases of deliberate self-harm referred to the general hospital in Oxford between 1976 and 1980. Only 20 per cent of this group had been injured in serious suicidal attempts by hanging, drowning, deep throat- or wrist-cutting, jumping from heights or in front of vehicles, or gunshot wounds. Almost all of these were suffering from serious psychiatric disorder.

The majority coming to the Accident Department did so after episodes of superficial self-cutting. Typically such patients are young, unattached and displaying many personality problems. Once regarded as a female behaviour it is now almost as common in men. Irritability of mood with impulsive tendencies to be aggressive, a disturbed background in childhood and difficulty in expressing emotions and needs, seem to be the foundation of repetitive self-laceration or other forms of mutilation. Following a period of mounting tension the wounding by razor, knife or broken glass is relatively painless, is accompanied by a need to draw blood and occasionally may be deep enough to damage arteries and nerves. Cutting, which is usually on the forearms but may be elsewhere on the body, is preceded by feelings of anger, extreme tension and misery, all of which usually disperse immediately to be replaced by embarrassment, shame and disgust. Many of the patients abuse alcohol and drugs, lack the ability to enjoy sexual relationships and are prone to eating disorders. Psychiatric management is invariably difficult but in time with maturation most patients abandon the behaviour.

Very rarely, self-mutilation or amputation of the genitals is encountered in the male. This has been reported in transexuals and in severe bereavement reactions but in most cases the patient is suffering from schizophrenia and responding to delusional ideas.

Aggressive behaviour

A potent source of anxiety in hospital staff is the aggressive or violent patient. Cultural and personality factors lead to a predisposition to react aggressively in crisis in some individuals especially if their self-esteem is threatened by insecurity, real or imagined criticism, lack of respect in others, or fear of losing control of their personal situation. Alcohol and drug intoxication as well as any medical or psychiatric condition where there is disinhibition and impairment of judgement or conscious awareness can release such behaviour. Acute organic reactions of any cause, severe depressive and hypomanic states, brain damage by injury or disease and schizophrenia may facilitate aggressive and assaultative propensities but only in a minority of patients. Contrary to popular belief aggression during seizures is exceedingly rare in those handicapped by epilepsy, although, as in acute organic reactions and dementia, restraint may evoke retaliatory aggression.

In the general population aggression and homicide occur usually in the setting of the family or other close relationships. In psychiatric states, especially severe depressive and paranoid ones, individuals may become the focus of a patient's delusions and their lives endangered. Morbid jealousy in a spouse may first come to light in a crisis and should always be given serious attention since it can lead to homicide. Such psychiatric conditions are fortunately not common. Much more frequently, battered wives (Gayford 1979), victims of rape (Bowden 1978) and child abuse come to the attention of doctors in emergency services.

Assessment of the aggressive or disruptive patient should proceed on the same lines as other emergencies with particular attention to the mental state and a rapid analysis of the situation. If possible an early decision should be reached on the likelihood of physical or mental illness being a primary contributing factor. Diffuse, generalized aggressive responses need to be differentiated from those directed at an individual or particular group.

Threats must be taken seriously and sufficient help summoned. The appearance of other staff or police officers in the background often has an inhibitory effect but intimidation, provocation or hostility must be avoided. Potential victims must be removed from the situation and no one should be left alone with the patient. An attempt should be made to encourage the person to talk and to ventilate their emotions and grievances. A calm, firm approach in which you make it clear that you cannot allow the person to cause harm is needed, and every opportunity taken to appeal to the mature adult part of their personality. Sudden movements which might be mis-interpreted must be avoided. If it becomes clear that restraint is required an experienced leader should take charge with assistants. Even the most dangerous and violent can be restrained with simple techniques (Perry and

Gilmore 1981). Medication should only be given against the patient's wishes for psychiatric or medical reasons in the interests of the patient's immediate health and safety and never simply to control or punish the behaviour. If the patient is not mentally ill or in need of observation, is not a danger to himself and is unresponsive to offers of appropriate help, he should be asked to leave the hospital premises and the police called to remove him if he refuses to do so.

The unco-operative patient

Implicit in the acceptance of the role of the sick patient is the assumption that advice and any treatment offered will be accepted and that co-operation with medical and other staff within the limits imposed by the illness will always be as full as possible. In return for the privileges of the sick role, expectations are created that certain attitudes and behaviours will be adopted and particular activities avoided. Patients who fail to comply are liable to be regarded as unco-operative, irresponsible or even mentally ill. To ignore advice, refuse an operation or treatment, threaten to leave hospital against advice or behave in some eccentric way, may arouse understandable concern and sometimes hostility.

Failures in communication and misunderstandings between patients and staff occur far more frequently than most physicians realize and these lead easily to false perceptions and expectations on both sides. In hospital settings where the expression of emotion is discouraged and the patient is unable to share with anyone their underlying problems they are liable to act-out their feelings, to show distrust, or to be reluctant to relinquish control. As Perry and Viederman (1981) have emphasized flexibility and understanding are required to detect and manage non-compliance as a defence against humiliation, helplessness, fears of emasculation or mistrust of others.

The clinician who is confronted with such a patient is well-advised to seek the assistance of a colleague, such as an experienced nurse, social worker or psychiatrist, to clarify the problems with the patient. In most cases, once the underlying difficulties have been exposed, it is possible to find a way of restoring the patient's self-esteem relieving the previously unexpressed fear or sense of insecurity, or correcting the misperceptions. Occasionally evidence of psychosis will be found and the services of a psychiatrist should then be sought urgently. On rare occasions mentally healthy individuals with well-considered views on the quality of their lives and the merits of the treatments offered, make rational decisions to refuse an operation or other treatment. While respecting the dignity and rights of such patients even the most senior of physicians is advised to obtain a second opinion from an experienced colleague as then they can share the inevitable emotions aroused as well as the ethical dilemma.

Munchausen syndrome and factitious illness

Since Asher (1951) first proposed that the name of Baron Von Munchausen, the subject of a book by Rudolf Raspe in 1786, should be used to describe the behaviour of those who feign serious illness to gain admission to hospital, the condition has attracted a surprising amount of attention considering its relative rarity. In Asher's descriptions the commonest presentations were with acute abdominal pain, evidence of recent visible blood loss, or neurological symptoms. However, since then a wide range of simulated medical and surgical emergencies has been reported. Not only physical illness may be shammed to gain the sick role but also feigned bereavement (Snowdon *et al.* 1978) and factitious psychosis (Hay 1983) have been recognized. Moreover, cases have been described where parents have induced illness in their children, the so-called Munchausen-by-proxy (Meadow 1977).

As Blackwell (1968) pointed out in a valuable review, the syndrome is a product of individual personality development influenced by life experiences involving gratification in the sick role and an established pathological response to mood swings and environmental set-backs. Carney (1980) has argued that these peripatetic patients are part of a larger group with similar psychopathology which includes people, often with pre-existing medical knowledge, who tamper with wounds, produce artefactual skin disorders, or are found to have factitious haematological or metabolic disorders. Their primary craving appears to be for medical rather than hospital attention. However, especially in wanderers, there may be subsidiary gains from receiving certain drugs, avoidance of the processes of law, gaining temporary accommodation, or the rewards of playing the central role in a dramatic situation. Admission reinforces the behaviour which may be extinguished eventually if this medical response is witheld repeatedly.

The essence of success in detecting these patients is to be alert for certain features of behaviour while adhering to the principles of assessment already outlined. They are often brought to the Casualty Department by concerned strangers having provoked a dramatic incident in a public place. They immediately express gratitude for attention and often set about gaining sympathy with a history of recent harrowing, stressful and dramatic events. Embedded in the medical history are fragments of genuine experiences in the sick role usually relating to investigations or operative procedures which appear to authenticate the account. Often on examination there is one or more physical signs such as an abnormal pupil, a cardiac arrhythmia, or murmur or an abnormal ECG.

Attempts to clarify the history and present problems produce uninformative and vague answers, a shift in the narrative with the introduction of more dramatic and attention-rivetting material, or behaviour to distract the clinician. These patients, who often appear out of normal working hours when the least experienced doctors are likely to be on duty, are skillful in creating the fear of missing some vital investigation or the necessity to provide urgent treatment. If their initially covert but later explicit demand for admission is not met they will endeavour to create guilt for neglecting their suffering, make veiled threats of suicide or become truculent and hostile. The clinician who is in the habit of routinely contacting the general practitioner in emergency situations will quickly realize that this is not possible, that the patient does not live locally and is itinerant. If admission is chosen as a seemingly sensible and reasonable short-term solution, the patient soon takes his discharge after consuming expensive resources, particularly if referral to a psychiatrist is suggested. Even when it has been possible to engage them in psychiatric treatment successful modification of the personality disorder has been rare.

Once the condition has been identified in the Casualty Department and any essential investigations to confirm the absence of a genuine medical emergency completed, confrontation should be avoided. Instead an attempt should be made to expose the current problems which have prompted the need to seek the sick role. In this way admission and reinforcement of this pathological behaviour pattern will be avoided and appropriate help may be possible. Measures designed to detect these individuals by photographing them, circulating their description to hospitals or constructing black-lists, not only raise ethical issues but in practice have proved naive and ineffective.

States of high arousal

Anxiety in varying degrees and manifestations is ubiquitous in the hospital environment and on occasions may be so acute and intense that it becomes the central feature of an emergency situation. Especially when it is episodic and accompanied by the physical manifestations of autonomic sympathetic over-activity in a personality which the hasty clinician may falsely assume is neurotic, there are pitfalls for the unwary and inexperienced. Such diverse conditions as hypoglycaemia, porphyria, temporal lobe seizures, carcinoid tumours, phaeochromocytoma, pulmonary embolism, pneumothorax, cardiac arrhythmias, asthma and pancreatitis have been mis-diagnosed initially as acute anxiety states and panic reactions. Hyperventilation in panic reactions is fairly common but should always be carefully assessed to exclude organic causes. The long-standing, traditional remedy of re-breathing into a paper bag should not be forgotten. In the majority of anxious patients adequate causes will be found in terms of their reactions to physical illness, current life problems or fears associated with their perception of the future. In many cases, expression of their feelings coupled with reassurance and explanation on the part of the clinician will be sufficient to relieve the anxious state. Occasionally, it will be necessary to give a benzodiazepine orally or systemically in the crisis situation but such treatment should always be regarded as a short-term tactic to be followed, if the symptoms persist, by comprehensive psychiatric evaluation and the introduction of psychotherapeutic and behavioural techniques of anxiety management. Patients with histrionic features in their personalities may become overwhelmed with anxiety and lose self-control completely. They usually respond to firmness, appeals to the more mature elements in their personality and the setting of limits beyond which such behaviours will not be tolerated.

In states of agitated depression some patients are so anxious and restless that they give a superficial impression of being in a highly aroused state. Diagnosis is rarely difficult since other classical features of depressive illness are to be found in the mental state. Very occasionally psychiatric patients on anti-psychotic medication will present themselves at casualty departments with the uncontrollable restlessness of akathisia, an extra-pyramidal side-effect of their medication.

In hypomanic states patients are excited, overactive, restless and distractable. They show an elevation of mood which gives a false impression of well-being and are often unhappy, irritable, sometimes impulsively self-destructive and occasionally suspicious, paranoid and hostile. Their behaviour and speech are meaningful to an alert observer and they show pressure of speech, flight of ideas and expansive ideation. The need for sleep is reduced, appetite and sexual drive are increased and persistent over-activity can lead to exhaustion. Unaware of the changes in their mental state these patients are self-neglectful, disinhibited and lacking in the normal regulation of their personal affairs. Grandiose, paranoid and other types of delusions may be expressed and hallucinations experienced.

In the fortunately rare schizophrenic excitement state there is a disintegration of the personality and, unlike the condition of the hypomanic patient, it is not possible to understand speech or behaviour. Onset is often acute and the patient may become homicidal, attacking indiscriminately anyone approaching them. Restraint and the immediate administration of intravenous haloperidol followed by admission to a psychiatric unit are necessary.

States of high arousal may occur in acute organic reactions. Severe anxiety and even hypomanic behaviour may be found. Abuse of hallucinogenic drugs or amphetamines may be responsible and should be considered especially in young patients.

Psychological withdrawal

In some cases of severe depressive illness the patient appears perplexed and indecisive, has difficulty in concentrating on the interviewer's remarks and is slow in marshalling and expressing ideas which are invariably pessimistic and may be self-reproachful or delusional. With patient and sensitive interviewing it is usually possible to obtain the history of psychological and biological symptoms and to establish the diagnosis. In paranoid psychotic states extreme suspiciousness allied to a delusional system may be responsible for evasiveness, hostility or mutism.

Hysterical aphasia and mutism are occasionally encountered. Usually, but not always, they occur in patients with a poor intellectual level. The ability to cough is unimpaired and it is clear from the non-verbal behaviour that the patient is in close touch with the environment.

Stupor is a condition in which there appears to be relative preservation of conscious awareness although the patient is immobile, mute and unresponsive to all but the strongest of painful stimuli. When the eyes are open they appear watchful and may follow moving stimuli. Before psychiatric causes are considered it is vital to exclude organic ones, although differentiation is not easy in many cases. An urgent task is to exclude raised intracranial pressure. Lesions in the posterior diencephalon or upper midbrain may be responsible. Extracerebral causes include hepatic and renal failure, hypoglycaemia, severe fluid and elecrolyte disturbance, myxoedema, Cushing's and Addison's diseases, hypopituitarism, hyperparathyroidism, severe alcohol or barbiturate intoxication, and nicotinic acid deficiency (Lishman 1978).

Functional stupors may be schizophrenic, depressive, manic or hysterical. In catatonic schizophrenia there may be echopraxia, negativism, waxy flexibility of the limbs, the adoption of awkward and strange postures or evidence of hallucinatory experiences. Depressive and manic stupors arise out of extreme forms of these illnesses and are exceedingly rare. In psychogenic stupor inconsistencies in the state of psychological withdrawal may be detected with fluctuation in responsiveness to environmental events suggesting an awareness of all that is going on and less dependency on others for personal nursing care. Secondary gains from the behaviour will usually become clear before long.

Acute organic reactions

Undoubtedly the commonest psychiatric syndrome found in the general hospital is the acute organic reaction. When presenting in a classical form, with obvious clouding of consciousness, disorientation in time and place, perceptual disturbances and restlessness, the diagnosis is rarely missed particularly if there is an obvious cause. However, in many cases, a fluctuating course with transient and much less florid symptomatology may lead to a failure to detect it or to misinterpretation in favour of a neurotic or a functional psychotic disorder. This is particularly liable to occur when impairment of consciousness is not obvious or only intermittently detectable by mild degrees of poor cognitive functioning of short duration. Onset may be preceded by inexplicable restlessness and insomnia and relatives or friends who know the patient well may be the first to realize the onset. The patient's pre-morbid personality, the immediate environment, the discomforts of the causative illness and treatment may all affect and determine the patient's perceptual experiences, emotional reactions and behaviour. While some patients are subdued, unnaturally quiet and withdrawn, others are irritable, restless, noisy and overactive. In struggling to understand their incomplete and distorted perceptions of environment and to relate such percepts to previous life experiences, there is a consistent tendency to misinterpret situations, other people and objects in favour of the familiar. As Stedeford (1978) has pointed out, it is often possible to understand the patient's seemingly psychotic experiences. When impairment of consciousness is not obvious, delusions of persecution or hallucinations may be misleading especially if no obvious cause has been found for an organic syndrome. It is a sound rule in clinical practice that if visual hallucinations are detected the most likely diagnosis is an organic one until proved otherwise. In the acute organic syndrome the experience of the patient is often a rich but frightening one with a mood state which is complex, unstable and constantly changing. An abnormal lability of mood is common with anxiety, fear, depression, suspiciousness, irritability or transient euphoria alternating with bewilderment. Purposeless movements are frequent and disinhibition may lead some patients to become aggressive or violent, cause embarrassment to others by their social indiscretions, or to inadvertently injure themselves. Paranoid components in the clinical picture are not uncommon. Evaluation of cognitive impairment must always be related to pre-morbid functioning and include the possibility of a pre-existing amnestic syndrome or dementia. The acute organic reaction runs a fluctuating and sometimes intermittent course, is worse in darkness, and may last for days or weeks. It often ends abruptly but there may be fleeting relapses for a time afterwards.

In most cases the underlying cause will be easy to find particularly if a careful history is obtained from reliable and relevant informants and the examination and preliminary investigations are systematic and thorough. In understanding the emergence of the reaction, assessment must be comprehensive and take account of individual vulnerability, any predisposing and facilitating factors, as well as the organic disease responsible (Lipowski 1980). Previous cerebral damage of any kind, addiction to alcohol or drugs and being over sixty years of age may be predisposing conditions. In addition, psychological stress, sleep deprivation and other disorders of the sleep-wakefulness cycle, sensory deprivation or overload and immobilization, may all facilitate this non-specific reaction. When evidence of organic disease is found it must not be assumed that it is solely responsible. Anaemia, infections, cardiac, renal or hepatic failure, respiratory insufficiency and fluid and electrolyte disturbances, may all act as the major factor in causation but in some cases are of secondary consideration. In every patient the possibility of central nervous system disease from degenerative processes, vascular disorder, infections, trauma or a space-occupying lesion should be entertained. Drug intoxication is an increasingly common cause in modern medical practice and withdrawal after dependence on alcohol or drugs must be constantly borne in mind (Davison 1980).

On occasions difficulty in finding an explanatory cause is encountered. Before embarking on further expensive and time-consuming investigations to identify any of the thousands of medical and surgical conditions which could be responsible, it is sensible to go back and question the validity of the information collected so far. In the author's experience failure to find a cause springs more often from lack of information about the patient's previous health, personality and environment than from a neglect to consider some obscure diagnosis. A further interview with a relative or close friend, a telephone conversation with the family practitioner and perusal of clinical notes, including those from hospitals where the patient has been treated previously, often pay dividends. While further investigations are being carried out regular physical examinations and accurate nursing observations must be maintained. In patients with intermittent disturbances of the mental state continuous electro-encephalographic recording may be helpful in exposing such conditions as complex partial seizures. For the patient and the relatives the acute organic reaction is a harrowing experience and as soon as it is recognized special measures in nursing care are needed. If possible, the patient should be moved away from other patients and sources of noise to a quiet room which can be kept dimly lit at night. As few staff members as possible should go to the bedside and every attempt made to help the patient to orientate himself and to understand what is happening. Drugs should be used sparingly and without further impairment of consciousness. Haloperidol is the drug of choice in the restless, psychotic patient. Benzodiazepines are valuable in reducing anxiety and encouraging sleep.

Loss of memory

From time to time individuals may be found in emergency situations who appear to have a gross disorder of memory without any impairment of consciousness. Several conditions need to be considered.

Patients with established dementia who wander away from their normal environment are encountered when they are brought to hospital from some public place. They show a generalized impairment of intellect as well as memory defects, disorientation in time and place and sometimes person. Powers of attention and concentration are usually grossly impaired and they are often perplexed, distractable and restless. They may be anxious, irritable and occasionally paranoid or hostile. Their mood may be abnormally labile and their behavioural repertoire limited and stereotyped. They are unable to give any account of themselves and may fall back on behaviour learned in social roles earlier in life in order to cope with the situation. Self-neglectful and with only partial or no insight into their condition, they may need the sanctuary of admission to protect and assess them. Patients with the amnestic syndrome with lesions in the posterior hypothalamus and adjacent structures or both hippocampi may present in a similar way. They are handicapped by impairment of recent memory and an inability to learn new material but there is preservation of remote memory and there is no generalized intellectual impairment. Disorientation in time is a prominent feature. Confabulation, in which the patient gives an unnecessarily detailed and elaborate explanation in response to a question, is common. Many, but not all, have been damaged by alcohol abuse and in some cases a history of the Wernicke–Korsakoff Syndrome due to thiamine deficiency, is obtained.

Transient global amnesia is a condition which commonly presents in an emergency situation. Essentially, it is a temporary but profound failure of the mechanisms of memory with preservation of other mental functions. It is commoner in men than women and occurs in late-middle or old age. It is abrupt in onset and lasts for an hour or two, or rarely, for several days. The sufferer appears bewildered and may be anxious, but is often capable of carrying out familiar tasks, often of considerable complexity such as driving a car, during an attack. There is loss of recall of memories of recent events stretching sometimes over several days and an inability to register in memory current experiences during the period of the attack. Recall of distant events remains intact and there is no clouding of consciousness. Knowledge of personal identity is retained throughout. Usually, no neurological signs can be found. Recovery is spontaneous and is followed by amnesia for the episode. The aetiology is uncertain but in many cases reported it has seemed likely to be due to cerebral ischaemia from insufficiency in the posterior cerebral circulation.

Hysterical amnesic states seem less common in casualty departments than they were several decades ago. Typically, the onset is sudden and the patient, like those who show Munchausen's Syndrome, is brought up by concerned strangers. There is no clouding of consciousness and, while the patient describes extensive memory disorder often with total loss of personal identity and disorientation in place and time, there is an absence of anxiety and their bewilderment seems contrived. The term fugue was originally applied to transitory abnormal behaviour with aimless wandering, more or less marked alteration of consciousness and usually, but not necessarily, followed by amnesia (Stengel 1943). Later the concept was broadened to include behaviour involving the mechanisms of escape from uncomfortable or threatening situations. Not all fugues with the impulse to wander are true dissociative states. Many patients on recovery from their putative loss of memory will admit later that they retained at least a peripheral awareness of playing a role throughout the episode. In most cases an obvious motive for, or gain from, the behaviour emerges. However, in evaluating states of hysterical amnesia and fugue the clinician must be cautious since, like all such dissociative behaviour, it may in itself be symptomatic of organic disease in the central nervous system. This is especially likely when arising during middle age or later in someone with a previously stable and well-adjusted personality devoid of histrionic features. When the hysterical nature of the condition has been established beyond doubt and neurological disorders excluded, it is still necessary to look further than the behaviour to underlying problems of a psychological nature which prompted it.

Drug abuse and dependence

With the widespread and increasing abuse of drugs especially by young people in the United Kingdom at the present time, it is necessary for all clinicians in emergency services to be familiar with the medical, psychological and social problems associated with the currently fashionable substances in use in their area. In the assessment it is important to differentiate the occasional abuser for recreational purposes from the person with established dependence and those who are genuinely seeking help from those whose prime purpose is to manipulate and deceive in order to obtain medication. Every emergency service should have clear policies for the management of these patients and established links with specialized psychiatric treatment centres.

Certain general signs may point to drug abuse and dependence. From relatives or friends there may be evidence of personality change with self-neglect, social withdrawal, unexpected absences from school, work or home, changes in sleeping habits and a poor appetite. Needle tracks, thrombosis of veins and bruising on the forearms, spots of blood on clothes and a reluctance to expose the arms even in hot weather, may be found. The occurrence of subcutaneous abscesses, cellulitis, serum hepatitis, pneumonia or other infections in young people should arouse suspicion.

Of the opiate group Heroin, diacetyl morphine, is the commonest drug available for illicit use. On injection it produces an immediate intensely pleasurable warm feeling leading to relaxation, euphoria, loss of appetite and libido and drowsiness. There may be itching of the skin and reddening of the eyes. Withdrawal symptoms occur some 4–6 hours after the last dose and may not reach a peak for 36–48 hours. The usual sequence is first anxiety, restlessness and insomnia, yawning, sweating, runnning eyes and nose and anorexia; then follow muscle and joint pains, pilo-erection, dilatation of the pupils, hot and cold flushes and tremors. Later, tachycardia increased blood pressure, a rise in the respiratory rate and fever develop. Finally, abdominal cramps, nausea, vomiting and diarrhoea with haemo-concentration, leucytosis, eosinopenia and increased blood sugar are found. Wherever possible, withdrawal should be carried out in hospital under the supervision of staff experienced in this field. For severe addiction, withdrawal may be achieved using diminishing doses of methadone by mouth. In milder dependence rapid withdrawal can be achieved by controlling symptoms with Lomotil (diphenoxylate hydrochloride and atroprine sulphate) and chlormethiazole.

Cocaine has become a drug of abuse because of its stimulating effect. It is taken by sniffing, chewing or intravenous injection. It causes euphoria, excitement, tremulousness, restlessness, dilatation of the pupils, dizziness and increased energy. A characteristic tactile hallucination of insects crawl-ing under the skin occurs occasionally. Complications of dependence include convulsions, depressive states and paranoid psychoses. The with-drawal syndrome is said to be mild.

In the United Kingdom only medical practitioners who hold a special licence issued by the Home Secretary may prescribe heroin or cocaine for addicts.

Barbiturate abuse, particularly in young people who may inject the drug intravenously having disolved it in water, causes dysarthria, ataxia, nystagmus, drowsiness, coma and respiratory depression. Dependence leads to personality deterioration, depression, impairment of cognitive functioning and malnourishment. Complications include serious local in-fections and ischaemic lesions at or near the site of injection and septicaemia. Stopping the drug suddenly in the addict is dangerous but the syndrome of withdrawal takes several days to develop. It includes anxiety, tension, restlessness, irritability, insomnia and tremulousness. Anorexia, nausea, abdominal pain and vomiting are common and fever, tachycardia and hypotension may be found. Acute organic reactions similar to those found with alcohol withdrawal as well as convulsions are liable to occur. For successful management admission to hospital is necessary and the drug withdrawn under the cover of benzodiazepines and anti-convulsants.

Amphetamines cause euphoria, excitement, insomnia, loss of appetite, increased energy output and signs of sympathetic over-activity. Withdrawal in those who are dependent leads to apathy, fatigue, irritability and depression. A paranoid pyschosis may result from chronic abuse. Although in medical practice amphetamines are used now only for the treatment of narcolepsy in adults and the hyperkinetic syndrome in childhood, their illicit use continues.

Lysergic acid diethylamide (LSD) and psylocybin-containing mush-rooms are the hallucinogenic agents most commonly abused in the United Kingdom. Taken orally they produce intense perceptual distortions in many individuals lasting up to twelve hours. In vulnerable personalities unpre-dictable and dangerous behaviour may lead to self-injury. In others, in-gestion produces intense fear and a sense of despair, the so-called 'bad trip'. During intoxication sympathetic over-activity may be observed. Following abuse, episodic recurrences of the psychedelic experience ('flashback') occasionally come to medical attention and may require treatment with benzodiazepines.

Solvent abuse, particularly by young adolescent boys, is increasing and causing considerable public concern (Black 1982). A wide range of solvents contained in adhesives, cleaning fluids and aerosols as well as petrol are inhaled from rags, plastic bags or other containers. Immediate intoxication with euphoria, light-headedness, blurring of vision, ataxia, disorientation and sometimes hallucinations may be followed by loss of consciousness. Sudden death may occur particularly with aerosols containing fluorocarbons or be due to accidental asphyxia, inhalation of gastric contents or trauma. Acute bronchospasm, polyneuropathy, hepatorenal damage, cardiac ar-rhythmias, aplastic anaemia and cerebral damage have been reported as complications. In accident and emergency departments abuse may be detected by the smell of the solvent on the breath or clothes, glue on the hands, a rash around the mouth and nose or excessive lacrimal and nasal secretions.

Drug-dependent individuals will often attempt to deceive clinicians in emergency situations to obtain medication. Many abuse more than one drug. Simulated pain is used to obtain analgesics especially dipipanone, pethidine and opiates. Pretending to have lost supplies of drugs on holiday may be the excuse to get barbiturates for epilepsy, amphetamines for narcolepsy, benzodiazepines for a host of reasons or methadone for the treatment of addiction. Psychiatric patients on long-acting antipsychotic depot injections may seek anticholinergic drugs for their mood-enhancing effects. While offering to arrange appropriate help the clinicians should firmly refuse to respond to such requests.

The Misuse of Drugs (Notification of and Supply to Addicts) Regul-ations 1973 require a medical practitioner to notify in writing the Chief Medical Officer, Drugs Branch, Queen Anne's Gate, London of any person he considers, or has reasonable grounds to suspect, is addicted to certain substances. A list of the drugs and the details of notification are to be found in the British National Formulary.

References and further reading

Asher R. (1951) Munchausen's Syndrome. *Lancet,* **i,** 339–41.

Bancroft J. (1979) Crisis Intervention. In Bloch S. *An Introduction to the Psychotherapies.* Oxford University Press, Oxford.

Bancroft J., Hawton K., Simkin S., Kingston B., Cumming C. and Whitwell D. (1979) The reasons people give for taking overdoses: A further enquiry. *British Journal of Medical Psychology* **52,** 353–365.

Black D. (1982) Misuse of solvents. *Health Trends* **14,** 27–28.

Blackwell B. (1968) The Munchausen Syndrome. *British Journal of Hospital Medicine* **1,** 98–102.

Bowden P. (1978) Rape. *British Journal of Hospital Medicine* **20,** 286–289.

Carney M.W.P. (1980) Artefactual illness to attract medical attention. *British Journal of Psychiatry* **136,** 542–547.

Davison K. (1980)Drug-induced psychiatric disorders. *Medicine,* **35,** 1823–1826.

Gayford J.J. (1979) Battered wives. *British Journal of Hospital Medicine,* **22,** 496–503.

Gelder M., Gath D. and Mayou R. (1983) *Oxford Textbook of Psychiatry.* Oxford University Press, Oxford.

Hawton K. and Catalan J. (1982) *Attempted Suicide: A Practical Guide to its Nature and Management.* Oxford University Press, Oxford.

Hay G.G. (1983) Feigned psychosis—a review of the simulation of mental illness. *British Journal of Psychiatry* **143,** 8–10.

Lipowski Z.J. (1980) *Delirium: Acute Brain Failure in Man.* Thomas. Springfield. Illinois.

Lishman W.A. (1978) *Organic Psychiatry.* Blackwell Scientific Publications, Oxford.

Meadow R. (1977) Munchausen syndrome by proxy. The hinterland of child abuse. *Lancet* **ii,** 343–345.

Perry S. and Viederman M. (1981) Management of emotional reactions to acute medical illness. *Medical Clinics of North America* **65,** 3–14.

Perry S.W. and Gilmore M.M. (1981) The disruptive patient or visitor. *Journal of the American Medical Association* **245,** 755.

Snowdon J., Solomons R. and Druce H. (1978) Feigned bereavement: twelve cases. *British Journal of Psychiatry* **133,** 15–19.

Stedeford A. (1978) Understanding confusional states. *British Journal of Hospital Medicine* **20,** 694–708.

Stengel E. (1943) Further studies on pathological wandering. *Journal of Mental Science* **89,** 224–241.

Index